Children with Emotional Disorders and Developmental Disabilities

CHILDREN WITH EMOTIONAL DISORDERS AND DEVELOPMENTAL DISABILITIES

Assessment and Treatment

Edited by

Marian Sigman, Ph.D.

Associate Professor
Departments of Psychiatry and Psychology
University of California at Los Angeles
School of Medicine
Los Angeles, California

G&S
GRUNE & STRATTON, INC.

(Harcourt Brace Jovanovich, Publishers)
Orlando San Diego New York
London Toronto Montreal Sydney Tokyo

Library of Congress Cataloging in Publication Data
Main entry under title:

Children with emotional disorders and developmental disabilities

Includes bibliographies and index.
1. Developmental disabilities—Complications and sequelae. 2. Mentally handicapped children—Rehabilitation. 3. Mentally ill children—Rehabilitation. 4. Child psychotherapy. I. Sigman, Marian. [DNLM: 1. Mental Disorders—complications. 2. Mental Disorders—infancy & childhood. 3. Mental Retardation—complications. WS 107 C536]
RJ135.C49 1985 618.92'89 85-958
ISBN 0-8089-1700-5

Grune & Stratton, Inc.
Orlando, FL 32887

Distributed in the United Kingdom by
Grune & Stratton, Ltd.
24/28 Oval Road, London NW 1

Library of Congress Catalog Number 85-958
International Standard Book Number 0-8089-1700-5
Printed in the United States of America
85 86 87 88 10 9 8 7 6 5 4 3 2 1

Contents

Foreword

All available evidence suggests that the incidence of emotional disturbance is substantially higher for mentally retarded persons than for the general population. Data have also been presented to indicate that disturbances in social and emotional adjustment frequently impede progress in the mainstreaming of mentally retarded children and in community placement of mentally retarded adults. The problem of emotional disturbance in mentally retarded individuals is thus an issue of paramount concern.

Until recently, however, this problem received little attention in the clinical or research literature. For example, in 1968, W. I. Gardner surveyed articles appearing in the *American Journal of Mental Deficiency* and found that less than eight percent dealt with either personality characteristics or psychopathology. The tendency has been for workers in the field of mental retardation to focus almost exclusively on the cognitive characteristics of retarded individuals, thereby excluding from study and awareness most other aspects of the functioning of the retarded. In so narrowing our perspective, we fail to recognize the full humanity of retarded persons. This limits our understanding and capacity to help, and our scientific work suffers as well. We know, for example, that many low-IQ individuals have experienced social deprivation, institutionalization, and repeated failure and ridicule. In work with nonretarded individuals, we would never overlook the consequences of such experiences for social and emotional development, or the impact that such consequences might have on behavior and test performance. Yet, a typical research paradigm used in studies of behavioral differences between retarded and nonretarded children involves the comparison of institutionalized retarded children, whose preinstitutional lives are frequently spent in the very lowest segment of the lowest socioeconomic status, with middle class nonretarded children who live at home. With respect to the retarded children, then, once we take note of a low IQ we tend to act as if we have nailed down all the variables of major import. Over the years the Yale group's research has been directed at the examination of the role of life experiences and personality variables in the functioning of retarded persons. Even with respect to IQ, an individual's score reflects the interaction of formal cognitive factors with achievement factors (what one has learned or been exposed to) and the attitudinal set one brings to the testing situation.

This book, which considers emotional disturbance in retarded children from the perspective of what we know about the social and emotional development of such individuals, is both timely and important. It represents one of a small handful of recent publications concerning individuals with the dual disabilities of mental retardation and emotional disturbance, and it provides a unique focus on these problems as they are manifested in childhood and adolescence. An important contribution is that the consideration of maladjustment and emotional disturbance is set within the framework of a broader examination of the social and emotional development of retarded children. Such a perspective recognizes the continuity between adaptive and maladaptive forms of functioning. Inasmuch as the literature on mental retardation has deemphasized both the typical problems faced by retarded children in social and emotional development and the issue of emotional disturbance, the present book, by considering both issues, consolidates our current knowledge and provides a systematic basis for further inquiry. Finally, given the third emphasis of the book, assessment and treatment, programming and intervention require an awareness both of typical problems and handicaps faced by mentally retarded children in their growth and development, and of specific forms of maladaptive behavior that some may manifest. For these reasons, I welcome this book as a needed and important contribution that should illuminate any issues concerning the social and emotional adaptation of mentally retarded individuals and serve as a foundation for further inquiry.

Edward Zigler
Sterling Professor of Psychology
Yale University
New Haven, Connecticut

Preface

Mental retardation is a common condition in childhood throughout the United States (President's Commission on Mental Retardation, 1972). Similarly, emotional disorders are also quite prevalent in childhood, with estimates that 10 percent of school-age children have adjustment difficulties that interfere seriously with academic and social development. In light of the difficulties of childhood for children of normal intelligence, adaptation must be that much more problematic for the mentally retarded child and adolescent. On this basis alone, the chances that children with cognitive limitations will develop emotional and behavioral disorders must be greater than the chances for children of normal intelligence, and the research literature bears this out (see Chapter 11).

Despite the high incidence of emotional disorders in mentally retarded children, relatively little attention has been paid in the scholarly or clinical literature to understanding or treating such disorders. In the last few years, a number of volumes have been published that have focused on the treatment of behavioral and emotional problems in mentally retarded individuals (Matson & Barrett, 1983; Syzmanski & Tanguay, 1983; Thompson & Grabowski, 1982). However, to my knowledge, there have been no volumes that emphasized the nature, assessment, and treatment of the child with dual disabilities. The purpose of this volume is to examine the issue of combined cognitive and emotional disorders in childhood from both developmental and clinical perspectives. The aims are two fold: first, to stimulate research investigations that will be useful for the prevention of emotional disorders in mentally retarded children and, second, to encourage assessment and intervention efforts directed at the treatment of such disorders.

The format of the book follows these two aims. The first section is devoted to understanding the emotional and social development of the mentally retarded child and adolescent. Without an examination of the patterns of such development, the breakdown of development and the formation of disorders cannot be understood. A chapter on the adaptation of the adult is included to elucidate the eventual goals to which the child's development is directed. Educational and training experiences in childhood should ideally be geared not only to aiding contemporaneous adaptation but also to facilitating the individual's adjustment to adult needs and roles. The second section of the volume examines childhood disorders in which a number of disabilities are manifested. The section ends with a review of dual disabilities in adulthood, with a view to encouraging the prevention of such conditions by intervention in childhood and/or treatment in the adult years. The third section reviews methods of assessment and treatment of cognitive and emotional disorders in the dual disability child and adolescent. A variety of assessment and intervention techniques utilized by clinical professionals from a number of different disciplines have been included in this section.

My interest in the child with dual disabilities stems from my experience as supervisor and co-administrator of an inpatient ward for dual disability adolescents, as well as my supervisory responsibilities in the outpatient treatment programs of the Department of Psychiatry at the UCLA School of Medicine. Unlike many treatment and research facilities, there is strong interest in understanding and treating mentally retarded children and adolescents in the Child Psychiatry Division at the UCLA Neuropsychiatric Institute and Center for the Health Sciences, under the leadership of James Simmons, M.D., Peter Tanguay, M.D., and George Tarjan, M.D. The cooperation of a large number of other professionals, particularly the staff of the ward for dual disability adolescents, and the sustained efforts of predoctoral and postdoctoral psychology trainees, were critical for my professional development in this area. The children and adolescents with whom I have worked, on both inpatient and outpatient services, have directly shaped the contributions to this volume through their difficulties, their strengths, their failures, and their triumphs.

This volume was prepared with the collaboration of many other individuals at UCLA. I am always grateful for the guidance provided by Leila Beckwith, Ph.D., Sarale Cohen, Ph.D., and Arthur H. Parmelee, M.D. The volume was completed during my sabbatical leave at the Laboratoire de Psychologie Expérimentale in the University of Paris. I am appreciative for the facilities made available to me by Marie-Germaine Pecheux and the supportive advice of Marc Bornstein during that period. Luisa Castillo not only typed several manuscripts but was responsible for collating materials from across the world in my absence from UCLA. As always, my husband, son, and daughter made many helpful suggestions. Finally, this book is dedicated to the memory of my father, who found himself facing some of the issues discussed in this book and did so with sensitivity and compassion.

Contributors

Robert Asarnow, PhD
Department of Psychiatry and Biobehavioral Sciences
University of California at Los Angeles School of Medicine
Los Angeles, California

Jeanne Brooks-Gunn, PhD
Institute for the Study of Exceptional Children
Educational Testing Service
Princeton, New Jersey

Steven R. Forness, PhD
Department of Psychiatry and Biobehavioral Sciences
University of California at Los Angeles School of Medicine
Los Angeles, California

Frederick Frankel, PhD
Department of Psychiatry and Biobehavioral Sciences
University of California at Los Angeles School of Medicine
Los Angeles, California

Irene Goldenberg, EdD
Department of Psychiatry and Biobehavioral Sciences
University of California at Los Angeles School of Medicine
Los Angeles, California

Tamar Heller
Illinois Institute for the Study of Developmental Disabilities
Chicago, Illinois

Anne E. Hogan, PhD
Mailman Center for Child Development
University of Miami
Miami, Florida

Martha Jura, PhD
Department of Psychiatry and Biobehavioral Sciences
University of California at Los Angeles School of Medicine
Los Angeles, California

Lorraine Luciano
Institute for the Study of Exceptional Children
Educational Testing Service
Princeton, New Jersey

Peter C. Mundy, PhD
Department of Psychiatry and Biobehavioral Sciences
University of California at Los Angeles School of Medicine
Los Angeles, California

Mary J. O'Connor, PhD
Department of Psychiatry and Biobehavioral Sciences
University of California at Los Angeles School of Medicine
Los Angeles, California

Steven Reiss, PhD
Department of Psychology
University of Illinois at Chicago Circle
Chicago, Illinois

Andrew T. Russell, MD
Department of Psychiatry and Biobehavioral Sciences
University of California at Los Angeles School of Medicine
Los Angeles, California

Jeffrey M. Seibert, PhD
Mailman Center for Child Development
University of Miami
Miami Florida

Tracy Sherman, PhD
Laboratory of Developmental Psychology
National Institute of Mental Health
Bethesda, Maryland

Marian Sigman, PhD
Department of Psychiatry and Biobehavioral Sciences
University of California at Los Angeles School of Medicine
Los Angeles, California

Douglas C. Smith, PhD
Fernald School, Department of Psychology
University of California at Los Angeles
Los Angeles, California

Ludwik S. Szymanski, MD
The Children's Hospital Medical Center
Boston, Massachusetts

Judy A. Ungerer, PhD
Department of Psychology
School of Behavioral Sciences, Macquarie University
New South Wales, Sydney, Australia

Denise Valenti-Hein
Illinois Institute for the Study of Developmental Disabilities
Chicago, Illinois

Peter M. Vietze, PhD
Mental Retardation and Developmental Disabilities Branch
National Institute of Child Health and Human Development
Bethesda, Maryland

Children with Emotional Disorders and Developmental Disabilities

SECTION I

The Social-Emotional Development of the Mentally Retarded Child

This section aims to describe normative developmental patterns in mentally retarded individuals and to define optimal rearing conditions, educational experiences, and developmental achievements for these persons. In order to be able to prevent emotional disorders from occurring or intensifying in childhood, an awareness of both typical and optimal life experiences is needed. Furthermore, pathology can only be understood in terms of normal behavior and adjustment. Emotional or behavioral patterns that represent adaptive responses by mentally retarded individuals to their life conditions should be recognized as such and encouraged. For these purposes, the chapters in this section examine the social, emotional, communicative, and vocational development and functioning of mentally retarded children and adults.

Jeanne Brooks-Gunn
Lorraine Luciano

1

Social Competence in Young Handicapped Children: A Developmental Perspective

Since the time of Seguin, when schools for educating the retarded were opened (Brooks-Gunn & Weinraub, 1983), adaptive behavior has been considered integral to the definition of retardation. Questions remain, however, as to the relative role of adaptive behavior and what skills this term encompasses (Bialer, 1977). Most recently, the AAMD Manual, following the "Heber paper" (Heber, 1961), used two criteria to define retardation: "significantly subaverage functioning," and "deficits in adaptive behavior" (Grossman, 1973). Age and cultural group also are taken into account in the AAMD Manual, stressing the relative nature of the term. For example, the label, "retarded," might not be appropriate for those individuals with subaverage IQ scores who are able to function independently in the community, nor for those disproportionately large numbers of minority and disadvantaged students placed in Educable Mentally Retarded classes (Greenspan, 1979; Mercer, 1975).

Of continuing debate is the issue of how to conceptualize adaptive behavior and what social skills are indicative of adaptive behavior (Meyers, Nihira, & Zetlin, 1979). Greenspan (1979) has suggested defining adaptive behavior as being a combination of conceptual, practical and social intelligence, similar to what Thorndike (1920) described over 60 years ago. Others have attempted to specify social skills for the mentally retarded (under the rubric of social

CHILDREN WITH EMOTIONAL DISORDERS AND DEVELOPMENTAL DISABILITIES ISBN 0–8089–1700–5

intelligence) and for children (under the rubric of social cognition). In the present chapter the term social competence is loosely analogous to social intelligence, and social skills include those abilities that enable one to analyze, understand, and respond to the behavior of other individuals as well as to initiate and maintain interactions with others. As we are concentrating on the young child, much of the research conducted on social intelligence or social cognition is not relevant, given developmental limitations, Therefore, social competence for the young child is characterized by the following five areas: social systems, social relationships and interpersonal interaction, social behaviors, social and self knowledge, and emotional expression (Lewis & Brooks-Gunn, 1979). All are critical for the early development of socially adaptive behavior (Emde, Kligman, Reich, & Wade, 1978; Kagan, 1978; Lewis & Rosenblum, 1979, 1981). We will review four of these features of social competence (the fifth, emotional development, is reviewed by Vietze in Chapter 2).*

SOCIAL SYSTEMS

Social Network Theory

The importance of the child's social network as the context in which the child behaves and develops has been recognized (Bronfenbrenner, 1977). From the moment of birth, the child is enmeshed in a social milieu, a network of people who, ideally, will offer security, love, and intimacy, but who will also demand the acquisition of an entire repertoire of social behaviors deemed appropriate by that particular group or culture. Social development requires growing up within a social system such that one is able to behave in socially acceptable ways. To explore the social ecology of the parent and child with regard to socialization, social networks are studied (Cochran & Brassard, 1979). Important attributes of social networks are their structural properties (i.e., size, interconnectedness, diversity of network membership), relational characteristics (i.e., content, direction, and intensity of each dyadic relationship), and location in time and space (i.e., geographic proximity of network members, continuity of network connections over time). Social networks are said to influence the child either directly, through the number and nature of persons with whom the child has contact, or indirectly, through the mediation of the parents (Lewis, Feiring, & Brooks-Gunn, in press).

*Most discussions of social competence in the handicapped have focused on mental retardation. This chapter focuses upon the handicapped young child, who, given the nature of tasks on preschool intelligence tests, is almost always cognitively delayed. With older handicapped individuals, this is not always the case.

The child's social network has been conceptualized in terms of the factors influencing the persons comprising the network and the possible social functions they could perform in the child's life (Lewis & Feiring, 1979). It has been suggested that the social network matrix of people and functions may change substantially over time, that the structure of the family may influence the contacts available to the child, and that sociocultural differences may have an impact on socialization. In addition, a child's socialization experience may be related to the family's interaction with network members (Crnic, Greenberg, Ragozin, Robinson, & Basham, 1983; Crockenberg, 1981). For example, mothers who experience stress related to the at-risk status of their child may provide the child with more positive parenting experiences if stress is mediated by contact with network members. In these families, contact with network members may provide important buffers for coping with stress due to such multiple factors as extra caregiving demands, stigmatization and parental grief (Beckman, 1983).

Social Networks of Handicapped Children

At least three topics germane to social systems have been studied in the handicapped young: family configuration, size of networks, and composition of networks. Having a handicapped infant is more likely to disrupt the family structure than would the birth of a nonhandicapped infant, if disruption is defined as father absence due to divorce or desertion (Price-Borham & Addison, 1978; Reed & Reed, 1965). How such change affects the family's social network, over and above the unavailability of the father, is unknown. In the only relevant study, Bristol & Gallagher (1982) found that the nonhandicapped but not the handicapped children had psychological problems following a divorce in families with a handicapped child.

Even when the birth of a handicapped child does not result directly in a change in the nuclear family structure, more and more children in general are spending time in single-parent families at some point in their childhood years. Indeed, it has been estimated that of all individuals born in 1977, 45 percent will spend part of their childhood in a single parent family (Glick & Norton, 1977). Thus, at least one-half of all children, including those with a handicap, will live in a single-parent family, typically with their mother.

The absence of the father may be problematic in that he plays a major role in the provision of material, emotional, and caregiving support to the wife and child. Fathers tend to help their wives with caregiving tasks more in families with a handicapped child than without (Gallagher, Cross, & Sharfman, 1981). Indeed, fathers feel that they should take more responsibility given the additional demands of handicapped children (Bristol & Gallagher, 1982). In addition, the father's influence may be indirect: maternal perceptions of paternal emotional support are related to mother's coping and acceptance of the handicapped child (Gallagher et al., 1981).*

Parents may be likely to have fewer children or to increase the spacing between children after the birth of a handicapped child. Whether or not a larger sibling network is beneficial to the child is not known. Some parents report that having more children reduces the demands of the handicapped child upon them (Turnbull, Summers, & Brotherson, in press).

In a recent study of the social network composition of 75 handicapped preschoolers and a matched sample of nonhandicapped children, networks of the former were found to be larger, not smaller, than the latter (Lewis et al. in press). Thus, the dysfunctional child is not isolated from contact outside the nuclear family. Not only are a number of service support personnel available, but parents elicit the help of kin and babysitters for childcare and emotional support to a greater degree if they have a handicapped than a nonhandicapped child. The larger network may be critical since mothers of handicapped children report that one of their major problems is the amount of child care required; intervention programs are valued for their help in this area, over and above education (Beckman, 1983).

Interestingly, the relative number of adults and peers within the children's networks differ as a function of being handicapped or not (Lewis et al., in press). Handicapped children's networks did not show an increase in the proportion of peer contacts from 3- to 6-years of age while the normal children's networks did. This is not surprising since handicapped children have typically been excluded from situations that would tend to promote peer interaction due to stigmatization and segregation (Beveridge & Evans, 1978; Brinker, in press).

RELATIONSHIPS WITHIN THE FAMILY

Young children enter into and maintain relationships, at least some of which are enduring over time and characterized by feelings of love and intimacy. Relationships arise from interactions with others in the social environment. The meaning of a relationship and the ability to interact in a complementary fashion with another individual is partially determined by one's cognitive skills. Thus, relationships may be defined not only by dimensions of interactions, but by

*Until recently, it was the mother who assumed major responsibility for the infant; consequently, few studies of father's interactions were conducted. However, fathers have been shown to be competent at early caregiving, to be just as nurturing as mothers, to receive satisfaction from such interchanges (Lamb, 1976, 1979; Hoffman, 1977). Given the rich data on fathers and infants, it is somewhat surprising that so few observational studies with handicapped infants have been conducted. In one, mothers of handicapped infants were more likely to take a managerial and teacher role than the fathers, similar to parent differences found with normal infants (Stonemen, Brody & Abbott, 1983).

developmental phenomena as well. Finally, relationships are embedded within social systems that expand as the child grows.

Early Parent-Child Interaction Patterns

By three weeks of age, mothers and infants are engaged in clearly describable reciprocal interactions. As Brazelton, Tronick, Adamson, Als, and Wise (1975) have observed, in the course of the interaction, mutual attentional and affective involvement occur in a sequence of dyadic phases including an initiation, mutual orientation, greetings, play–dialogue, and, eventually, disengagement. The cyclic quality of approach/withdrawal and attention/nonattention underlying this sequence of social events is made possible both by the caregiver's sensitivity to the cues of the infant's involvement and by the infant's active participation in the maintenance or discontinuance of the exchange (Stern, 1977). This kind of rhythmic interaction and rudimentary turn-taking is considered by some to be the basis for later social and linguistic communication (Bates, 1976; Stern, 1977).

Early asynchrony in social interchanges has been associated with a number of etiologic factors, including infant characteristics such as a handicapping condition, inattentiveness, unattractiveness, or irritability. For example, premature infants who smiled late or who exhibited reduced responsivity were found to have mothers who were less likely to interact with them (Cohen & Beckwith, 1979; Field, Tong, & Shuman, 1979; Field, 1979).

By three months of age the child should be firmly entrenched within the family system. By this time, parents usually have established definite perceptions of their children based partially on their infant's individual characteristics and partially on their own expectations and belief systems. A basic individual characteristic attributed to infants is temperament, with several dimensions being studied: sociability, distractibility, intensity of mood, activity, and persistence (Carey, 1970, 1972; Thomas & Chess, 1977).

Handicapped infants with difficult temperaments experience different maternal interaction patterns and less time in interaction with their mothers than "easy" babies with less difficult temperaments. Moreover, mothers are less apt to vocalize to handicapped infants who are active and distractible (Brooks-Gunn & Lewis, 1982c). Perceptions alone can influence interactions. Mothers of babies sick at birth treat their infant more carefully and interact with them less, even at three months of age when the infants are completely well, than mothers of three-month-old babies who are healthy at birth. It is as though the parents believe the children are still fragile or sick long after recovery (Fox & Lewis, 1981).

Through the first year of life, mother–infant interactions become more consistent, predicting later interactive styles. Not only are response styles descriptive of the infants' concurrent behavior, but they predict later emotional adjustment and self-concept (Ainsworth, Blahar, Waters, & Wall, 1978). In fact, attachment and social interaction may be more predictive of later functioning than cognitive skills (Sroufe, 1979; Lewis & Coates, 1980). The second half of the first year heralds the formation of an attachment style (Ainsworth & Bell, 1970; Ainsworth et al., 1978).

Maternal Interactions With the Handicapped

Maternal interaction with handicapped and non-handicapped infants has been studied extensively. In general, mothers with handicapped infants are more directive in their play sequences, more controlling of interactions, and take the initiation in interaction sequences more than mothers of normal infants (Buckhalt, Rutherford, & Goldberg, 1978; Buium, Rynders, & Turner, 1974; Jones, 1977; Kogan, Wimberger & Bobbitt, 1969; Shere & Kastenbaum, 1966). Few studies have examined age-related changes or differences between handicapped groups. In a recent study of 111 young handicapped children ranging in age from 3 to 36 months, mothers became more responsive to their infants as a function of the infants' age. In addition, mothers of developmentally delayed infants were more responsive than mothers of Down's syndrome and cerebral palsied infants (Brooks-Gunn & Lewis, 1984). One major issue has to do with the effect of the infants' mental functioning as separate from chronological age. In the findings just presented, it is not clear whether mothers' interactions are influenced by unique group characteristics or more general functional levels. For example, maternal responsivity was also related to infants' mental as well as chronological age. Partial correlational analyses revealed that the infant's developmental, not chronological age, was related to maternal responsivity. Thus, mothers were sensitive to their children's level of functioning. In addition, the difference between mothers of developmentally delayed and other handicapped groups also were accounted for by mental age.

Other studies have examined the effects of specific age-related developmental abilities, in particular sensorimotor functioning and linguistic competence, on mother–infant interaction. Dividing retarded and normal children into those functioning at sensorimotor stage IV and those at stage V (based on the Uzgiris-Hunt scales), mothers of stage V infants were more responsive than those of stage IV infants, in both samples (Dunst, 1980). Comparing two samples of Down's syndrome infants, one matched for chronological age and one matched for mean length of utterance with a normal sample, Leifer and Lewis (1983) and Rondal (1977) found that maternal vocalization patterns are related to the child's expressive language ability rather than chronological age. Buckhalt et al. (1978) report a similar finding for complexity of maternal language. Mothers repeatedly have been shown to adjust their speech in accordance with their normal children's developing linguistic competence (Moerk, 1974; Shatz & Gleitman, 1973; Snow, 1972).

At the same time, handicapping condition also affects maternal responsivity. For example, mothers exhibited more proximal behavior (but were not more responsive) to cerebral palsied than Down's syndrome infants (Brooks-Gunn & Lewis, 1984). In all likelihood, they were responding to their children's difficulties in interacting with the mothers as well as with toys by exhibiting more proximal behavior (Brooks-Gunn & Lewis, 1982b).

Maternal Affective Exchanges With the Handicapped

Not only may mothers of handicapped children differ with respect to responsivity, directives, control, and initiation, but they may exhibit different affective patterns, as compared to mothers of normal children. One of the mother's major socialization tasks is to help the child manage his or her emotions, as well as to interpret and attach meaning to the expressed emotions of the child. In terms of emotional management, the mother may modulate the child's emotional responses and facilitate emotional expression.

Modulating emotions includes such processes as inhibition of a response or dampening of a response. Modulation may be especially important for the handicapped or high-risk infant, who often has difficulty in this aspect of emotional expression. For example, premature infants tend to exhibit disorganized sleep–wake patterns (Dreyfus-Brisac, 1970), a high degree of irritability and dampening deficits (Brachfeld, Goldberg, & Sloman, 1980). Down's syndrome infants have longer latency to cry in free play settings but, once negative affect is elicited, take much longer to calm down. Serafica and Cicchetti (1976; Cicchetti and Serafica, 1981) suggest that Down's syndrome infants have deficits in dampening and arousal mechanisms. Given these problems, we might expect mothers of high-risk infants to alter their behavior to help their infants. Typically however, mothers do not spontaneously alter their behavior. With intervention, mothers tend to change their styles of interaction. For example, Bromwich and Parmelee (1979) found that parental involvement in a program for high-risk infants increased maternal enjoyment and responsivity to the infant.

Facilitation of emotions is another area in which mothers may be of assistance to their children. Handicapped infants exhibit less positive affect than same-age normal infants (Brooks-Gunn & Lewis, 1982a). However, mothers do not seem to facilitate positive emotional expression as evidenced by their responsivity to infant smiles. If anything, mothers of handicapped infants are *less* responsive to their children's smiling behavior (Brooks-Gunn & Lewis, 1982a). Similar findings are reported by Bromwich and Parmelee (1979) for premature infants whose smiling is delayed. Maternal disappointment, frustration, or expectations may be mediating factors. The point here, however, is that mothers of handicapped infants may be less facilitative of their infants' positive affect than are mothers of normal infants, if specific intervention is not initiated.

Negative affective exchanges are not seen very frequently in observational studies given the social undesirability of such behavior (if initiated by adults). However, extreme instances of negative affect or behavior such as child abuse and neglect may be more common with at-risk than normal young children (Sameroff & Chandler, 1975). Another way to look at negative exchanges is to examine mothers' responses to their children's negative behaviors. Maternal responsivity to infants' frets and cries in a free play setting decreases with age. Mothers of handicapped children became less responsive to cries after the first six months of life, regardless of the infant's overall amount of fretting (Brooks-Gunn & Lewis, 1982a). Perhaps mothers interpret fretting differently in the first half of the first year than in the second, the former being interpreted as a biological need (hunger, fatigue, gas, dampness), regardless of the developmental status of the child.

Interactions with Siblings

Sibling relationships, often ignored for the young child, are now seen as developing early and potentially having an impact on the socialization of the child (Bandura, 1977; Hartup, 1978a; Zajonc & Markus, 1975). Brody and Stoneman (1983) have proposed that siblings contribute to one another's social development by reinforcing certain patterns of behavior while discouraging others; by serving as models who furnish information about the appropriateness or inappropriateness of many kinds of responses in a variety of settings; and by providing a forum in which children participate in the formation of rules that govern their conduct. Older siblings are potentially teachers and younger siblings students (Lamb, 1978; Zajonc & Markus, 1975).

Research with handicapped children and their siblings has examined the attitudes of as well as stress and caregiving responsibilities placed on the normal sibling. For example, the more accepting parents are of a handicapped child, the more normal siblings like his/her brother or sister and the more time they spend in interaction with the handicapped sibling (Grossman, 1972). Also having a same sex retarded sibling causes more embarrassment to the normal sibling than does an opposite-sex sibling. Finally, the more information children have about the specific handicapping condition and the limitations imposed by the condition, the better able they are to interact successfully with their siblings (Chinitz, 1981; Grossman, 1972).

The handicapped child may be perceived as a burden by the normal sibling. Especially difficult is the situation where the handicapped family member is an older sibling. At some point, the younger sibling experiences a role reversal and must, in fact, assume the position in the family normally delegated to the older sibling (Farber & Ryckman, 1965). Girls assume more responsibility for their retarded siblings living at home than boys and may experience stress as a result of this. The caregiver role of female siblings, in many instances, extends to adulthood as well (Trevino, 1979).

SOCIAL BEHAVIORS AND PEERS

Typically, social behavior in older children is studied via such constructs as empathy, aggression, cooperation, conformity, and competition. These socially-directed behaviors are believed to evolve, in a large part, through peer interaction. That peers may be as important as parents vis-a-vis socialization has, until recent years, leaned heavily on the classic studies of Anna Freud and Harry Harlow. Following World War II, Freud and Dann (1952) described a group of young children who, while living together in a concentration camp, lost their parents and came to rely exclusively on one another for nurturance and affection. When brought to England after the war, the children refused to interact with others. Only with a great deal of patience and encouragement from their caregivers did they eventually form other attachments. Their responsivity to one another and displays of protection and concern suggested that peers could very well provide for many of the needs usually thought to be the province of parents. In a radically different context, Harlow demonstrated that motherless monkeys, when reared in groups of peers, could grow up to be effective adults and could demonstrate appropriate social behavior (Harlow, 1969). Harlow also referred to the substitution of peers as love objects for the young.

Typically, peers are not considered substitutes for parents but are believed to perform different functions than adults or even siblings (Hartup, 1978b). Peers may influence social behavior in several ways. First, peer relations are critical for the learning of role taking, different perspectives, and empathy. A child learns that life is a series of "give and take" situations calling for mutual cooperation as well as interchangeable roles of "teacher" and "student" (Gottman, Gonso, & Rasmussen, 1975). Second, children learn to master aggressive impules within the context of peer relations. Studies have shown that peers are a viable mechanism for establishing appropriate and socially acceptable boundries for aggressive feelings and behaviors (Hartup, 1974; Patterson, Littman, & Bricker, 1967). Third, peers serve as reinforcers of the culturally determined expressions of gender-appropriate behavior and gender identification (Fagot & Patterson, 1969). Fourth, peers may directly influence the moral reasoning process of and the moral judgements made by a child or adolescent (Keasey, 1971; Piaget, 1932).

Early Peer Interactions

Early peer interactions may be described as follows: in the first months of life, infants exhibit a visual interest in one another, just as they do for other objects, people, and mirror images (Bridges, 1933; Vincze, 1971). By the sixth month, the looking-and-touching infant who takes the initiative of adding a coo or a gurgle to his or her repertoire of peer-directed behaviors is able to elicit a smile response from the age-mate (Durfee & Lee, 1973). It is not until approximately the ninth month that such differences are observed and that infant-infant interactions may be described as unique. At this time, the infant's interaction may be considered as social in nature: infants are seen offering and taking objects and playing reciprocal games such as rolling a ball back and forth (Bronson, 1975). By 12 months of age, infants have been shown to interact differently with adults and peers, and strangers and familiar persons (Brooks-Gunn & Lewis, 1979; Lewis, Young, Brooks, & Michalson, 1975). In a series of studies, these investigators found that three quarters of all infants offered a toy to their mothers and to their same-age peers, but only 15 percent did so to unfamiliar adult females (in this case, the other infants' mothers).

Mueller and colleagues (Mueller & Brenner, 1977; Mueller & Lucas, 1975), using a Piagetian framework, have described the development of early peer relationships in terms of three stages. In the first stage, the one-year-old focuses on object-centered contacts when interacting, with interest being maintained by the action on the object around which the interaction is taking place (not the reverse). In the second stage, toddlers actively initiate interactions, seemingly in terms of the contingencies that children receive from one another. Children respond to a social initiation by a peer in a variety of ways and attempt to keep the interaction going. While in Stage I, the behavioral sequences that maintained an interaction were rigid and formalized and the interchange usually ended with a single response. In the second stage, the interchange is more extensive: a child's laughing at a peer's antics, joining in, or acting silly, all of which can prove engaging for the peer and prompt a sequential response. By Stage III, the interchanges are complementary and reversible, with role switching occurring for the first time.

The careful descriptive research of Guralnick (1981a) has demonstrated that peer interaction in retarded infants follows the same sequence as described earlier. Little is known about the development of peer relationships in physically impaired children. Physical disabilities in and of themselves may impose restrictions on the availability of peers, the type of interactions possible, and by inference, on the quality of the interaction.

Preschool Peer Interactions

Opportunities to practice social skills blossom in the preschool and kindergarten years. Children are introduced into a nonfamilial setting that has a relatively fixed routine and is primarily social in nature. By preschool, the child's social network has changed with the inclusion of more peers. In addition, more nonrelated adults are added, in the form of teachers. Both groups, teachers and peers, expect a different set of behaviors from the child than do the parents. Also, frequency of contact with any one person may be lower, as teachers have many students and are unable to be as responsive to any one child as the parent. The number of peers in school settings is much greater than the number of siblings at home. By preschool, children are able to become mutually engaged in complex social exchanges for extended periods of time, can readily accommodate to the social behavior of a peer, and can form important relationships with them (Garvey & Hogan, 1973). In the past, handicapped children had less opportunity for expanded peer contact. When placed in school, their classmates were children who, like themselves, were delayed. When both members of an interactive dyad are delayed, the chances for successful interactions are limited (Beveridge & Brinker, 1980). As variability among handicapped children became recognized, mainstreaming became accepted, at least for mildly retarded individuals (Guralnick, 1978a; Tjossem, 1976; Zigler & Trickett, 1978). Integration is thought to be beneficial as it provides a more challenging environment, offers opportunity for observational learning, and increases the likelihood of receiving adaptive consequences from peers (Guralnick, 1978a, 1981b). Both teachers and administrators have endorsed these basic goals of integration (Allen, 1980; Guralnick, 1978b; Turnbull & Blacher-Dixon, 1981). However, integration with normal peers does not always result in more peer interaction. Children with mild to moderate retardation show improvement in developmental functioning and appropriate social behaviors as a result of interactions with normal children (Bricker & Bricker, 1972; Field, Roseman, DeStefano, & Koewler, 1981; Galloway & Chandler, 1978; Guralnick, 1981c; Ispa & Matz, 1978). Severely handicapped children often do not show such obvious improvement.

Developmental Age and Peers

When referring to a child's peers, we mean those individuals who share with the child a common or comparable developmental level of behavior complexity (Rubin, 1980; Vandell & Mueller, 1980). Peers compliment each other; there is a reciprocity inherent in such relationships (Hartup, 1978b). Peers share play, friendship, learning of skills, practicing of roles, competition, and cooperation.

Peers may or may not be the same ages, although in our culture the former appears to be the norm. For the handicapped young, this age segregation may prove to be detrimental to the acquisition of appropriate social behavior. When handicapped children are placed in a setting that includes younger nonhandicapped peers who are at approximately the same developmental stages, interactions resemble those occurring between normal, nonhandicapped peers more than when placed with same-age, more advanced peers. Even when controlling for developmental age, however, peer interactions are somewhat less mature than those of normal children at a comparable developmental level. As earlier interactions between parents and handicapped children tend to be somewhat delayed, subsequent relations with peers may be more difficult to establish (Cunningham, Reuler, Blackwell, & Deck, 1981; Terdal, Jackson, & Garner, 1976). Older children function in the roles of surrogate parent, caregiver, teacher and role model. Typically, the more able child will modify various behaviors to accommodate for deficiences of the other in order to allow an interaction to take place, just as adults will. For example, children, like adults, use speech patterns that take into consideration the cognitive and linquistic capabilities of the listener (Gelman & Shatz, 1977; Masur, 1978; Shatz & Gelman, 1973).

SOCIAL KNOWLEDGE

Knowledge of Others

Part of the concept of social competence involves what has been called social cognition, or knowledge about others. With somewhat older children, this includes role taking, social inference about the behavior of others, understanding of social institutions and social processes, comprehension of consistent personality characteristics and motivations of other individuals, moral judgment, and referential communication about one's perceptions, thoughts, and feelings. The study of many of these aspects of social cognition has not been extended downward to the early years, with the exception of empathy and role-taking.

What has been studied in the early years is the process by which infants learn to differentiate among different persons or classes of persons. Typically, four different categories are thought to be salient cross-culturally and developmentally: familiarity, kinship, gender, and age (Brooks-Gunn & Lewis, 1978).

By the end of the first year, infants interact differentially with father than mother, recognize siblings and other salient figures, and respond differently to strangers. Parents accelerate this process by the manner in which they interact with their children: fathers are more likely to engage in play, mothers in caregiving and nurturance (Lamb, 1976). The child, recognizing that interaction patterns are unique to specific individuals, can utilize this information and differentiate among persons. Additionally, interactive differences, if tied to social roles, teach the infant about the various functions of persons, thereby contributing to social knowledge. For example, by 18 months, gender, age, and familiarity are dimensions of the social world that the child can and does utilize to differentiate among others. Between 9 and 18 months of age, infants respond more positively to children and infants than to adults, to women than to men, and to parents than to other adults (Brooks-Gunn & Lewis, 1981). Very little is known about differentiation of people in the handicapped young, although it is clear that most handicapped infants do differentiate between mother and others in the early months (as inferred from mother-infant interaction studies). However, studies comparable to those described earlier have not been conducted with handicapped young children.

Knowledge of Self

The acquisition of self-knowledge is perhaps the most important aspect of social knowledge. Two aspects of self knowledge are typically distinguished (Cooley, 1912; Mead, 1934). One, which has been called the subjective self (the self as "me"), is simply that "cognitive understanding" that enables the child to differentiate the self from the other. The second feature of the self is the objective self (the self as "I"). This feature, called the categorical self, represents the emergence of particular attributes of the self. Whereas the cognitive processes underlying the first feature result in the differentiation of the self from the other, the processes associated the second feature provide the means by which the child acquires specific features of the self.

The young infant may be interacting with others in an organized fashion, but, until he or she has acquired a concept of self, truly reciprocal relationships in the sense we have described are not possible. The young infant must first distinguish between self and others by learning that the self is separate from other people. This occurs probably around 3 to 6 months of age, the age at which Mahler, Freud, and Spitz suggested the self was differentiated. At 8 to 9 months of age, rudimentary knowledge that one exists across space probably develops. Like object permanence, self permanence allows children to conceptualize themselves as separate from others and lays the groundwork for self-identity (Lewis & Brooks-Gunn, 1979).

Emerging around the same time in a sequential but parallel fashion is the categorical self, comprised of the features that the child attributes to himself or herself. These features are determined primarily by the social environment. Self-recognition in the 15- to 18-month period represents the emergence of an active self-concept. At this time, infants rapidly accumulate knowledge about themselves related to relevant social categories such as age, sex, size, competence and effectance, and they come to view themselves as perceptually unique, as evidenced by their recognition of visual self representations and facial features.

In the second and third years of life, self categorizations facilitate the development of complex social behaviors, social knowledge, and emotional expressions and experiences. The acquisition of the sense of self in the second year not only facilitates the acquisition of social knowledge, but underlies social competence, peer relationships, gender identity, and empathy. For example, the preference for same-sex playmates is a function of the child's self identity (Lewis & Weinraub, 1979). Likewise, the child's knowledge of age distinctions (derived from the perception of facial and bodily features) contributes to the development of social knowledge about social roles (Edwards & Lewis, 1979). In the emotional domain, the emerging self-concept enables children to reflect on their own emotional state, a condition necessary for the acquisition of emotional experience (Lewis & Michalson, 1983). The emergence of the self also facilitates the development of social emotions, such as empathy and deceit. For example, emphatic behavior cannot emerge until the child has a concept of self and is capable of taking the role of another or being influenced by someone "like me." Thus, the self stands between the early social interactions of the child and his or her world and later complex social behavior, social knowledge and emotional development.

By preschool, persons like the self are preferred (especially in terms of same-sex and same-age persons), constancy develops, and self categories are added at a rapid rate. The child's growing sense of self is necessary, but not sufficient, for the development of relationships (Youniss, 1980) that require for their initiation and maintenance the negotiation of two separate and distinct selves. At the same time, as Mead, Cooley, Sullivan, and others have pointed out, it is through the development and experience of relationships that the child's notion of self is enhanced.

Regrettably, little information on the process of acquiring self-knowledge exists for the handicapped young. Self-recognition in mirrors, the most frequently studied aspect of the early self, has been examined for the handicapped. In general, handicapped young with a developmental age of more than 15 to 18 months and with adequate motoric control, exhibit self-recognition (Cicchetti & Sroufe, 1978; Lewis & Brooks-Gunn, 1982). Autistic preschoolers with adequate cognitive ability (over 18 months) also exhibit mark recognition (Ferrari & Matthews, 1983). Thus, a developmental competence seems to be a prerequisite for at least some aspects of self-knowledge.

Self-concept has been studied in older retarded children. In general, mentally retarded children either have unrealistic self-concepts (Fine & Caldwell, 1967) or negative self-concepts (Lambeth, 1966; Pier & Harris, 1964). Measuring self-concepts in severely handicapped children is difficult, given the reliance on verbal explanations or comprehension of verbal requests (e.g., "point to the picture that is most like you").

SUMMARY

While this review of literature on social competence in the handicapped young is not exhaustive, it does emphasize the importance of five social skill areas. Not only are they believed to lay the foundation for later social competence (Anderson & Messick, 1974), but they are thought to be interrelated. The role of social interaction in the development of emotional expression and the mother's influence on the management of emotions were discussed. Knowledge of others, which may be translated into empathy and social perception later on, is acquired through interaction with others as well as through knowledge of self (as Merleau-Ponty, 1964, and Mead, 1934, have argued, knowledge of self and other are reciprocal processes, both mediated through interaction). The challenge is to see in what ways the developmental processes underlying the acquisition of these social competencies differ for the handicapped, the ways in which they are similar, and to discover which skills or processes are related to later social skills.

Acknowledgments

We would like to thank Drs. Linda Michalson and Richard Brinker for their assistance on an early draft of the chapter, and Rosemary Deibler for her help in manuscript preparation. The research reported in this chapter was supported by the Special Education Program, U.S. Department of Education under the auspices of an Early Childhood Research Institute.

REFERENCES

Ainsworth, MDS, & Bell, S. (1970). Attachment, exploration and separation: Illustrated by the behavior of one-year-olds in a strange situation. *Child Development, 41*, 49–67

Ainsworth, MDS, Blahar, MC, Waters, E, & Wall, S. (1978). *Patterns of attachment: A psychological study of the strange situation*. Hillsdale, NJ: Erlbaum

Allen, KE (1980). Mainstreaming: What have we learned? *Young Children, 35*, 54–63

Anderson, S, & Messick, S. (1974). Social competency in young children. *Developmental Psychology, 10*(2), 282–293

Bandura, A. (1977). *Social learning theory*. Englewood Cliffs, NJ: Prentice-Hall.

Bates, E. (1976). *Language and context: The acquisition of pragmatics*. New York: Academic Press

Beckman, PJ (1983). The influence of selected child characteristics on stress in families of handicapped infants. *American Journal of Mental Deficiency, 88*(2), 150–156

Beveridge M, & Brinker, R. (1980). An ecological-developmental approach to communication in retarded children. In M Jones (Ed.), *Language disorders in children*. London: MTP Press

Beveridge, M, & Evans, P. (1978). Classroom interaction: Two studies of severely educationally subnormal children. *Research Education, 19*, 39–48

Bialer, I. (1977). Mental retardation as a diagnostic construct. In I Bialer & M Sternlicht (Eds.), *The psychology of mental retardation: Issues and approaches*. New York: Psychological Dimensions

Brachfeld, S, Goldberg, S, & Sloman, J. (1980). Parent-infant interaction in free play at 8 and 12 months: Effects of prematurity and immaturity. *Infant Behavior and Development, 3*, 289–305

Brazelton, TB, Tronick, E, Adamson, L, Als, H, & Wise, S. (1975). Early mother-infant reciprocity. *Parent-Infant Interaction*. Ciba Foundation 33. New York: Elsevier

Bricker, D, & Bricker, W. (1972). *Toddler research and intervention project report: Year II*. IMRID Behavioral Science Monograph 21, Institute on Mental Retardation and Intellectual Development. Nashville, TN: George Peabody College

Bridges, KMB. (1933). A study of social development in early infancy. *Child Development, 4*(1), 36–49

Brinker, RP. (in press). Curricula without recipes: A challenge to teachers and a promise to severely retarded students. In D Bricker & J Filler (Eds.), *Serving the severely retarded: From research to practice*. Reston, VA: Council for Exceptional Children

Bristol, MM, & Gallagher, JJ. (1982). A family focus for intervention. In C Ramey & P Trohanis (Eds.), *Finding and educating the high-risk and handicapped infant*. Baltimore: University Park Press

Brody, GH, & Stoneman, Z. (1983). Children with atypical siblings: Socialization outcomes and clinical participation. In BB Lahey & AE Kazdin (Eds.), *Advances in clinical child psychology*, Vol. 6. New York, Plenum, pp. 285–327

Bromwich, R, & Parmelee, A. (1979). An intervention program for pre-term infants. In T Field, A Sostek, S Goldberg, & H Shuman (Eds.), *Infants born at risk: Behavior and development*. New York: SP Medical & Scientific Books

Bronfenbrenner, U. (1977). Toward an experimental ecology of human development. *American Psychology, 32*, 513–531.

Bronson, W. (1975). Peer-peer interaction in the second year of life. In M Lewis & LA Rosenblum (Eds.), *Friendship and peer relations*. New York: Wiley

Brooks-Gunn, J., & Lewis, M. (1978) Early social knowledge: The development of knowledge about others. In H. McGurk (Ed.), *Childhood social development*. London: Methuen

Brooks-Gunn, J., & Lewis, M. (1979) The effect of age and sex on infants' playroom behavior. *Journal of Genetic Psychology, 134*, 99-105

Brooks-Gunn, J, & Lewis, M. (1981). Infant social perception: Responses to pictures of parents and strangers. *Developmental Psychology, 17*(5), 647–649

Brooks-Gunn, J, & Lewis, M. (1982a). Affective exchanges between normal and handicapped infants and their mothers. In T Field & A Fogel (Eds.), *Emotion and interaction: Normal and high risk infants*. Hillsdale, NJ: Erlbaum

Brooks-Gunn, J., & Lewis, M. (1982b) Development of play behavior in handicapped and normal infants. *Topics in Early Childhood Special Education, 2*(3), 14–27

Brooks-Gunn, J, & Lewis, M. (1982c). Temperament and affective interaction in handicapped infants. *Journal of The Division of Early Childhood, 5*, 31-41

Brooks-Gunn, J, & Lewis, M. (1984). Maternal responsivity in interactions with handicapped infants. *Child Development, 55*, 782–794

Brooks-Gunn, J, & Weinraub, M. (1983). Origins of infant intelligence testing. In M Lewis (Ed.), *Origins of intelligence* (2nd ed.). New York: Plenum

Buckhalt, J, Rutherford, R, & Goldberg, K. (1978). Verbal and nonverbal interaction of mothers with their Down's Syndrome and non-retarded infants. *American Journal of Mental Deficiency, 82*(4), 337-343

Buium, N, Rynders, J, & Turner, R. (1974). Early maternal linguistic environment of young Down's syndrome language learning children. *American Journal of Mental Deficiency, 79*(1), 52–58

Carey, WB. (1970). A simplified method for measuring infant temperament. *Journal of Pediatrics*, 77, 188

Carey, WB (1972). Measuring infant temperament. *Journal of Pediatrics, 81*, 414

Chinitz, SP. (1981). A sibling group for brothers and sisters of handicapped children. *Children Today. 10*(6), 21-23, 33

Cicchetti, D, & Serafica, FC. (1981). Interplay among behavioral systems: Illustrations from the study of attachment, affiliation, and wariness in young children with Down's syndrome. *Developmental Psychology, 17*, 36–49

Cicchetti, D, & Sroufe, LA. (1978). An organizational view of affect: Illustration from the study of Down's syndrome infants. In M Lewis & L Rosenblum (Eds.), *The development of affect: The genesis of behavior*, (Vol. 1). New York: Plenum

Cochran, MM, & Brassard, JA. (1979). Child development and personal social networks. *Child Development, 50*, 601-616

Cohen, SE, & Beckwith, L. (1979). Preterm infant interaction with the caregiver in the first year of life and competence at age two. *Child Development, 50*, 767-776

Cooley, CH. (1912). *Human nature and the social order*. New York: Charles Scribner & Sons

Crnic, KA, Greenberg, MT, Ragozin, AS, Robinson, NM, & Basham, RB. (1983). Effects of stress and social support on mothers and premature and full-term infants. *Child Development, 54*, 209–217

Crockenberg, SB. (1981). Infant irritability, mother responsiveness and social influences on the security of infant-mother attachment. *Child Development, 52*, 857-865

Cunningham, CE, Reuler, E, Blackwell, J, & Deck, J. (1981). Behavioral and linguistic developments in the interactions of retarded children with their mothers. *Child Development, 52*, 62-70

Dreyfus-Brisac, C. (1970). Sleep ontogenesis in human prematures after 32 weeks of conceptional age. *Developmental Psychobiology, 3,* 91–121

Dunst, C. (1980, April). *Developmental characteristics of communicative acts among Down's syndrome infants and nonretarded infants.* Paper presented at the biennial meeting of the Southeastern Conference on Human Development, Alexandria, VA

Durfee, JT, & Lee, LC. (1973, August). *Infant-infant interaction in a day care setting.* Paper presented at the American Psychological Association Meetings, Montreal

Edwards, CP, & Lewis, M. (1979). Young children's concepts of social relations: Social functions and social objects. In M Lewis & L Rosenblum (Eds.), *The child and its family: The genesis of behavior* (Vol. 2). New York: Plenum

Emde, RN, Kligman, DH, Reich, JH, & Wade, TD. (1978). Emotional expression in infancy: I. Initial studies of social signaling and an emergence model. In M. Lewis & L. Rosenblum (Eds.), *The development of affect.* New York: Plenum

Fagot, BI, & Patterson, GR. (1969). An in vivo analysis of reinforcing contingencies for sex-role behaviors in the preschool child. *Developmental Psychology, 1*(5), 563–568

Farber, B, & Ryckman, DB. (1965). Effects of severely mentally retarded children on family relationships. *Mental Retardation Abstracts, 2,* 1-17

Ferrari, M, & Matthews, WS. (1983). Self-recognition deficit in autism: Syndrome specific or general cognitive delay? *Journal of Autism and Developmental Disorders, 13*(3), 317–324

Field, T. (1979). Interaction patterns of preterm and term infants. In T Field, A Sostek, S Goldberg, & H Shuman (Eds.), *Infants born at risk: Behavior and development.* New York: SP Medical & Scientific Books

Field, T, Roseman, S, DeStefano, L, & Koewler, JH. (1981). Play behaviors of handicapped preschool children in the presence and absence of nonhandicapped peers. *Journal of Applied Developmental Psychology, 2,* 49–58

Field, T, Tong, G, & Shuman, HH. (1979). The onset of rhythmic activities in normal and high risk infants. *Developmental Psychobiology, 12,* 97–100

Fine, MJ, & Caldwell, TE. (1967). Self evaluation of school related behavior of educable mentally retarded children: A preliminary report. *Exceptional Children*

Fox, N, & Lewis, M. (1981). The role of maturation and experience in preterm development. In J Gallagher (Ed.), *New directions in special education.* San Francisco: Jossey-Bass

Freud, A, & Dann, S. (1952). An experiment in group upbringing. *The Psychoanalytic Study of the Child, 6,* 127–168

Gallagher, JJ, Cross, A, & Sharfman, W. (1981). Parental adaptation to a young handicapped child: The father's role. *Journal of the Division for Early Childhood, 3,* 3–14

Galloway, C, & Chandler, P. (1978). The marriage of special and generic early education services. In MJ Guralnick (Ed.), *Early intervention and the integration of handicapped and nonhandicapped children.* Baltimore, MD: University Park Press

Garvey, C, & Hogan, R. (1973). Social speech and social interaction: Egocentrism revisited. *Child Development. 44,* 562–568

Gelman, R, & Shatz, M. (1977). Appropriate speech adjustments: The operation of conversational constraints on talk to two year-olds. In M Lewis & L Rosenblum (Eds.), *Interaction, conversation and the development of language.* New York: Wiley

Glick, CP, & Norton, AJ. (1977). Marrying, divorcing, and living together in the U.S. today. *Population Bulletin, 32,* 5–20

Gottman, J, Gonso, J, & Rasmussen, B. (1975). Social interaction, social competence, and friendship in children. *Child Development, 45*(3), 709–718

Greenspan, S. (1979) Social intelligence in the retarded. In NR Ellis (Ed.), *Handbook of mental deficiency research: Psychological theory and research* (2nd Ed.) Hillsdale, NJ: Erlbaum

Grossman, FK. (1972). *Brothers and sisters of retarded children.* Syracuse, NY: Syracuse University Press

Grossman, HJ. (1973). *Manual on terminology and classification in mental retardation.* Washington, DC: American Association on Mental Deficiency

Guralnick, MJ. (Ed.) (1978a). *Early intervention and the integration of handicapped and nonhandicapped children.* Baltimore, MD: University Park Press

Guralnick, MJ. (1978b). Integrated preschools as educational and therapeutic environments: Concepts, design, and analysis. In MJ Guralnick (Ed.), *Early intervention and the integration of handicapped and nonhandicapped children.* Baltimore, MD: University Park Press

Guralnick, MJ. (1981a). The development and role of child-child social interactions. *New Directions for Exceptional Children, 5,* 53–80

Guralnick, MJ. (1981b). Programmatic factors affecting child-child social interactions in mainstreamed preschool programs. *Exceptional Education Quarterly, 1*(4), 71–91

Guralnick, MJ. (1981c). The social behavior of preschool children at different developmental levels: Effects of group composition. *Journal of Experimental Child Psychology, 31,* 115–130

Harlow, HF. (1969). Age-mate or peer affectional system. In DS Lehrman, RA Hinde, & E Shaw (Eds.), *Advances in the study of behavior* (Vol. 2) New York: Academic Press

Hartup, WW. (1974). Aggression in childhood: Developmental perspectives. *American Psychologist, 29*(5), 336–341

Hartup, WW. (1978a). Children and their friends. In H McGurk (Ed.), *Issues in childhood social development.* London: Methuen

Hartup, WW. (1978b). Peer interaction and the process of socialization. In MJ Guralnick (Ed.), *Early intervention and the integration of handicapped and nonhandicapped children.* Baltimore, MD: University Park Press

Heber, R. (1961). *A manual on terminology and classification in mental retardation.* Washington, DC: American Association on Mental Deficiency

Hoffman, LW. (1977). Changes in family roles, socialization, and sex differences. *American Psychologist, 32,* 644–647

Ispa, J, & Matz, RD. (1978). Integrating handicapped preschool children within a cognitively oriented program. In MJ Guralnick (Ed.), *Early intervention and the integration of handicapped and nonhandicapped children.* Baltimore, MD: University Park Press

Jones, OHM. (1977). Mother-child communication with pre-linguistic Down's syndrome and normal infants. In HR Schaffer (Ed.), *Studies in mother-infant interaction.* London: Academic Press

Kagan, J. (1978). On emotion and its development: A working paper. In M Lewis & L Rosenblum (Eds.), *The development of affect.* New York: Plenum

Keasey, CB. (1971). Social participation as a factor in the moral development of preadolescents. *Developmental Psychology, 5*(2), 216–220

Kogan, K, Wimberger, H, & Bobbitt, R. (1969). Analysis of mother-child interaction in young mental retardates. *Child Development, 40,* 799–812

Lamb, ME. (Ed.). (1976). *The role of the father in child development* (Vol. 1). New York: Wiley

Lamb, ME. (1978). The development of sibling relationships in infancy: A short-term longitudinal study. *Child Development, 49,* 1189-1196

Lamb, ME. (1979). The effects of the social context on dyadic social interaction. In ME Lamb, S. Suomi, & G. Stephenson (Eds.), *Social interaction analysis.* Madison, WI: University of Wisconsin Press

Lambeth, HD. (1966). *The self concept of mentally retarded children in relation to educational placement and developmental variables.* Unpublished doctoral dissertation, University of North Carolina, Chapel Hill, NC

Leifer, J, & Lewis, M. (1983). Maternal speech to normal and handicapped children: A look at question-asking behavior. *Infant Behavior and Development, 6,* 175–187

Lewis, M, & Brooks-Gunn, J. (1979). *Social cognition and the acquisition of self.* New York: Plenum

Lewis, M, & Brooks-Gunn, J. (1982). Developmental models and assessment issues. In N Anastasiow, W Frankenberg, & A Fandal (Eds.), *Identifying the developmentally delayed child*. Baltimore, MD: University Park Press

Lewis, M, & Coates, DL. (1980). Mother-infant interactions and cognitive development in twelve-week-old infants. *Infant Behavior and Development, 3*, 95–105

Lewis, M, & Feiring, C. (1979). The child's social network: Social object, social functions and their relationship. In M Lewis & L Rosenblum (Eds.), *The child and its family: The genesis of behavior*. (Vol. 2). New York: Plenum

Lewis, M, Feiring, C, & Brooks-Gunn, J. (in press). The social networks of handicapped and nonhandicapped young children. In S Landesman-Dwyer & PA Vietze (Eds.), *Living with retarded people*

Lewis, M, & Michalson, L. (1983). *Children's emotions and moods: Development, theory, and measurement*. New York: Plenum

Lewis, M, & Rosenblum, L. (Eds.). (1979). *The child and its family: The genesis of behavior* (Vol. 2). New York: Plenum

Lewis, M, & Rosenblum, L. (Eds.). (1981). *The uncommon child: The genesis of behavior* (Vol. 3) New York: Plenum

Lewis, M, & Weinraub, M. (1979). Origins of early sex-role development. *Sex Roles, 5*(2), 135–153

Lewis, M, Young, G, Brooks, J, & Michalson, L. (1975). The beginning of friendship. In M Lewis & L Rosenblum (Eds.), *Friendship and peer relations: The origins of behavior* (Vol. 4). New York: Wiley

Masur, EF. (1978). Preschool boys' speech modifications: The effect of listeners' linguistic levels and conversational responsiveness. *Child Development, 49*, 924–927

Mead, GH. (1934). *Mind, self, and society: From the standpoint of a social behaviorist*. Chicago: University of Chicago Press

Mercer, JR. (1975). Sociocultural factors in educational labeling. In MJ Begab & N Hobbs (Eds.), *Issues in classification of children* (Vol. 1). San Francisco: Jossey-Bass

Merleau-Ponty, M. (1964). *Primacy of perception* (J Eddie, Ed., and W Cobb, (Trans.). Evanston, NJ: Northwestern Universities Press

Meyers, CE, Nihira, D, & Zetlin, A. (1979). The measurement of adaptive behavior. In NR Ellis (Ed.), *Handbook of mental deficiency: Psychological theory and research*. (2nd Ed.). Hillsdale, NJ: Erlbaum

Moerk, E. (1974). Changes in verbal mother-child interaction with increasing language skills of the child. *Journal of Psychological Research, 3*, 101–116

Mueller, E, & Brenner, J. (1977). The growth of social interaction with a toddler play group: The role of peer experience. *Child Development, 48*, 854–861

Mueller, E, & Lucas, T. (1975). A developmental analysis of peer interaction among toddlers. In M Lewis & L Rosenblum (Eds.), *Friendship and peer relations: The origins of behavior* (Vol. 4). New York: Wiley

Patterson, GR, Littman, RA, & Bricker, W. (1967). Assertive behavior in children: A step toward theory of aggression. *Monographs of the Society for Research in Child Development, 32* (Whole No. 113)

Piaget, J. (1932). *The moral judgment of the child*. Glencoe, IL: The Free Press

Pier, E, & Harris, D. (1964). Age and other correlates of self-concept. *Journal of Educational Psychology, 55*, 91–95.

Price-Borham, S, & Addison, S. (1978). Families and mentally retarded children: Emphasis on the father. *The Family Coordinator, 3*, 221–230

Reed, EW, & Reed, SC. (1965). *Mental retardation: A family study*. Philadelphia: Saunders

Rondal, J. (1977). Maternal speech and normal and Down's syndrome children. In P Mittler (Ed.), *Research to practice in mental retardation. Education and training* (Vol. 2). Baltimore, MD: University Park Press

Rubin, Z. (1980). *Friendship*. Cambridge, MA: Harvard University Press

Sameroff, AJ, & Chandler, MJ. (1975). Reproductive risk and the continuum of caretaking causality. In FD Horowitz, M Hetherington, S Scarr-Salapatek, & G Siegel (Eds.), *Review of child development research* (Vol. 4). Chicago, IL: University of Chicago Press

Serafica, F, & Cicchetti, D. (1976). Down's syndrome children in a strange situation: Attachment and exploration behaviors. *Merrill-Palmer Quarterly, 22,* 137–150

Shatz, M, & Gelman, R. (1973). The development of communication skills: Modifications in the speech of young children as a function of listener. *Monographs of the Society for Research in Child Development, 38*(5)

Shatz, M, & Gleitman, R. (1973). The development of communication skills: Modifications in speech of young children as a function of the listener. *Monographs of the Society for Research in Child Development, 38* (5, Serial No. 152)

Shere, E, & Kastenbaum, R. (1966). Mother-child interaction in cerebral palsy: Environmental and psychosocial obstacles to cognitive development. *Genetic Psychology Monographs, 73,* 255

Snow, C. (1972). Mother's speech to children learning language. *Child Development, 43,* 549–565

Sroufe, LA. (1979). The coherence of individual development: Early care, attachment, and subsequent developmental issues. *American Psychologist, 34,* 834–841

Stern, D. (1977). *The first relationship: Infant and mother.* Cambridge, MA: Harvard University Press

Stoneman, Z, Brody, GH, & Abbott, D. (1983). In-home observations of young Down's syndrome children with their mothers and fathers. *American Journal of Mental Deficiency, 87,* 591–600

Terdal, L, Jackson, RH, & Garner, AM. (1976). Mother-child interactions: A comparison between normal and developmentally delayed groups. In EJ Mash, LA Hamerlynck, & LC Handy (Eds.), *Behavior modification and families.* New York: Brunner/Mazel

Thomas, A, & Chess, S. (1977). *Temperament and development.* New York: Brunner/Mazel

Thorndike, EL (1920). Intelligence and its uses. *Harper's Magazine, 140,* 227–235

Tjossem, TD. (Ed.). (1976). *Intervention strategies for high risk infants and young children.* Baltimore, MD: University Park Press

Trevino, F. (1979). Siblings of handicapped children: Identifying those at risk. *Social Casework: The Journal of Contemporary Social Work, 60*(8), 488–492

Turnbull, AP, & Blacher-Dixon, J. (1981). Preschool mainstreaming: An empirical and conceptual review. In P Stain & MM Kerr (Eds.), *Mainstreaming of children in schools: Research and programmatic issues.* New York: Academic Press

Turnbull, AP, Summers, JA, & Brotherson, MJ. (in press). The impact of young handicapped children on families: Future research directions. In *Parents' roles in the rehabilitation of their handicapped young children.* Washington, DC: National Institute of Handicapped Research

Vandell, DL, & Mueller, EC (1980). Peer play and friendships during the first two years. In HC Foot, AJ Chapman, & JR Smith (Eds.), *Friendship and social relations in children.* New York: Wiley

Vincze, M. (1971). The social contacts of infants and young children reared together. *Early Child Development and Care, 1*(1), 99–109

Youniss, J. (1980). *Parents and peers in social development: A Sullivan-Piaget perspective.* Chicago: University of Chicago Press

Zajonc, RB, & Markus, GB. (1975). Birth order and intellectual development. *Psychological Review, 82,* 74–88

Zigler, E, & Trickett, PK. (1978). IQ, social competence, and evaluation of early childhood intervention programs. *American Psychologist, 33,* 789, 798.

Peter M. Vietze

2

Emotional Development in Retarded Children

As has been documented for many years, (Menaloscino, 1970; Reiss, Levitan, & Szyszko, 1982) mentally retarded individuals may often experience emotional problems and psychopathology. Professionals holding psychoanalytic views, as well as those who are not of the psychoanalytic school, contend strongly that emotional development in the first 6 or 7 years of life may determine an individual's emotional wellbeing later in life. It is not yet clear whether this belief is supported by well controlled observations, because observations to demonstrate its truth are difficult to obtain. However, many practitioners and researchers assume that it is true. Whether it is also the case that the early emotional development of retarded children contributes to their later emotional health is unknown. The present chapter is based on the assumption that early emotional development is important for both retarded and nonretarded children. To substantiate the early experience hypothesis would require carefully controlled longitudinal investigations of retarded children. Hopefully, this chapter will contribute to the planning of such studies (Lewis & Rosenblum, 1978).

In approaching the topic to be addressed in this chapter, we are faced with an interesting problem. The development of emotions has been a central issue in the study of human behavior since such study was first undertaken at the end of the 19th century. And yet, in the 1980s, more than 100 years later, we are barely further along in our knowledge about emotional development. We have no real theory of the development of emotions and we have precious little data, although currently there is wide interest in the development of emotions and data are accumulating rapidly. We do have theories about personality develop-

CHILDREN WITH EMOTIONAL DISORDERS AND DEVELOPMENTAL DISABILITIES ISBN 0–8089–1700–5

ment that incorporate ideas about emotions and emotional wellbeing. But we do not have any widely accepted, well-integrated theory about how emotions themselves develop. One of the problems that interferes with the formulation of an integrated theory is that emotions are expressed on a variety of levels: motor, cognitive, physiological, verbal, and perceptual. The task of integrating these various levels of behavior is monumental and often the evidence on one level contradicts that on another. There are several theoretical positions on emotional development and these will be reviewed here.

One approach to understanding emotional development in retarded children is to apply what is known about emotional development in general, that is the several recent formulations, to retarded children. There is a danger in doing this. It is conceivable that such generalization is not supported by the evidence. We will therefore attempt to review recent data on emotional development in retarded children and come to some conclusion about whether generalization from normal to retarded children is justifiable. In order to make this task manageable and to be able to bring some focus to the task at hand, the major part of the discussion will be limited to infancy and early childhood. Furthermore, although it may seem that temperament is an important concept to consider in discussing emotional development, it was decided that temperament is a surrogate for personality and therefore will not be discussed here.

One of the goals of the present chapter will be to identify aspects of emotional development that might have implications for prevention of emotional problems among retarded children. Studying emotional development in retarded infants and children may lead to important insights into their emotional wellbeing as well as revealing a new understanding of the relationship among the levels of behavior on which emotional behavior may be experienced. For example, much has been written about the relationship between cognition and emotions. Piaget and Inhelder (1969) have stated that affect and cognition are inseparably intertwined. Studying emotional development in retarded children whose cognitive development is delayed or arrested may thus clarify the relationship between cognition and emotions.

THEORETICAL POSITIONS ON EMOTIONAL DEVELOPMENT

A number of theoretical positions on the development of emotion have emerged in the last decade. Izard (1971) has developed a position based on the Darwinian notions about emotions as interpreted by Tomkins (1962). For Izard, emotional development can be understood best by studying facial expressions. He and Ekman (Ekman & Friesen, 1975) working separately have developed observational systems for studying facial expressions in both adults and children. Izard claims the facial expression itself transmits the particular emotional state to the individual expressing it. There is some evidence, though it is scanty, that this may be the case. However, it is difficult to validate that part of the theory. Both Izard and Ekman have conducted cross-cultural studies in which members of different cultures have identified particular facial expressions in similar ways (Ekman, 1973; Izard, 1977). The purpose of these demonstrations was to show that expression of emotional states is a human characteristic influenced little by culture. Izard's position states that newborn infants are capable of experiencing several discrete emotions and that these are shown through specific facial expressions. The specific emotions that neonates are thought to experience are distress, interest, and disgust. According to Izard, these emotions are necessary for the infant to function adaptively and this illustrates the principle that emotions emerge only when they provide an adaptive advantage for the infant. Thus, distress and disgust are necessary for the neonate to communicate discomfort to the caregiver. Interest is also important for the infant to attend to relevant features of the environment. Following the newborn period, joy, anger, and surprise emerge. These expressions may serve to communicate reactions to the environment to the people around the infant. Anger also may serve to facilitate action in relation to frustrating obstacles and hence may be a way of motivating voluntary action. Expression of joy of course stimulates reactions from the social objects and elicits protection from caregivers.

During the second half of the first year, according to Izard, expressions of fear and shyness develop. Both of these expressions emerge as the infant begins to differentiate familiar from strange persons. These expressions do not come out until the infant is capable of locomotion and voluntary actions that allow adaptive responses to strangers. Shyness emerges toward the end of the first year when the infant's sense of self or self awareness begins. Finally, Izard discusses the emergence of guilt. Guilt is of necessity tied to an understanding of the culturally imbued values, which are learned. In order to express guilt or to feel guilt, the child must have an awareness of right and wrong. This does not begin to emerge until the second year. Thus, guilt expression may develop only after the cognitive capacity to understand transgression is present. To summarize Izard's position, differential emotions theory is mainly concerned with the development of emotions as facial expression. The different emotions are correlated with changes in perceptual, cognitive, and motor capacities, but for the most part are not a consequence of these changes. The adaptive significance of emotion expressions seems to account for their emergence at different periods.

Izard's viewpont has some appeal in that it is tied to observable behavioral changes and is tied to biologic phenomena in two different realms. On the one hand, facial expressions are made up of activation of different facial muscles controlled by the facial nerves. Secondly, Izard has suggested that the emergence of the different emotions is governed by their adaptive value for the infant. There are problems with Izard's theory, however. There is ample evidence to indicate that emotional development depends on cognitive and motoric development. Izard seems to deny this without offering counter evidence. It is also likely that environmental and cultural factors play an important role in the timing of emotional development. Nevertheless, the contribution of differential emotion theory may well be for the rich descriptive material on facial expressions and the methods for measuring such expressions. With one exception, this approach awaits testing in retarded populations.

A second approach to the development of emotions is offered by Sroufe (1979). Sroufe's theory includes a description of how specific emotions develop in the first three years of life, the development of affect, which encompasses more than the specific emotions, and the relationship between cognition and affect. Each of these will be briefly described. Sroufe first reviews the classic theory of emotion development, that of Katherine Bridges (1932). In her theory, she postulates that emotions are differentiated with age beginning with a basic emotional state called excitement. Her scheme for the development of emotions is like a tree, with branching of emotions as one gets higher. Sroufe, on the other hand, proposes that all emotions spring from three basic complexes that are evident at birth: pleasure–joy, wariness–fear, and rage–anger. He also labels eight stages or periods of emotional development and locates the emergence of different emotions along this continuum.

According to Sroufe (1979), these two developmental schemes are derived from the empirical literature. He states that logic partly dictates which emotions emerge and that there must be an orderly unfolding of emotions one from the other. We find only weak empirical support for these two descriptions of the development of specific emotions. Sroufe's proposed eight stages of affective development conform better to empirical findings. The stages he proposes are: (1) absolute or passive stimulus barrier, (2) turning toward, (3) positive affect, (4) active participation, (5) attachment, (6) practicing, (7) emergence of self-concept, and (8) play and fantasy. These eight stages are presented in parallel with Piaget's (1952) sensorimotor levels of cognitive development and with Sander's (1977) stages of social development. Although Sroufe's stages of affective development have better empirical support than the development of specific emotions, they are illustrated by only sketchy references to empirical findings. Nevertheless, these ideas have an intuitive appeal. In the third part of Sroufe's theory of emotional development he argues that there is an inseparable interrelationship between affect and cognition. This is predicated on notions from the adult literature on emotions (Lazarus, 1984; Schachter & Singer, 1962) that cognition underlies emotion, and on evidence from his own laboratory that emotional expression promotes cognitive development. He cites other empirical evidence pointing to the importance of affect for cognition but doesn't seem to make more of a case than that affect and cognition are correlated. In order to determine that affect and cognition are truly reciprocal, as Sroufe wants us to believe, one would have to examine both systems longitudinally and attempt to construct causal models between affect and cognition using some methodologically sound variant of cross-lag analysis. If the causal modeling failed but the correlations in both directions remained strong, then perhaps we could have greater confidence that cognition and affect are inextricably intertwined. Another alternative would be to study individuals in whom either affective development or cognitive development were blocked or delayed and show that in either case, there was a delay in the other system. We will return to this notion later.

Another factor Sroufe introduces into his theory of emotion is the construct of tension. He suggests that this is necessary in order to account for the range of emotions, strength of affective expression, and continuity in emotional development. This is an important contribution conceptually, but it does not add to our understanding of how affect may influence cognitive development.

A third approach to the study of emotional development is outlined by Campos, Barrett, Lamb, Goldsmith, and Stenberg (1983). These authors also recognize the importance of cognition for the development of emotions. However, they do not accord it the great significance that Sroufe asserts. They suggest seven features that must be represented in a theory of emotional development although they do not propose a specific theory themselves. Perhaps the most important postulate held by this group is that differentiated emotional states are evident in early life, perhaps even in the neonate and exist throughout the lifespan. These include the basic emotions of joy, anger, sadness, fear, and interest. They also acknowledge the role of cognitive development as being necessary for the emergence of more "complex inter-coordinated emotions" such as shame, guilt, envy, and depression. A third principle is that as the infant develops, different circumstances will elicit specific emotional states and expressions. The implication of this is that if the appropriate eliciting situation is encountered at a particular age, a variety of emotional expressions may result. This supports the view that all of the basic emotions may be present from birth.

Another postulate proposed by Campos et al. (1983) is that emotional expressions may not reflect a corresponding emotional experience at all ages, and that the correspondence, when it does exist, may change with development. They specifically point out that very early emotional displays may not reflect the corresponding emotional experience and that cultural norms may dictate the emotional expressions children show, with a period of close correspondence coming between the early period and the onset of cultural conformity. The way in which the infant and child handles a particular emotion may change with development. This principle reflects the fact that infants increase their ability for self-regulation as they gain a variety of skills. Thus, elicitation of a negative emotional state such as fear may lead to physical withdrawal from the eliciting situation when the infant is capable of locomotion and crying before the child is capable of crawling away. The influence of culture or socialization on the expression and even the experience of emotions is the subject of another principle postulated by Campos et al. (1983). Specifically, they assert that emotions are subject to socialization as the child becomes older. This includes how emotions are expressed and under what circumstances, how emotions are labelled, which emotions involve social comparison, how we respond to the emotion displays of others, and even rules for how we should feel under different circumstances, or the appropriateness of feelings. These aspects of how socialization influences emotional expression and experience may be especially important in understanding emotional development in retarded children. The last postulate proposed by Campos et al. (1983) is that infants change their responses to the emotional displays of others as they develop. They refer to a formulation outlined by Klinnert, Campos, Sorce, Emde, and Svejda (1982) in which several levels of response to facial expression are suggested. The first level lasts from birth to 6 weeks and consists of the infant's merely orienting and scanning facial displays and features but not responding to emotional information. The second stage lasts until about 5 months and is marked by the ability to discriminate among facial displays differing in emotional content. At this stage, it is asserted that the infant shows no appreciation for the meaning of such emotional expressions. At the third stage, the infant shows differential emotional responsiveness to facial displays of others. The third level lasts from 5 to 8 months and allows for the possibility of emotional communication between the infant and some other individual. The fourth level, which begins at 8 or 9 months permits the infant to share in the emotional significance of an external event with another person. Beyond the infancy period, there is little description of further development of emotional communication.

Campos et al. (1983) point out that much of the focus of their formulation as well as that of others is on facial expression, but that voice and gesture may be equally important in understanding the development of emotions. Unfortunately there has been little empirical work on the emotional significance of vocal or gestural expression of emotions that might be used in outlining a theory of emotion development.

Perhaps the most complete and well organized of the recent formulations of emotional development is presented in a recent volume by Lewis and Michalson (1983), though it is not as well supported empirically as the others. In their book they first present what they refer to as the "structure of emotion," which includes five components: elicitors, receptors, states, expressions, and experiences. A brief description of each of these factors follows, ending with an outline of Lewis and Michalson's model. An *emotional elicitor*, according to these authors, always induces an internal physiological state change and is necessary for an emotion to occur. They note that elicitors may change in significance with the development of the child and that some events may elicit internal physiological states but may not trigger an emotional response. It is admitted that there is a circularity in the way an emotional elicitor is defined but no way out of the circle is offered.

Emotional receptors refer to the physiological pathways that mediate between the elicitor and the organism's response mechanisms in order for the organism to respond to the eliciting event. The existence of emotional receptors per se is questionable, but there is evidence that the hypothesized neural pathways that might serve as receptors are subject to developmental changes during the first few years of life, since there are substantial changes in CNS structure. Both specific and general receptor systems are discussed rather vaguely since little evidence exists to tie the development of specific pathways to specific emotional states.

Emotional states are the resulting internal set of physiological changes arising from the triggering of emotional receptors by emotional elicitors. These states are the real substance of emotions. Lewis and Michalson (1983) raise the possibility that an organism is always in some emotional state, which makes sense if one considers the range of labels that emotion theorists and researchers have included. If one wants to include "no emotional state" as an emotional state, then it becomes difficult to define emotional states apart from states of wakefulness or arousal.

Several models of the development of emotional states are discussed. These include the three positions previously described. Both the origin of emotional states and how they develop are included in this discussion. The alternatives include development from one or two states that become differentiated as a result of socialization, maturation, and mental development, as well as the speculation that emotions arise entirely out of maturation of brain structures and systems. Finally, it is recognized that at this point, there is no adequate way for measuring emotional states. There is some success in measuring emotional expression, although it is not yet clear that emotional expressions are isomorphic with emotional states.

Emotional expressions are the behaviors that we observe from which we infer that an individual is in a particular emotional state. These expressions are evident in the face, voice, posture, and movements of the individual. As indicated above, much of the empirical work on emotional expressions has centered on facial emotional expression. No attempts have been made to integrate these different channels of emotional expression, although this will probably be necessary before we have a full understanding of emotions and their development. The fact that we can control how we express emotions makes the correspondence between emotional expression and the underlying state it represents difficult. As we have seen with the other theoretical positions reviewed above, there is no general agreement on even the mere description of the development of emotions. This is due to the fact that the criteria for labeling emotional expressions are still being developed. Elaborate measurement systems for labeling facial expressions have been developed recently and extended to infants. However, no consensus has been reached regarding the defining characteristics of each different expression. This is essential in understanding the specifics of the development of emotional expressions, our window into the developing emotions. The measurement of emotional expression in faces is receiving major attention, although as mentioned earlier, other modalities of expression are being neglected. It should be possible to clearly define the features of different facial expressions of emotions and then chart the course of their development.

The last major feature of Lewis and Michalson's model of emotions is *emotional experience*. Emotional experience is the individual's awareness of his or her own emotional state. Psychoanalytic writers have suggested that both conscious and unconscious awareness of emotional experience are possible. Nevertheless, in order for an individual to have an emotional experience, some interpretation of his or her emotional state and expression may be necessary. This is decidedly cognitive and this is where it may become difficult to see how emotional development is purely maturational. The development of emotional experience is most difficult to understand. It is clear that a certain level of cognitive skill is necessary in order to experience one's emotions, but in addition, there must be self awareness and clear differentiation of the self. Since we know so little about retarded children's self awareness and self conceptualization, this may make the emotional development of retarded individuals hard to predict and difficult to study.

Lewis and Michalson (1983) describe how the five components of emotion may be incorporated in a model of emotional development. However, their formulation is incomplete, as they indicate. They suggest that there are not sufficient empirical data to provide more specific details of how emotional development really works. Nevertheless, they describe two alternative approaches to emotional development, the biological approach and the socialization approach. The specific derivations of each of these approaches from their model is too complex for the present discussion. Suffice it to say that their model appears to provide the most comprehensive description of emotional development presented in this chapter. It seems quite evident that they have proposed a model that can be used to generate important hypotheses about the development of emotions in infants and young children. The model could also guide research attempting to understand emotional development in retarded children and contribute to the treatment of emotionally disabled children as well.

Four theoretical approaches to the development of emotions have been described. They vary from Izard's view that emotional development can be understood by focusing on facial expressions alone, through Sroufe's notion of the strong interdependence of emotional and cognitive development, Campos et al.'s (1983) eclectic approach, to Lewis and Michalson's (1983) more traditional formulation of a multilevel, multidetermined construct that ranges from emotional elicitation to emotional experience. None of these approaches includes truly developmental parameters in their formulations. It is of course impossible to derive many general principles from these formulations in their incomplete states. Nevertheless, there are some generally accepted milestones of emotional development that are often used to determine whether a young child is emotionally normal. These will be considered briefly, in the following section.

MILESTONES IN EMOTIONAL DEVELOPMENT

At birth, it is generally acknowledged that infants experience two undifferentiated emotional states, neutral and negative. The negative state is expressed by crying and the neutral state is expressed by quiet alertness. Occasionally, newborns smile and sometimes joy is attributed to this expression. Until the infant begins to smile reliably at other people at 2 to 3 months, the expression of joy or happiness is not acknowledged. People, especially the infant's caregivers, are the major elicitors of joy in young infants. However, as the infants get older they also begin to show positive affect to inanimate objects and to various successful performances. There is also considerable evidence that they show enjoyment at certain incongruities they view. The negative state that is present from birth is often described as anger. The anger is seen to arise from extreme discomfort, hunger, or pain. It should be mentioned that from the newborn period infants exhibit what Izard (1971) considers to be interest. This is an engaged, involved, bright-eyed look usually directed at a visually presented stimulus, but sometimes in response to a sound. Other workers in this area do not generally acknowledge this as an emotional state per se. By seven months, some signs of fear become evident although it has been described as wariness as early as four months of age (Bronson, 1972). Fear of strangers is generally acknowledged to be full-blown by nine months of age. Fear of unfamiliar objects or incongruous situations may also be evident by then, although this is not as widely observed. Certainly unexpected onset of a loud noise will sometimes elicit a fear response. By one year of age, most infants begin to show negative emotional reactions to being separated from their mothers or other primary caregivers. This is often called separation anxiety, since the infant is upset about the mother's absence. Sadness in infancy expressed in response to ordinary circumstance is unusual. However, when infants are separated from their mothers or primary caregivers, they often will show prolonged evidence of sadness and even grief and depression. Other emotions such as jealousy, shame, and guilt, which are considered social emotions, develop during the second year of life and are usually dependent on their social events such as experience with peers. These emotions are also dependent on the development of self, which emerges during the second year.

It is rare that failure for any one of these milestones to emerge will be seen as an indicator of emotional disturbance. It is more likely that emotional disturbance will be considered only if such failure is accompanied by other signs such as severe motor handicap or failure to walk or talk. It is unlikely that failure to develop stranger fear or separation anxiety would be seen generally as a sign of emotional disturbance unless accompanied by absence of other developmental milestones or presence of unusual behaviors. There are other signs of emotional disturbance however that often are used as indicators that a child is not developing normally. Such things as gaze aversion associated with a lack of smiling at people or existence of extreme behavioral stereotypes would be seen as risk factors for behavioral disturbance. In addition, general lack of activity, lethargy, and lack of interest in visual exploration might also be taken as a sign of emotional disorder. However, it would be unusual for any of these signs alone to be seen as danger signals.

It is obvious that our general knowledge about emotional development in the first years of life is severely limited. Furthermore, it will be evident that research on emotional characteristics of retarded youngsters is limited. Perhaps one reason that emotional factors are given little credence in early childhood in characterizing disabilities is that there are limited criteria for normal emotional development.

RESEARCH ON EMOTIONS WITH RETARDED CHILDREN

Research on emotions in retarded children may be divided into two groups of studies. The first group consists of investigations of emotional development in infants. These studies consist largely of investigations of positive or negative affective responses to a variety of experimental situations using infants with Down's syndrome as participants. The second group of studies includes a handful of reports on affective and emotional responses in children, ranging widely in age from middle childhood to adolescence. The research is so sparse it is difficult to make any developmental generalizations.

Emotional Development During Infancy

Most of the studies of emotions in infancy have included infants with Down's syndrome. One reason for this, of course, is that Down's syndrome is easily identified early in infancy. Only two of the studies to be discussed include other handicapped infants. We will see therefore, that any conclusions we may draw must be largely limited to Down's syndrome. The other limitation of the studies to be discussed is that they are based on experimental situations rather than naturalistic observations. This means that the findings may only reflect what is possible with these children, not what is typical.

One of the earliest efforts in which affect was examined in retarded infants was carried out by Serafica and Cicchetti (1976). This study utilized the "strange situation" (Ainsworth, Blehar, Waters, & Wall, 1979) in which infants are exposed to a series of trials of mother and a stranger leaving and entering a room where the infant is left. The reactions of the infants are recorded and used to infer how securely the infant is attached to the mother. Behaviors used to make these inferences include the infants' emotional responses to these comings and goings. In this particular study, 12 infants with Down's syndrome and 12 normal comparison children were studied. The median ages for the two groups were 33.5 months for the Down's infants and 32.8 months for the normal infants. For our purposes here, the results indicate a difference in the number of children in each group who cried during any of the episodes of the strange situation, though no differences in smiling were found. The retarded infants showed almost no crying at all, and this was statistically significant during periods when the mother was not in the room. Vocalization was also recorded and this was shown to differ in all episodes, with the normal children vocalizing significantly more than the Down's syndrome children. In general, these findings reflect a lower emotional reactivity of the retarded children to environmental events to which most young children are responsive. This is consistent with the general view that children with Down's syndrome show less emotional intensity than do normal children.

A second report from these investigators provided data on an additional 30 children with Down's syndrome (Cicchetti & Serafica, 1981). Unfortunately, there is no normal comparison group examined for this second report. In this study, the authors focus on affective behavior and other behaviors directed to the mother and the stranger during the different episodes of the strange situation procedure. In episode 3, when the mother and stranger are both present with the child, the children were found to smile more to the stranger than to the mother, though the smiles directed to the mother were more intense than those directed to the stranger. The children were likely to avert their gaze after smiling at the stranger, though not so with the mother. It is not clear what this means, from the authors' account. It could be coyness or it could reflect ambivalent affect. Since episode 3 is the only one in which both mother and stranger are present, it is the only episode in which a direct comparison can be made. However, it is possible to compare infant responses to mother and stranger alone in episodes 7 and 8. The children smiled more to the mother in episode 8 than at the stranger in episode 7. They also showed more gaze aversion to the stranger than to the mother when this comparison was made. In general, there was little crying shown by the children in any of the situations. Thus, it is difficult to evaluate the children's fearfulness or wariness as evidenced by crying. However, the gaze aversion and the fact that the children often turned their backs to the strangers does suggest that they were trying to avoid contact with the stranger. The authors point out that the Down's syndrome children showed less distress at having been left alone with a stranger than did the normal children. They suggest that this may be due either to lower intellectual capacity or to higher arousal threshold. Here we see, then, that these retarded young children show less evidence of fear than normal children would, but about the same level of positive affect shown to their mothers in this experimental situation. Thus, in general, with the exception of fear, the Down's syndrome children do not seem to show lower levels of affect expression than normal children. It is also noteworthy that, as with normal young children of a similar developmental level, different situations lead to different levels of emotional expression and different patterns of such expression.

Another set of studies are more directly relevant to the development of emotions and affect in retarded infants. These studies emanate from a longitudinal project in which a relatively large number of infants with Down's syndrome were followed over a period of several years. The first report relates the results from a cohort of 14 infants with Down's syndrome, tested when they were 4 months old and each month thereafter to 18 months, using a set of procedures designed to elicit emotional responses (Cicchetti & Sroufe, 1976). The test consists of 30 items that provide auditory, visual, social, or tactile stimulation to the infant. The test was administered in the infant's home with the mother as the social agent for the items. The infant's behavior was coded using a six point scale, which ranged from crying to laughter. The results obtained with this sample of Down's syndrome infants were compared with previously collected data on normal infants (Sroufe & Wunsch, 1972). The Down's syndrome infants were seen to show a similar course of development of positive affect (laughing and smiling) to that of the normal infants studied earlier. However, this developmental course was delayed with laughter appearing 6 to 7 months later in the Down's group than it did in the normal group. Smiling also appeared later in the group of Down's syndrome infants than in the normal infants. The authors point out that there is some heterogeneity in the Down's group with regard to hypotonicity and, similarly in emotional reactions to the 30 items. They maintain that a certain amount of tension is necessary to produce the positive affect responses and that this tension depends on the infant's ability to process the information provided by the stimulus situation. The tension is produced by the effort expended in such information processing and the resulting laughter or smiling releases this tension. The various indices of affective expression are also shown to correlate with both mental and motor scales of the Bayley Scales of Infant Development as well as object permanence and causality scales of the Uzgiris-Hunt Scales. These data are used as evidence that emotional and cognitive development are closely intertwined. In fact, the data seem to suggest that level of cognitive development predicts level of emotion expression.

In another report from this study, Cicchetti and Sroufe (1978) compared normal and Down's syndrome infants in their reactions to a looming stimulus, impending collision, visual cliff, and the assessment of positive affect described above. In their presentation of the looming and impending collision procedures, Cicchetti and Sroufe describe the behavioral reactions of both groups of infants without much interpretation of the affective significance of the reactions. The quantitative analyses of reactions to these procedures indicated little noteworthy differences between the normal and Down's syndrome infants. An exception to this was the proportion of infants in each group who cried in relation to these situations. The normal infants began crying at 4 months of age while the Down's infants only began at 12 months. Thus the Down's infants seemed to be about 8 months delayed in the onset of crying to the looming and impending collision situations. The investigators also reported that once the Down's syndrome infants began to cry, they showed very intense and prolonged reactions. The reactions to the visual cliff also seemed delayed with little heart rate acceleration and few infants showing fearful responses, although they do not venture out over the deep end of the visual cliff. In comparing reactions to the visual cliff and to the looming stimulus the investigators reported a fair amount of consistency. The results for the "laughter assessment" are comparable to those reported above; in the earlier study; not surprising considering that this is mostly the same sample. Again, these authors conclude that their data support an "organizational view of development" and that even when the infants may have had the cognitive requisites to understand the stimulus situations, they do not necessarily show the appropriate emotional reactions.

Some separate analyses are done to examine the relationship between hypotonicity and emotional reactions. These analyses reveal that the most hypotonic of the Down's syndrome infants show the most delayed affective reactions. In addition, those infants who were diagnosed with mosaicism were shown to have the least delayed emotional reactions, including crying on the visual cliff. This is taken as evidence for some basic physiological differences between infants with Down's syndrome, and normal infants, that interfere with the normal development of affect.

Since the infants in this study have continued to be studied longitudinally, another report describes a cross sectional study of their symbolic play (Motto, Cicchetti, & Sroufe, 1983). In this sudy, 31 children who had been studied earlier in the looming stimulus situation and the "laughter assessment" were seen at either 3, 4, or 5 years of age in a laboratory assessment of free play. Results of this investigation revealed that children who showed more mature levels of symbolic play were more likely to have cried to the looming objects at 16 months or laughed prior to 10 months in the earlier assessments. They also reported that the more mature their symbolic play, the earlier children had smiled to complex social and visual stimuli in the earlier assessment. Again, this is taken as evidence for the interrelationship between emotional and cognitive development.

In order to investigate the relationship between affect and cognition, Gunn, Berry, and Andrews (1981) studied the affective responses of a group of infants with Down's syndrome. Their sample consisted of 10 one-year-old infants and 7 two-year-olds. First, the Bayley Scales of Infant Development were given. Then each infant was introduced to an experimental procedure in which the doll used in the Bayley Scales was made to appear from behind a screen, squeaked, and disappeared. This was repeated ten times in relatively short order. The child's facial expressions were videotaped and coded for the presence of affective behaviors, active smile, smiles, cry face, crying, and neutral. The younger children were retested periodically at 5 month intervals. When the younger children's behavior on their first session was compared with that of the older children, it was found that 70 percent of the former kept a neutral expression throughout the ten trials while only 14 percent of the older ones remained neutral. As the behavior of the younger children was observed on repeated occasions, it was revealed that most of them did not show any affective response before 16 months. Significant correlations between onset of affective behavior and the Mental Development Index of the Bayley Scales were also found. These results seem to provide support for the notion that the affective and cognitive systems are highly correlated, although these authors admit that the nature of the relationship is unclear.

Using a different methodology from those reported thus far, Emde and his colleagues have been studying the emotional expressions of infants with Down's syndrome (Emde, Katz, & Thorpe, 1978; Sorce & Emde, 1982). They have judges sort mothers' descriptions of their Down's syndrome infants and photographs of these infants. The results of these studies indicate that there is a great deal of ambiguity in the emotional signaling of these infants as compared to that of normal infants. Further, the social smile shows much lower intensity than that of normal infants observed at similar or earlier ages. Intensive study of a number of families with Down's syndrome infants reveals that the parents show deep disappointment at the dampened affect shown by their infants. These results are quite in keeping with those reported by the other investigators reviewed here in that there seems to be a higher threshold for affective expression in infants with Down's syndrome.

Gallagher, Jens, and O'Donnell (1983) studied a group of multiply handicapped and mentally retarded infants using the "laughter assessment" devised by Cicchetti and Sroufe (1976). These investigators were interested in the relationship between affect expression and physical status, with the latter measured using a rating scale to measure muscle tonus. They found high negative correlations between muscle tone impairment and the number of laugh responses, though no relationship between muscle tone and smile responses were seen. Developmental age as measured by the Bayley Scales, on the other hand, was correlated with smiling, though not with laughing. These results imply that although the physical status of the children in the study may have prevented them from producing sufficient laughter in appropriate situations, they may not be delayed in affective or emotional development.

EMOTIONAL DEVELOPMENT IN OLDER CHILDREN

As indicated earlier, research on the emotional development and behavior of retarded children school age and older is very diverse and sparse. Often these studies include participants ranging in chronological age from 7 years to adulthood although their mental ages are usually lower than 10 years. In this section research on various aspects of emotional development among subjects whose mental age is below 10 years will be reviewed.

Izard has devised a coding system to code facial expressions (Maximally Discriminative Facial Movement Coding System). Few studies have been carried out with retarded subjects using this system or his earlier measures of emotion recognition. One exception is a recent study that compared 14 children with Down's syndrome, ranging in age from 2 to 7 years, with an equal number of MA and CA matched controls. The research examined emotional reactions to experimentally presented skits designed to elicit specific emotions (Nakhnikian, 1983). The three skits were short puppet shows that portrayed either a happiness theme, a fear theme or a neutral theme. Ratings were made of the children's facial expressions, behaviors exhibited by the children indicating approach or avoidance, and children's self report. Results indicated first that the Down's syndrome children were more likely to approach the stage during the fear condition than the other children and that this tendency was found in the lower MA Down's syndrome children rather than in the higher MA children in that group. Nevertheless, in general, the entire sample showed appropriate behavior in the three conditions. The results for the facial expressions indicated that all the children showed a preponderance of happiness expressions during the happiness condition, though the Down's syndrome children showed somewhat less than the two other groups. For the fear condition, however, all the children tended to show happiness expressions. The Down's syndrome children showed the least happiness during the fear condition compared with other groups. The author suggested that all the children were, in fact, experiencing fear in the fear condition, but were trying to "cover up" their fear by smiling. Perhaps the Down's children were less able to "cover up" and this accounted for their expressing less happiness in the fear condition. In general then, this study found, as has been reported above, that children with Down's syndrome may express appropriate emotions but their expressions are less intense.

Most of the research reviewed thus far concerns emotion expression in various groups of retarded children. However, one can also learn about the development of emotions from knowing how well an individual can identify emotions when shown examples of different facial expressions. Izard (1969) developed the Differential Emotion Scale in order to study emotion recognition in children from different cultural and subcultural groups. He has reported (Izard, 1971) that although there are similarities across national cultures in the way they label specific facial expressions, children from disadvantaged backgrounds performed poorly on the task. Simpson and Izard (unpublished observations, 1979) reported a study using the Differential Emotion Scale with retarded children and adults. The 33 residents of a state institution for the mentally retarded ranged in mental age from 4 years 5 months to 9 years 8 months. The results are unfortunately not reported in detail. The authors indicate that there was a low correlation between mental age and ability to recognize emotions and that the retarded subjects in their study seemed to show poorer ability to recognize emotions when compared to age-matched normal individuals. However, there is no information given regarding whether there was differential recognition of emotions. It is clear that this procedure might be very useful in beginning to understand how retarded persons are able to recognize emotional expressions in the faces of others. This might serve as a diagnostic instrument useful for predicting future emotional problems in retarded persons. Simpson and Izard (1979) do suggest that such study might be useful in determining the impact of length of institutionalization on emotional maturity.

A number of studies have been conducted that examine fears in mentally retarded children. Three different approaches have been taken. The first one used the Lousville Fear Survey for Children (Guarnaccia & Weiss, 1974). This instrument was given to the parents of 102 trainable retarded persons attending a day school but living at home. The age range of the retarded individuals was 6 to 21 years with IQs ranging from 15 to 65 with a mean IQ of 43. It should be noted that this study examined the parents' perceptions of their children's fear and that the parents' responses may not reflect the true fears felt by their children. The results were factor analyzed and this analysis yielded four independent factors labeled Separation, Natural Events, Physical Injury, and Animals. According to the authors, this factor structure corresponded with the factor structure based on nonretarded populations. No attempt was made to provide any descriptive developmental information regarding the specific items for different ages or IQ levels.

A second study exploring the fears of retarded children compared trainable mentally retarded, educable mentally retarded, specific learning-disabled, and normal children (Derevensky, 1979). The age range in the different groups varied from 7 to 18 years in the educable group to 9 to 19 years in the trainable group. In this investigation, the children themselves were given an opportunity to tell what fears they had. Specifically, they were asked, "What are the things to be afraid of?" Their answers were taperecorded and transcribed and then classified as Animals, People, Dark, Spooks, Natural hazards, Machinery, Death and injury, and Miscellaneous. Although the data are not presented, it is stated that the exceptional children gave more responses than the normal children and that this tendency decreased with age. All four groups showed the highest proportion of fear responses as Animals, ranging from 30 percent in the normal group to 58 percent in the learning-disabled group. The second highest category varied by group and was not necessarily very distinct from any of the other categories. When the groups were broken down by age it was found that the fear of animals decreased with age among the three groups of exceptional children, though not for the normal children. Almost none of these data were subjected to any sort of statistical evaluation, which makes drawing conclusions difficult. Nevertheless, this study provides some normative data by age and classification, which should make a contribution to research on children's fears.

Another approach that has been taken in studying fears of retarded children is a more applied one. Matson (1981) successfully treated three moderately retarded girls who had been referred for debilitating fearfulness. They were assessed for fear of strangers in a laboratory setting and then given an intervention consisting of training in meeting strangers. The training was conducted by the child's mother first in the laboratory and later at home. This was a multiple baseline study in which three dependent variables were measured: rating of fear made by the child herself, number of words spoken, and distance to the stranger. Results of this intervention study were immediate and dramatic especially when compared to matched nonfearful children's behavior over the same time period. Follow-up data as late as 6 months after the initial baseline period showed maintenance of the intervention effect for all three children. This study demonstrated that retarded children's fearfulness can be modified by well-designed intervention procedures documented by data taken over the whole period of the intervention. It is not clear that the self ratings of fearfulness are accurate measurements of the child's fearfulness, although without taking psychophysiological data it would be difficult to determine this.

A few investigations have examined affective responses of retarded children to task performance in experimental settings. Harter (1977) explored "pleasure" expressed during and after working on jigsaw puzzles of varying difficulty. She used a 4-point scale to rate smiling in 11-year-old "familial" retarded children and a six-year-old comparison group who were matched for mental age. Retarded children tended to smile more to the easier puzzles than to the harder ones while the reverse was true for the comparison group. It was also found that in general, the retarded children showed less smiling, hence pleasure, than the nonretarded children in the present situation.

In two similar studies retarded children were asked to rate how they felt upon completing experimental tasks by selecting photographs depicting children expressing a variety of affective expressions after completing a motor task. These two investigations illustrate an approach that might be used with retarded children, by utilizing pictures of emotional expressions, thus eliminating the need for verbal descriptions that might be difficult for the participants to understand. The first of these studies (Miller & Gottlieb, 1972) examined how affect related to performance following completion of a ring toss game. The children were asked to pick the photo showing how they felt, how they wish they felt and how the child in the picture felt after completing the task. Findings indicated that retarded children attributed positive feelings to themselves and negative feelings to the child in the photo after completing the task. The nonretarded children showed opposite results. When asked how they wished they felt, both groups indicated that they wished they had felt positively. Results relating performance to the affect ratings indicated a high positive correlation for the nonretarded children between performance and self ratings. For the retarded children the only significant correlation was a moderate one between performance and positive affect for the "other" child and no correlation for the self ratings. The fact that the retarded children respond that they feel positively after the task, and that this is not highly related to their performance suggests that their expressed feelings are not necessarily realistic. The authors suggest that the retarded children are responding in terms of how others will feel about their performance. This may be an indication of the "outerdirectedness" often attributed to retarded children (Zigler & Balla, 1981). In order to explore the idea that retarded children are more sensitive to the way other people feel about them, Hayes and Prinz (1976) asked mildly retarded and nonretarded youngsters to select facial expressions similar to those used by Miller and Gottlieb (1972) to indicate how they thought their teachers would feel, how they felt, and how they wished they felt, about their performance on a simple motor task. The experimenters provided feedback to the children about their task performance. Results indicated that both groups indicated positive affect after success for both the self and teacher ratings. However, younger retarded children attributed less positive ratings to the teacher than did nonretarded children. This indicates that as retarded children get older, they may be more likely to deny their actual feelings. Failure led to more positive ratings for the retarded children than for the nonretarded children. Retarded children thus have different affective reactions to success and failure, which is perhaps in keeping with the realities of their lives. It is possible to utilize these findings and paradigms to further study affect in retarded children.

These latter three investigations indicate that there is a complex relationship between affective reactions and various types of task performance for all children. Furthermore, it is evident that the degree of mental retardation, the type of task, and the level of the child's performance all interact in determining affective response to the task. It would be difficult to sketch out a developmental scheme to describe changes in affect, or affective reactions to different tasks for retarded or nonretarded children. However, it is possible to see that retarded children have affective responses to challenging tasks, and that these responses may not always reflect their true feelings. It is possible that the apparent dampened or distorted affect shown by the retarded children is realistic in relation to their life experience. The methods utilized by these three studies should prove useful in continued investigation of the relationship between affect and performance on challenging tasks.

CONCLUSIONS

We began with brief descriptions of four recent theoretical formulations of early emotional development. The focus on early emotional development was taken because it is widely acknowledged that early emotional experience has great influence on later development. It was noted that there are many empirical holes in these formulations that await further data. It was suggested that these developmental formulations might be models of emotional development in retarded children, although there are few studies that suggest the wisdom of such an assumption.

Following presentation of these four conceptualizations, we reviewed much of the empirical literature available from recent years on emotional and affective behavior in retarded children. The majority of these studies focus on infants and young children with Down's syndrome. One reason for this is that Down's syndrome can be identified early with fairly good reliability. Down's Syndrome children are also reputed to be emotionally easy-going, and this has made them the subject of studies on emotional and affective behavior. The conclusions that can be reached from these reports are that the retarded children who have been studied seem to go through similar stages of emotional development as nonretarded children and that physical limitations such as hypertonia or hypotonia may influence their ability to communicate emotions and affect to the people around them. When we examined the scanty research on older children we learned that fears held by retarded children and adolescents may depend on the degree of retardation, age of the retarded individuals, and research methodology. There was a lack of consistency in the few findings reported.

There was one study to indicate that excessive fearfulness in retarded children could be successfully modified and essentially eliminated. The single study of facial recognition in retarded persons showed that they were not as good at identifying a variety of facial expressions as nonretarded persons. Finally, research was reviewed in which affective behavior was studied as a response to various challenging tasks. These investigations also revealed that affective responses in retarded children, as with nonretarded children, depend on chronological age, mental age, and situational factors.

In general, we might conclude that retarded children are less likely to express emotions when they are very young (less than 5 years) and are less likely to voluntarily express negative emotions at older ages. It is not clear whether this is a result of socialization or an attempt at optimal self presentation. These conclusions must be qualified by the caveat that the developmental level or mental age of the retarded person may influence the degree to which emotions are and can be expressed.

This last notion brings us to one of the central themes in the theorizing and research on emotions and emotional development. The relationship between cognition and emotions has been debated widely and often (Lazarus, 1984; Zajonc, 1980, 1984). Sroufe (1979) has argued forcefully that affect and cognition are intertwined and interdependent. It is of interest to note that neither Zajonc (1984) nor Lazarus (1984) cite Sroufe at all, although Sroufe has presented data on retarded infants in which he studied both cognition and affect (Cicchetti & Sroufe, 1978). As indicated in the beginning of this chapter, studying the emotional and affective behavior of retarded children might give us insight into the relationship of affect and cognition in humans. Of course, as could be seen in the present review, there is not sufficient data from the study of retarded children to impact on how affect and cognition are related in children. Further, well-planned studies may decide this controversy. It seems that research on mentally retarded children could play a major role in this research.

Finally, what is the importance of studying emotions in mentally retarded children for understanding dual diagnosis? If we believe that mental illness and behavior disturbances are truly the result of dysfunctional emotional development then it is essential that we understand the developmental course of emotions in retarded persons. This understanding, based on empirical findings, will contribute to the development of optimal treatment programs for mentally retarded persons who are suffering from mental illness. Perhaps by understanding the developmental course of emotions in retarded children, we can prevent the double jeopardy of being mentally ill and retarded in our modern, industrial society.

REFERENCES

Ainsworth, MDS, Blehar, M, Waters, E, & Wall, S. (1979). *Patterns of attachment: A psychological study of the strange situation.* Hillsdale, NJ: Erlbaum

Bridges, KMB. (1932). Emotional development in early infancy. *Child Development, 3,* 324–341

Bronson, GW. (1972). Infants' reactions to unfamiliar persons and novel objects. *Monographs of the Society for Research in Child Development, 37* (3, Serial No. 148)

Campos, JJ, Barrett, KC, Lamb, ME, Goldsmith, HH, & Stenberg, C. (1983). Socioemotional development. In P Mussen (Ed.), *Handbook of Child Psychology* (Vol. 2). New York: Wiley

Cicchetti, D, & Serafica, FC. (1981). Interplay among behavioral systems: Illustrations from the study of attachment, affilitation, and wariness in young children with Down's syndrome. *Developmental Psychology, 17,* 36–49

Cicchetti, D, & Sroufe, LA. (1976). The relationship between affective and cognitive development in Down's syndrome infants. *Child Development, 47,* 920–929

Cicchetti, D, & Sroufe, LA. (1978). An organizational view of affect: Illustration from the study of Down's syndrome infants. In M Lewis & LA Rosenblum (Eds), *The development of affect.* New York: Plenum

Derevensky, JL. (1979). Children's fears: A developmental comparison of normal and exceptional children. *The Journal of Genetic Psychology, 135,* 11–21

Ekman, P. (1973). Cross-cultural studies of facial expression. In P Ekman (Ed.), *Darwin and facial expression.* New York: Academic Press

Ekman, P, & Friesen, WV. (1975). *Unmasking the face.* Englewood Cliffs, NJ: Prentice-Hall

Emde, RN, Gaensbauer, TJ, & Harmon, RJ. (1976). *Emotional expression in infancy.* New York: International Universities Press

Emde, RN, Katz, EL, & Thorpe, JK. (1978). Emotional expression in infancy: II. Early deviations in Down's syndrome. In M Lewis & LA Rosenblum (Eds.), *The development of affect.* New York: Plenum

Gallagher, RJ, Jens, KG, & O'Donnell, KJ. (1983). The effect of physical status on the affective expression of handicapped infants. *Infant Behavior and Development, 6,* 73–77

Guarnaccia, VJ, & Weiss, RL. (1974). Factor structure of fears in the mentally retarded. *Journal of Clinical Psychology, 30,* 540–544

Gunn, P, Berry, P, & Andrews, RJ. (1981). The affect response of Down's syndrome infants to a repeated event. *Child Development, 52,* 745–748

Harter, S. (1977). The effects of social reinforcement and task difficulty level on the pleasure derived by normal and retarded children from cognitive challenge and mastery. *Journal of Experimental Child Psychology, 24,* 476–494

Hayes, CS, & Prinz, RJ. (1976). Affective reactions of retarded and nonretarded children to success and failure. *American Journal of Mental Deficiency, 81,* 100–102

Izard, CE. (1969). *Differential emotion scale.* Unpublished test, Vanderbilt University

Izard, CE. (1971). *The face of emotion.* New York: Appleton-Century-Crofts

Izard, CE. (1977). *Human emotions.* New York: Plenum

Jens, KG, & Johnson, NM. (1982). Affective development: A window to cognition in young handicapped children. *Topics in Early Childhood Special Education, 2,* 17–24

Klinnert, MD, Campos, JJ, Sorce, JF, Emde, RN, & Svejda, M. (1982). Emotions as behavior regulators: Social referencing in infancy. In R Plutchik & H Kellerman (Eds.), *Emotions in early development.* New York: Academic Press

Lazarus, RS. (1984). On the primacy of cognition. *American Psychologist, 39,* 124–129

Lewis, M, & Michalson, L. (1983). *Children's emotions and moods.: Developmental theory and measurement.* New York: Plenum

Lewis, M, & Rosenblum, L. (1978). *The development of affect.* New York: Plenum

Matson, JL. (1981). Assessment and treatment of clinical fears in mentally retarded children. *Journal of Applied Behavior Analysis, 14,* 287–294

Menaloscino, FJ. (1970). *Psychiatric approaches to mental retardation.* New York: Basic Books

Miller, MB, & Gottlieb, J. (1972). Projection of affect after task performance by retarded and nonretarded children. *American Journal of Mental Deficiency, 77,* 149–156

Motto, F, Cicchetti, D, & Sroufe, LA. (1983). From infant affect expression to symbolic play: The coherence of development in Down's syndrome children. *Child Development, 54,* 1168–1175

Nakhnikian, E. (1983, April). *Facial expressions of emotion in Down's syndrome and non-retarded children.* Paper presented at the biennial meeting of the Society for Research in Child Development, Detroit

Piaget, J. (1952). *The origins of intelligence in children.* New York: International Universities Press

Piaget, J, & Inhelder, B. (1969). *The psychology of the child.* New York: Basic Books

Reiss, S, Levitan, GW, & Szyszko, J. (1982). Emotional disturbance and mental retardation: Diagnostic overshadowing. *American Journal of Mental Deficiency, 86,* 567–574

Sander, LW. (1977). Infant and caretaking environment: Investigation and conceptualization of adaptive behavior in a system of increasing complexity. In EJ Anthony (Ed.), *The child psychiatrist as investigator.* New York: Plenum

Schachter, S, & Singer, J. (1962). Cognitive, social and physiological determinants of emotional state. *Psychological Review, 65,* 379–399

Serafica, CS, & Cicchetti, D. (1976). Down's syndrome children in a strange situation: Attachment and exploration behaviors. *Merrill-Palmer Quarterly, 2,* 137–150

Simpson, RG, & Izard, CE. (1979). Emotion recognition in the severely mentally retarded. Unpublished manuscript, University of Delaware

Sorce, JF, & Emde, RN. (1982) The meaning of infant emotional expressions: Regularities in caregiving responses in normal and Down's syndrome infants. *Journal of Child Psychology and Psychiatry, 2,* 145–158

Sroufe, AL. (1979). Socioemotional development. In JD Osofsky (Ed.), *Handbook of infant development.* New York: Wiley

Sroufe, LA, & Wunsch, J. (1972). The development of laughter in the first year of life. *Child Development, 43,* 1326–1344

Tomkins, SS. (1962). *Affect, imagery, consciousness: The positive affects* (Vol. 1) New York: Springer

Zajonc, RB. (1980). Feeling and thinking: Preferences need no inferences. *American Psychologist, 35,* 151–175

Zajonc, RB. (1984). On the primacy of affect. *American Psychologist, 39,* 117–123

Zigler, E, and Balla, D. (1981). Issues in personality and motivation in mentally retarded persons. In M Begab, HC Haywood, & HL Garber (Eds.), *Psychosocial influences in retarded performance.* Baltimore: University Park Press

Peter C. Mundy
Jeffrey M. Seibert
Anne E. Hogan

3

Communication Skills in Mentally Retarded Children

Deficiencies in the ability to communicate effectively with adults and peers pose a significant problem for the optimal development of mentally retarded children. Several approaches have therefore been employed in attempts to understand and intervene with these deficiencies. One important approach has been to devote attention to the role of speech and hearing impairments in communication dysfunction. Exemplifying this approach are studies of speech discrimination (Niswander & Kelley, 1975) and articulatory deficits (Dodd, 1975) in the mentally retarded. Another important approach has been to focus on language development in order to understand the problems encountered by mentally retarded children in the acquisition of a vocabulary and syntactic and semantic functions (Layton & Sharifi, 1978; McLeavey, Toomey, & Dempsey, 1981).

Recently a third approach has begun to emerge from varied sources including the literature on sociolinguistics (Hymes, 1974), pragmatics, (Bates, 1976) and referential communication (Glucksberg, Krauss, & Weisberg, 1966). This approach is predicated on the assumption that communication is a social process. It is assumed that, in addition to the adequate development of speech, hearing, and language, a distinct aspect of communication competence involves knowing how to use gestural and linguistic signals to accomplish different communicative functions in social interactions. The domain of inquiry concerned with examining the ability of individuals to use different types of communicative acts in social interactions has been referred to as communication skills research (Dickson, 1981).

CHILDREN WITH EMOTIONAL DISORDERS AND DEVELOPMENTAL DISABILITIES ISBN 0–8089–1700–5

In research with mentally retarded children this approach is typified by the general question of whether or not these children are limited in producing or responding to specific types of communicative acts. Such acts include greeting others, asking questions to gain information, maintaining a topic of conversation, directing others, requesting objects or events, or referring to objects or events. Developing the ability to accomplish different types of communicative acts is affected by how well children can utilize their cognitive resources to solve problems presented by the social interactive demands of communicative situations (Shatz, 1983). Moreover, social factors have an effect on communicative competence (Hymes, 1974). The characteristics of communicative partners such as the age, sex, or status relationships among partners can affect the tendency of individuals to use particular types of communicative acts. Therefore, research in this area is also concerned with understanding the cognitive and social factors that affect the frequency and quality of the different types of communicative acts used by mentally retarded children.

The goals of this chapter are to acquaint the reader with specific aspects of the communication skills literature and to discuss the relevance of this research to issues of concern regarding intervention with retarded children. An overview of research examining the capacity of mentally retarded children to use different types of communicative acts in social interaction will be presented. Of course, the space constraints of a chapter do not permit the inclusion of all of the areas of research that may be considered relevant to this topic. The literature on role taking and other social cognitive skills in retarded children (Greenspan, 1979; Simeonsson, 1978), the communication of emotional states and the development of social inference skills in retarded children (Emde, Katz, & Thorpe, 1978; Greenspan, 1979), the cognitive factors involved in the development of communication skills in normal children (Ammon, 1981; Shatz, 1983) are all germane to the present discussion. However, as these topics have been reviewed in detail elsewhere they will not be of central concern here.

Research on the use of gestures, eye contact, and vocalization by prelinguistic children to communicate in interactions with caregivers and adults will be discussed first. This includes the presentation of a preliminary model concerning how deficits in prelinguistic communication skills may contribute to developmental delays in retarded children. A discussion of research and hypotheses regarding the strengths and weaknesses of mentally retarded children's verbal communication skills and of the implications of communication skills research for intervention with retarded children will follow. This research suggests the need to broaden the content of behavioral targets of intervention. The potential of communication skills training as an avenue of approach to intervention with the more general behavioral domain of social competence is also included in this discussion. Finally, we shall argue for the need to consider the social psychology of the intervention process with mentally retarded children. It is important to consider the effects of partner characteristics and the style of interaction between participants in the context of intervention with communication skills.

STUDIES OF COMMUNICATION SKILLS

Prelinguistic Skills

According to current research and theory on pragmatics, or the social functions of communicative acts, an appreciation of the communicative functions of behavior begins to emerge early in infancy (Bates, Benigni, Bretherton, Camaioni, & Volterra, 1979; Bruner, 1977; Seibert, Hogan, & Mundy, 1982). Prior to the development of speech, normal infants develop the capacity to use and respond to gestures, eye contact, and vocalizations in order to refer to objects, share experiences, and socially interact with caregivers. Two general periods may be distinguished in the development of these prelinguistic communication skills. In the first period, infants produce acts, such as reaching to objects or crying when hungry, that have signal value for caregivers. In this period it is not clear, however, whether infants use behaviors purposefully to convey information to caregivers. Between the eighth and twelfth month of life, though, the intent of normal infants to convey specific needs and wants with nonverbal acts becomes more apparent (Bates et al., 1979; Harding, 1982).

This second period is marked by the emergent ability to use conventional gestures like pointing, showing, or giving to request objects and events or to direct an adult's attention to interesting objects or events (Bates et al., 1979; Murphy, 1978; Rheingold, Hay, & West, 1976). Moreover, infants develop the capacity to divide attention between two entities, such as when they devote visual attention to an adult while gesturing to an object or event. This capacity enables the intent of their behavior to be made more explicit (Sugarman-Bell, 1978). In addition, increases in the capacity of infants to comprehend and respond to communicative acts parallels the development of early gestural, productive communication skills. After eight months of age infants become increasingly capable of following adult initiated referential gestures such as pointing or the direction of eye gaze (Butterworth & Jarrett, 1982; Lempers, Flavell, & Flavell, 1977). Normal infants also become increasingly capable of complying with simple gestural and/or verbal requests and commands (Benedict, 1979; Miller, Chapman, Branstow, & Reichle, 1980).

Recently, developmental measures of these types of behaviors (Seibert & Hogan, 1982; Snyder, 1978) have been used to examine associations between prelinguistic communication and cognition in young mentally retarded children. One such study indicates that developments in prelinguistic communication are associated with visual information processing abilities in mentally retarded infants and infants "at-risk" for retardation (Mundy, Seibert, Hogan, & Fagan, 1983). Other studies (Mundy, Seibert, & Hogan, 1984; Seibert, Hogan, & Mundy, 1984) indicate that developments in prelinguistic communication skills among retarded and "at risk" children are asssociated with performance on a psychometric measure of infant mental development (Bayley, 1969).

An important framework for other studies of this kind has been provided by Piaget's (1952) theory of sensorimotor/cognitive development. Several studies indicate that there is a strong association between sensorimotor and prelinguistic communication development in retarded and at risk children (Greenwald & Leonard, 1979; Lobato, Barrea, & Feldman, 1981; Mundy et al., 1984; Seibert et al., 1984). This association appears to be independent of chronological age or the motor ability of the children (Lobato et al., 1981; Seibert et al., 1984). The relationship is also particularly strong for the sensorimotor abilities involved in understanding means–end relationships (e.g., tool use) and being able to represent the social–conventional uses of objects in play with toys (Mundy et al., 1984). These last findings are consonant with research on normal infants (Bates et al., 1979) and they suggest that the cognitive factors specific to understanding means–end relationships and the conventional use of objects are also particularly important to the acquisition of prelinguistic communication skills in developmentally young mentally retarded children.

Researchers have also begun to compare the prelinguistic skills of young normal and mentally retarded children. Greenwald and Leonard (1979) reported that 16- to 26-month-old Down's Syndrome children used conventional gestures and coordinated acts directed to an adult and a referent in order to request objects or share attention. However, a comparable level of competence was exhibited by younger normal infants between the ages 9 and 13 months. In another study Blacher (1982) examined "social-communication" in mentally retarded and normal children ranging in age from 24 to 92 months. Included here were measures of showing skills and the ability to follow an adult's direction of gaze and pointing. Blacher found that the sophistication of gestural communication increased with the social age (Doll, 1965) of the mentally retarded children, but at a slower pace than in the normal sample.

Jones (1980) has examined the prelinguistic communication skills used by normal and Down's Syndrome infants in interactions with their mothers. The 8- to 24-month-old Down's Syndrome infants were more likely to present vocalizations to their mothers in rapid succession than were the developmentally matched normal infants. This pattern of closely phased vocalizations appeared to restrict the opportunity of mothers to respond to their infant's vocalizations and to enter into turn-taking vocal dialogue.

Jones also compared Down's Syndrome and normal infants' use of referential eye contact. Referential eye contact was defined as a transition of visual attention from an object or event to mother's face and then back to the object or event. This pattern of alternating eye contact often serves to direct adult attention to an object or event (Jones, 1980) and may be viewed as a behavior pattern that developmentally precedes more overt forms of referential gesture such as pointing (Seibert & Hogan, 1982). Jones found that the Down's syndrome infants exhibited proportionately less referential eye contact but more simple face-to-face gazing with caregivers than did normal children. This is not an isolated finding. Disproportionately high levels of face-to-face gazing have also been reported in other comparisons of Down's Syndrome and normal infant–caregivers' interaction (Berger & Cunningham, 1981; Gunn, Berry, & Andrews, 1982). Although this pattern of eye contact may be beneficial to the establishment of a mother–child bond (Berger & Cunningham, 1981), it provides less of an opportunity for the use of referential eye contact (Gunn et al., 1982).

Berger and Cunningham (1981) and Jones (1980) favor a cognitive hypothesis in explaining this pattern of eye contact. They refer to research that indicates that Down's Syndrome infants have difficulty in processing and/or inhibiting responding to visual information. One consequence of this may be that Down's Syndrome infants are less likely to turn their attention away from a given source of visual information. These infants may thus not engage in referential eye contact to the extent that normals do because information processing deficits attenuate their capacity to alternate looking between two sources of information.

It is difficult to draw strong conclusions from a small literature such as the one comparing the prelinguistic communication skills of mentally retarded and normal children. Furthermore, this literature has methodological problems, not the least of which is that many of these studies focus only on Down's Syndrome children. Therefore, it is not possible to determine if these findings are unique to Down's Syndrome children or are representative of mentally retarded children in general. Nevertheless, these studies do suggest that young mentally retarded children experience delays and disturbances in the use of gestures, vocalization, and eye contact to communicate with caregivers and other adults.

The supposition that visual information processing deficits may help to explain problems in the early development of the communicative use of eye contact has been briefly discussed. Consistent with this notion are data that indicate that variability in visual information processing is related to variability in the rate of acquisition of intentional prelinguistic communication skills among developmentally delayed infants (Mundy et al., 1983). In addition, developments in understanding cause and effect relationships (Piaget, 1952), representational skill (Bates et al., 1979), and the ability to attend to more than one entity simultaneously (Trevarthen & Hubley, 1978) have all been implicated in explanations for the acquisition of intentional prelinguistic communication. It therefore appears likely that delays in the acquisition of early communication skills in retarded children may be linked to one or more of these cognitive factors.

Current theory also suggests that certain cognitive skills are acquired as part of the process of prelinguistic communication development. Bruner (1977), for example, suggests that an understanding of the mechanics of shared attention and turn-taking emerges as part of early communication development. Moreover, the cognitive skills that emerge as part of early communicative development are thought to provide a foundation for the subsequent acquisition of language (Bruner, 1977). Deficits in the development of prelinguistic communication may thus play a significant role in the delayed language acquisition of mentally retarded children. Also, as part of a transactional process (Sameroff, 1975) these deficits may affect aspects of mother–child interaction that feedback to influence the cognitive and linguistic development of mentally retarded children. To illustrate the latter point we present the following tentative model.

Within the first 18 months of life cognitive deficits in mentally retarded children contribute to impairments in the use of basic prelinguistic communication skills such as referential eye contact, pointing, or showing. According to the transactional facet of the model, these impairments are hypothesized to affect child–caregiver interactions negatively by restricting the opportunities of mentally retarded children to experience contingent caregiver responding.

This restriction on interactions is assumed to result from two factors. First, prelinguistic communication skills comprise a set of behaviors that appear to be prepotent elicitors of responding from caregivers. Studies suggest that caregivers respond contingently more often to conventional referential gestures like pointing and showing than they do to other infant behaviors such as reaching to objects or exploring novel objects (Masur, 1981; West & Rheingold, 1978). Therefore, deficits in the use of these types of behaviors are likely to lead directly to reduced opportunities to experience contingent caregiver responding. Furthermore, because of deficits in early communication skills, caregivers of mentally retarded children encounter difficulties in interpreting the behavior of their children (Jones, 1980). Consequently, these caregivers may not come to perceive their children as "partners" in social interaction to the degree that caregivers of normal children do. This perception is hypothesized to be an important precipitating factor in the caregiver's adoption of a particular style of interaction with mentally retarded children. This style is characterized by a more directive approach to interaction, which affords children fewer opportunities to experience caregiver responsivity (Brooks-Gunn & Lewis, 1982; Cunningham, Rueller, Blackwell, & Deck, 1981; Eheart, 1982).

The restricted experience of contingent caregiver responding is hypothesized to adversely affect the development of young mentally retarded children. Socially interactive experiences that involve contingent caregiver responsivity are thought to be important to the cognitive development of young children (see Stevenson & Lamb, 1981, for review). Therefore, reduced opportunities to experience these types of social interactions may contribute to cognitive delay in mentally retarded children.

In addition, reductions in certain types of contingent caregiver–child interactions may also have a particularly deleterious effect on language development. Caregivers typically respond to referential gestures like pointing or showing by commenting on or labeling the object or event referred to by the child (Masur, 1981; West & Rheingold, 1978). Also, the extent to which caregivers provide labels in response to referential gestures has been associated with subsequent developments in children's vocabulary (Masur, 1981). That this type of interaction is an important context for lexical development should not be surprising. It capitalizes on the child's momentary interest in some object/event and the shared caregiver–child attention initiated by the child regarding this object/event (Bruner, 1977). However, delays or disturbances in the development of prelinguistic forms of reference among mentally retarded children may reduce the occurrence of this type of caregiver–child contingent interaction. This, in turn, may contribute to delays in the transition from gestural to linguistic modes of communication.

More generally a responsive caregiver style of interaction has been associated with optimal language development, whereas a more directive and less responsive style of interaction has been associated with impeded language development (Nelson, 1973). Therefore, if deficits in prelinguistic skills contribute to the caregiver's adoption of a directive interactive style, these deficits may play a role in the formation of a disadvantageous developmental milieu with respect to language acqusition.

Verbal Referential Speaker Skills

In the previous section we discussed research on the prelinguistic communication skills of mentally retarded children and speculated on how deficits in this area may affect subsequent developments in language. In the following section we begin the discussion of research on the verbal communication skills of developmentally older retarded children.

It is probably safe to say that more research on the communication skills of verbal mentally retarded children has been conducted using the referential communication paradigm (Glucksberg, Krauss, & Weisberg, 1966) than with any other paradigm. The goal of this type of paradigm is to examine one specific type of communicative function, that of exophoric reference or directing the attention of other people to objects or events in the perceptual field. Inasmuch as this paradigm involves the examination of a particular communicative function, it is part of the larger domain of studies on the pragmatics of communication. Typically in this paradigm child–child or child–adult dyads are presented with matched sets of stimuli. One member of the dyad is designated as the speaker, and the other member is the listener. A barrier may separate the members of the dyad so the listener cannot see the speaker's stimulus set and vice versa. On a given trial there is a designated target item(s) and the speaker's task is to construct a verbal message that enables the listener to distinguish the target item from other items in the stimulus set.

A seminal finding in research with this paradigm has been that the ability of normal children to provide listeners with unambiguous messages about target items increases between the ages of 6 and 11 years (Krauss &

Glucksberg, 1969). Moreover, in this study the developmental increment in communicative performance was not a simple function of advances in linguistic factors like breadth of vocabulary. Instead Krauss and Glucksberg concluded that the data reflected a developmental shift in children's "ability to employ language in a functional setting."

Recently several researchers have begun to use variations of this paradigm to examine the ability of mentally retarded children to use language in a functional setting. Longhurst (1974) examined the referential communication skills of retarded adolescents. Communicative effectiveness was positively associated with the IQs of both listeners and speakers. However, even a group of borderline children (mean IQ, 78) had considerable difficulty on the task. In this group, listeners were able to correctly identify the target, based on speakers messages on only 54 percent of the trials. Although direct comparisons with a normal sample were not provided, this level of competence is lower than one might expect from normal children of comparable developmental age (Krauss & Glucksberg, 1969).

One important issue with respect to this finding was whether ineffective referential communication was a consequence of inadequate speaker skills, listener skills, or both. In exploring this issue, Longhurst (1974) found that retarded listeners did much better on referential tasks when presented with normal adult speaker messages than when presented with messages from retarded adolescents. Retarded listeners thus performed reasonably well on this type of task when provided with messages from normal speakers. On the other hand, Rueda and Chan (1980) found that normal adult listeners were as poor as retarded listeners in identifying referents on the basis of messages from retarded speakers. This finding indicated that retarded speaker messages were indeed ambiguous. Together the results of these studies suggest that speaker rather than listener skills constituted a primary factor in the ineffective performance of mentally retarded children on the referential communication tasks.

At this time the nature of the inadequacies of mentally retarded speaker messages are not completely clear. The referential competence of mentally retarded speakers varies to some degree with performance on measures of syntactic and lexical development (Longhurst, 1974). However, research indicates that even where samples are quite homogeneous with respect to IQ and expressive language level, there still is considerable variability among mentally retarded children in the production of clear messages on referential tasks (Beveridge & Tatham, 1976; Beveridge, Spencer, & Mittler, 1979). Longhurst (1974) has suggested that, instead of linguistic level, an important factor is that developmentally young children, such as the mentally retarded adolescents in his study, perform egocentrically on referential tasks. They therefore generate messages with personal meaning but with limited conventional referential utility. In support of this hypothesis, Longhurst (1974) noted that when retarded speakers were given their own messages after a two week interval, they were able to identify the correct referent more often than were independent listeners.

Longhurst interpreted these data to indicate that indeed speaker messages were in fact laden with personal meaning. However, the possible confounding effects of memory for the stimuli make it difficult to draw conclusions from these data.

An alternative possibility proposed by Rueda and Chan (1980), following Rosenberg & Cohen (1966), is that mentally retarded children have difficulty in critical feature analysis. They therefore experience difficulty in formulating discriptions that are useful to listeners in distinguishing referents from nonreferents. Rueda and Chan demonstrated that when referent and nonreferent pictures could be distinguished on the basis of a simple label (e.g., bear versus bell), moderately retarded adolescents had minimal difficulty on a referential task. However, when distinguishing between items requiring more detailed feature analysis and articulation, such as, "clown with a round hat," versus "clown with a triangular hat" the mentally retarded children had considerable difficulty. Consistent with these findings, analyses of structured speech samples also indicate that mentally retarded children experience difficulty in modifying nouns with adjectives (Bliss, Allen, & Walker, 1978). Moreover, difficulty in describing the discriminant features of objects may be the result of more basic deficits in the ability of mentally retarded children to attend to two or more aspects of an entity at one time.

In another study Beveridge and Tatham (1976) presented mentally retarded adolescents with action pictures such as "girl cutting a cake" on a referential task. Speakers made more errors when referent and nonreferent pictures were distinguishable on the basis of action, than when the agent of action or object of action was the critical feature. The type of comparison needed to distinguish referents and nonreferents thus affected referential effectiveness. These results may also be explained by a variation on the critical feature hypothesis. That is, mentally retarded children may exhibit a tendency to process particular types of information (e.g., agents of action) and neglect other types of information (e.g., action) when analyzing and describing pictures and events.

The literature discussed above suggests that mentally retarded children experience difficulty in formulating messages that unambiguously direct a listener's attention to a particular referent. This type of communication skill deficit may stem from an egocentric orientation and/or deficits in less socially oriented cognitive factors such as the ability to identify the discriminant features of objects. However, if the latter is true and this type of deficit is directly the result of a basic cognitive problem, can it truly be regarded as a communication skills deficit? In our view the answer to this question is yes. The successful completion of any communicative act may be reduced to the operation of a circumscribed set of basic cognitive abilities. The capacity to employ specific cognitive abilities in a noninteractive context is, however, likely to be different from the capacity to employ the same abilities in an interactive social-communicative context. This assumption follows from theory that maintains that cognitive skills and the context of application are not necessarily independent and separable components (Fischer, 1980). The ability to effectively perform a specific type of communicative act in social interaction, although dependent on basic cognitive abilities, is thus nevertheless a communication skill. Questions regarding the relationship between cognition and communication, however, are far from being resolved. They remain at the core of present attempts to articulate a more precise definition of communication skills (Ammon, 1981). Ultimately, however, the answer to this question will most probably be relativistic depending upon one's theoretical perspective and the level of analysis of research.

Another issue concerns whether, in addition to having difficulty with exophoric reference, mentally retarded children also have difficulty with making reference to propositions occurring earlier in discourse. This is endophoric reference and this form of reference appears to be more difficult for young normal children than exophoric reference (Shatz, 1983). Therefore, it would not be surprising to find that endophoric reference also presents problems for the mentally retarded. To our knowledge this issue has yet to be examined. On the other hand, researchers have begun to examine other aspects of speaker skills in retarded children. We shall discuss some of this research in the following section.

Other Verbal Speaker Skills

Studies of speaker skills in mentally retarded children are not limited to those involving the referential communication paradigm. Several other studies employing a variety of paradigms have also begun to contribute to this area of research.

Naremore and Dever (1975) compared the child–adult conversation skills of low intelligence children (IQs 74 to 84) and developmentally matched average IQ children. The average children used more filled pauses as in, "I'm, *ah*, six years old," and more false starts, such as, "*I'm six*, no, seven years old," than did the borderline children. Naremore and Dever suggest that filled pauses and false starts function as discourse spacers to allow time for cognitive monitoring of ongoing speech acts. They thus hypothesize that low intelligence children use false starts and filled pauses less often than normals do because they also cognitively monitor the content of their ongoing speech less often. We are not aware of any attempts to follow up on this interesting hypothesis. Considering the state of research on cognitive monitoring of communication in normal children (Flavell, 1981), an examination of the hypothesis should be feasible in future research with low intelligence and retarded children.

In a study of developmentally young children, Owens and MacDonald (1982) compiled a taxonomy of nine functions of early speech acts. They then compared groups of six Down's Syndrome children and six normal children on the use of the nine types of speech acts in caregiver–child interactions. These groups were partitioned into two language levels: Mean Length of Utterance (MLU) 1.0 to 2.0 morphemes, and MLU 2.5 to 3.0 morphemes. Although the sample size attenuated the power of comparisons, group differences in the use of specific types of communicative acts were observed. In normal children, the posing of questions (i.e., requests for information and verification) and the use of declaratives (i.e., extensions of replies, commentaries, or exclamations) increased with language level. The Down's Syndrome children did not exhibit similar increases. Thus, at the higher language level, large though not significant group differences were observed in the use of questions and declaratives. Additional research is obviously necessary before any conclusions can be drawn concerning these data. Nevertheless, the data suggest that young normal and Down's Syndrome children differ in the use of specific types of communicative acts during caregiver–child interaction.

If these differences are in fact reliable, they may reflect the styles of caregiver–child interaction experienced by retarded and normal children. As previously discussed, caregivers of young retarded children tend toward more dydactic patterns of interaction. Therefore, it follows that retarded children may have fewer opportunities to use communicative acts like questions or declaratives, which serve to direct the focus of communicative interactions. This hypothesis exemplifies the need to consider the interactive features of the communicative context when interpreting comparative data on the communication skills of normal and retarded children.

Other studies have indicated that the information gathering quality, or function of questioning in retarded children is relatively poor. Denny (1974) and Borys (1979) found that mentally retarded children have difficulty in phrasing questions in the most informative manner and in using information that is provided in response to questions. Nevertheless, developmentally delayed children and adults often come to rely on questions to initiate social exchanges and to obtain goals in social interactions (Abbeduto & Rosenberg, 1980; Bedrosian & Prutting, 1978; Hurtig, Ensrud, & Tomblin, 1982; Weiss & Weinstein, 1968). For example, in one study (Bedrosian & Prutting, 1978) severely retarded young adults were observed to control interactions by "chaining" or asking successive questions, and by "arching" or responding to questions with questions. Moreover, the use of these interrogative interactional strategies varied to some extent depending on the situation and conversational partner. The mentally retarded adults were more likely to use questions to control interactions with a young normal child as opposed to interactions with peers, parents, or clinicians. Like the results of Owens and MacDonald (1982) this finding raises the possibility that the characteristics of the listener and/or situation affect the mentally retarded individual's use of certain types of communication acts. We shall return to this point later in the chapter.

Listener Skills

Communicative interactions involve listeners or receivers of messages as well as speakers of messages. While it may be that speaker skills are central to the communication problems of retarded children in certain situations, such as referential tasks, this does not mean that mentally retarded children do not also experience difficulties in listener skills. In fact, even after intervention, the listener skills of mentally retarded children, although improved, still tend to be worse than those of normal children (Ross & Ross, 1972). What we know of the listener skills of mentally retarded children derives for the most part, however, from studies of the effects of syntactic and semantic factors on comprehension (Dewart, 1979; Duncham & Erickson, 1976). Relatively few studies have addressed what we would consider to be issues of central concern regarding the communication skills of mentally retarded listeners. To illustrate the type of issues we have in mind, we will briefly discuss two areas that could be explored in future research.

The first area involves the listener's ability to interpret the elocutionary force of speaker utterances. A single utterance can have a variety of meanings. The sentence, "Do you want to put those toys away?" for example may be spoken by an adult to a child as an offer, as a request for information, or perhaps as a warning. The intent of the speaker is referred to as the elocutionary force of the utterance (Austin, 1962). Interpretation of the elocutionary force of utterances by listeners often depends on the listener's ability to relate the utternace to the context (e.g., preceding events) in which the utterance is presented. At an early age normal listeners appear to be capable of adjusting their responses to similar utterances based on differences in context (Shatz, 1983). However, the degree to which young mentally retarded listeners are capable or incapable of context-based interpretations has yet to be determined.

A second potentially useful area of research is suggested by a recent anecdotal finding. Rueda and Chan (1980) observed that young moderately and severely retarded listeners rarely asked speakers for clarifications or modifications of ambiguous messages in a referential communication paradigm. There may be several reasons why these children adopted passive roles as listeners. One important possibility is that retarded children may be deficient in comprehension monitoring skills (Markman, 1981). In other words, just as retarded children may be deficient in the cognitive monitoring of their own speech (Naremore & Dever, 1975), they may also have difficulty understanding whether or not a message is informative or if they have understood the message. A recent study that indicates that retarded adolescents fail to understand when referential errors are due to ambiguity in the speaker's message (Beveridge et al., 1979) supports this hypothesis. However, it may also be that mentally retarded children have difficulty spontaneously adopting the role of speaker in a situation where they have been asked by an adult to play the role of listener. The failure of listeners to ask questions concerning ambiguous messages in a referential communication paradigm may thus be more a function of social constraints rather than a cognitive deficit. This aspect of retarded listeners' communication skills also remains open to examination.

Interactions Between Speakers and Listeners

Communication is an interactional process. As was alluded to in the preceding discussion, speaker's and listener's roles may be interchanged during the course of an interaction to allow for clarification and elaboration of the content of discussion. For example, a speaker must become a listener when presented with feedback concerning the adequacy or inadequacy of his or her message. Also, because communication involves interactions with others, an individual's understanding and perception of the characteristics of his partner(s) can affect the content and quality of the communicative exchange. An illustration of this point is provided by Shatz and Gelman (1973), who found that young normal children modify their speech as a function of the age of the listener. Recently studies have begun to examine issues related to interactional processes in the communication of mentally retarded children.

Longhurst and Berry (1975) examined how well low IQ and retarded adolescents responded to different types of listener feedback that indicated failure to understand the referential message. Mentally retarded speakers were paired with adult listeners who responded to some descriptions with gestural or verbally implicit indices of uncertainty, such as as quizzical facial expression or "I don't understand." Sometimes the adult also responded with verbally explicit prompts for additional information, such as, "tell me something else about it." Explicit feedback elicited more redescription of the referent than did implicit verbal feedback, which in turn elicited more redescription than did gestural feedback. The group of children with low IQs (mean IQ, 78) provided significantly more redescriptions of the referent in the implicit and gestural condition than two groups of retarded children with mean IQs of 63 and 47. Moreover, the most frequent type of response to feedback among the two retarded groups was silence across all feedback types. This was not the case for the low IQ group. Again it is unfortunate that a normal comparison sample was not included in this study. However, by way of comparison, data from Peterson, Danner, and Flavell (1972) indicate that seven-year-old normal children are quite responsive to implicit verbal requests in this type of situation.

How the young child's awareness of the information available to the listener affects communication has been examined in a recent study. Leonard, Cole, and Steckol (1979) presented young mentally retarded children, who had single word speech, with a series of toys and the children were asked to name each toy. The results indicated that the children provided the name for a toy significantly more often when the toy was novel as opposed to when it had been seen before in the series. Leonard et al., interpreted these data to suggest that mentally retarded children exercise selectivity in responding to requests for labels. More specifically, Leonard et al., suggest that these children take into account what information has previously been presented in an interaction and name a toy when the label has the greatest potential for providing new information to the listener.

In another study on a similar topic Hoy and McKnight (1977) examined whether or not mentally retarded children would adapt their referential communication to accommodate mentally retarded listeners. Listeners and speakers were either similar or dissimilar in chronological and mental age. Two age groups of children were involved in this study. One group had a mean MA of 6.6 years and a mean CA of 15.5 years and the other group had a mean MA of 3.7 years and a mean CA of 11.2 years. Speakers were instructed on the rules of a simple board game and subsequently instructed listeners in the play of the game. The results indicated that the speakers at both levels adjusted their communications to accommodate listeners of different developmental levels. Speakers explained as many game items to low- and to high-level listeners, but used verbal descriptions alone less often and combined verbal descriptions with manipulation of some pieces more often with low-level listeners. The functional types of speech acts also differed across the groups with low-level listeners receiving more attention-getting speech acts, such as "look," "see," "watch," and more imperative acts.

The data also indicated that low-level speakers were reserved in their communications with high-level speakers. Low-level speakers used significantly fewer total utterances, explained fewer items, and used fewer imperatives and attention getters when speaking to high-level listeners as opposed to low-level listeners.

This study exemplifies a sociolinguistic approach to research on communication skills in the retarded. That is, it is concerned with the relationship between the characteristics of the individuals participating in an interaction, and both the form and function of communicative expressions. Other sociolinguistic studies on the communication of the mentally retarded agree with the findings of Hoy and McKnight. Rosenberg, Spradlin, and Mabel (1961) found that the frequencies of vocal and gestural communication were similar for dyads composed of two low IQ children and dyads composed of higher IQ children. However, the frequency of communication was considerably lower for dyads composed of one low-level and one high-level child. Also, as noted earlier, data from Bedrosian and Prutting (1978) suggests that mentally retarded adults are more likely to use conversation control strategies with a young child as opposed to peers, caregivers, or clinicians.

The results of these studies have implications for how data on the communication skills of mentally retarded children are interpreted. The finding that mentally retarded children are capable of adapting their communications to accommodate the developmental level of the listener (Hoy & McKnight, 1977) is not consistent with the argument that mentally retarded children are particularly egocentric in communication with others (Longhurst, 1974). Furthermore, the developmental level or social status of the listener may affect the extent to which mentally retarded children use different functional types of speech such as imperatives and attention getters (Hoy & McKnight, 1977), or questions (Bedrosian & Prutting, 1978). Therefore, as previously noted, in interpreting apparent deficits in specific types of speech acts among the retarded (Owens & McDonald, 1982), it is important to consider the potential effect of social partners on children's communicative interactions. The possible effects of social partners on mentally retarded children's communication also has implications for intervention, which will be discussed in the following section.

INTERVENTION IMPLICATIONS

The foregoing review was intended to provide an illustration of the types of studies that comprise the burgeoning literature on communication skills in mentally retarded children. These studies embrace a common concern with understanding how well mentally retarded children produce and respond to different types of communicative acts, such as referring to object and events. Although this literature is in its formative stage with respect to both methodology and theory, it is already of value in that it suggests several hypotheses that have implications for intervention.

Research suggests that the communicative difficulties experienced by mentally retarded children are not restricted to language but are also manifest in early forms during the prelinguistic phase of development. Furthermore, current developmental theory postulates that intentional prelinguistic skills embody cognitive factors such as the ability to divide attention between a referent and another person. These cognitive factors presumably provide a foundation for later developments in linguistic communication (Bruner, 1977). It therefore may be effective to begin language intervention programs at an early age by targeting prelinguistic communication skills for training (Seibert & Oller, 1981; Yoder & Reichle, 1977). This type of early intervention may be a particularly useful supplement to extant sensorimotor intervention programs (Bricker, Dennison, & Bricker, 1976). Both types of intervention aim to develop cognitive skills that are important to language acquisition. However, since prelinguistic training would presumably focus on interpersonal exchange, it may be effective in fostering the use of cognitive abilities in social interactions. Moreover, according to our transaction model, if it is possible to increase children's use of higher level (i.e., less ambiguous) prelinguistic acts, this should enhance caregiver–child interactions and help to create a developmentally more positive social milieu.

The communication skills literature also holds useful suggestions for the content or targets of intervention with older children. Until recently, intervention on communication problems among verbal mentally retarded children most often focused on goals related to lexical, syntactic and semantic functioning (Yoder & Reichle, 1977). The communication skills approach suggests that these are important but intermediate goals for language intervention. The ultimate goal is the appropriate use of language in social interactions (Hecht,

Conant, Budoff, & Morse, 1983; Seibert & Oller, 1981). In accordance with this view, several communication programs have expanded their goals to include the training of specific types of acts and processes important to communicative effectiveness, such as referential messages, turn-taking, topic maintenance and topic switching, responding to questions, or use of eye contact during verbal exchanges (Conant, Budoff, & Hecht, 1983; Leger, Groff, Harris, Finfrock, Weaver, & Kratochwill, 1979; MacDonald, 1982; Miller, 1978). Communication skills may also be regarded as a subset of cognitive skills, which are defined by their goals and domain of utilization—problem solving and information exchange in social interactions (Ammon, 1981). Therefore, aspects of communication skill deficits in mentally retarded children may be amenable to treatment with some form of cognitive behavior therapy. For example, it was previously suggested that mentally retarded children may be poor at monitoring the content of their own speech and their understanding of others' speech. If this is correct, cognitive behavior therapy may be an appropriate means by which to help these children to develop a system of rules for interactions, which may help to offset this problem.

Communication skills training may also be a particularly useful means of intervention in the broader domain of social competence in mentally retarded children. Social competence has been advocated as a target both for early intervention programs (Zigler & Trickett, 1978) and for programs that attempt to integrate or mainstream mentally retarded children with normal peers (MacMillan, Jones, & Meyers, 1976). However, a variety of behavioral components may be gathered together under the rubric of social competence (Anderson & Messick, 1975). Progress toward targeting social competence in intervention programs has therefore been impeded by lack of consensus on an operational definition of this factor. The issue is further complicated when one considers that the kinds of skills that lead to successful or adaptive social interactions change throughout the lifespan (Keane & Conger, 1981; Simeonsson, 1978). Therefore, an operational definition of social competence needs to be defined with sufficient plasticity to accommodate developmental shifts in behavioral content.

While it may be difficult to define social competence operationally in its entirety, recent reviews and position papers propose that communication skills play a central role in the development of social competence in mentally retarded children (Blount, 1969; Greenspan, 1979; Schiefelbusch, 1981; Simeonsson, 1978). Furthermore, the utility of a communication skills approach to the assessment and intervention of social competence is supported by a number of points. First, communication skills comprise a set of behaviors that may be well defined operationally. Second, these types of skills also may be targeted for intervention at different developmental levels while maintaining a degree of continuity in the behavioral content of the intervention across age groups. Moreover, the intervention objective of communication skills training is to increase children's functional use of gestures or language to achieve goals in social interactions. This objective dovetails with recent attempts to define social competence. For example, Weiss and Weinstein (1968) define social competence as, "the ability to manipulate others' responses." O'Malley (1977) defines this construct as the ability to engage in, "productive and mutually satisfying interactions between a child and peers or adults," where "productive interactions attain personal goals of the child." Thus, there is an affinity between the goals of communication skills intervention and the apparent nature of what is meant by the term social competence.

Several studies have also found associations between performance on communication skill measures and extant indices of social competence. Previously it was noted that Blacher (1982) found that gestural communication skills increased with performance on a measure of social maturity (Doll, 1965) in a sample of mentally retarded children. Similarly, Halpern and Equinozzi (1969) have shown that the degree to which verbal mentally retarded children can converse coherently with an adult in the context of dyadic interaction is also related to the children's performance on the Vineland Social Maturity Scale (Doll, 1965). Furthermore, this relationship was independent of IQ and chronological age within the sample. In another study, Beveridge et al. (1979) found that mentally retarded children who produce less ambiguous messages on a referential task tended to interact more frequently and initiated more social (i.e., task unrelated) exchanges in classrooms than did children with relatively poor referential communication performance. These findings were obtained from a sample which was quite homogeneous with respect to performance on a standardized measure of expressive language skill. The result of this study were therefore independent of the general level of linguistic competence of the children. Moreover, studies have demonstrated that referential communication task performance is associated with sociometric status (i.e., number of friends) in classrooms of grade school children (Gottman, Gonso, & Rasmussen, 1975; Rubin, 1972). Thus, the rational underpinning the hypothesized utility of a communication skills approach to social competence intervention with mentally retarded children is also supported by research that documents the concurrent validity of communication skill measures as an index of social competence.

One last but very important hypothesis to be discussed derives from research indicating that the perceived characteristics of social partners, such as informational needs (Leonard et al., 1979) or developmental level (Hoy & McKnight, 1977), affect both the quality and content of mentally retarded children's communication interactions with adults or peers (Bedrosian & Prutting, 1978; Hoy & McKnight, 1977). This research suggests that in order to maximize the effectiveness of communication training, it is important to consider the social psychology of the intervention process. That is, the accustomed social roles established between adults and retarded children in communicative interactions may have important influences on what children learn about the communication process and about themselves as communicators.

What are the accustomed social roles established between adults and retarded children? Research indicates that these roles are often characterized by a didactic relationship between the adult and child, which is lacking in reciprocal turn-taking opportunities and serves to predominantly confine the child to a listener/responder role. It was previously noted that these social roles are characteristic of caregiver–child interactions involving mentally retarded children (Brooks-Gunn & Lewis, 1982; Cunningham et al., 1981; Eheart, 1982). Other studies indicate that this is not an isolated experience, but is one that is present in classrooms (Beveridge & Hurrell, 1980) and institutions (Prior, Minnes, Coyne, Golding, Hendy, & McGillivary, 1979; Veit, Allen, & Chinsky, 1976). For example, Prior et al. (1979) found that the most frequent type of interactive initiation between institutional staff and young mentally retarded residents was instructional, as in "go sit down," while the least frequent type of initiation was conversational, as in "What did you do today?" However, conversation-type initiations were also found to be the strongest elicitors of verbal responses from the institutional residents. Thus, as Prior et al. concluded, "the most favorable form of communication for the promotion of verbal responses from residents is the least evident in the habitual milieu of the residents." Moreover, results from this study indicated that residents initiations were ignored approximately one-third of the time by staff members.

A highly didactic approach is also common to many intervention programs that specifically target language and communication skills (Hecht et al., 1983; Yoder & Reichle, 1977). Because of a focus on a training agenda, the interventionist in many of these programs may be so intent on eliciting a specific response that initiations on the part of the child are missed or ignored (Seibert & Oller, 1981). Common intervention practices may also often violate the child's role as a communicative partner in the interaction. For example, intervention programs based on learning theory may incorporate the use of positive social reinforcement, such as responding to the children's verbal initiations with, "that's good talking." Although the use of social reinforcement may have positive effects on the frequency of social behaviors (Mayhew, Enyart, Anderson, 1978), the use of reinforcers in this type of situation may serve to disrupt the children's understanding of the communicative functions of behavior since the reinforcer is usually discontinuous with the children's communicative intent (Seibert & Oller, 1981).

Potential problems with lexical drilling strategies such as holding up desired objects out of reach and asking, "What is this?" or "What do you want?" have also been noted. Such a situation is characterized by an abitrary demand for talking (Hecht et al., 1983), which violates the validity of the communicative context for the child, since the adult knows the name of the object, the adult knows that the child wants the object, and the child is aware of all of this (Seibert & Oller, 1981). This argument is supported by research that suggests that even among very young mentally retarded children, responding to requests for labels is affected by whether the label is likely to provide information to the adult listener (Leonard et al., 1979).

As part of a transactional process, a directive and didactic style of adult–child interaction may arise in response to adult's perception of the behavioral and communicative disorganization of mentally retarded children. Furthermore, this style of interaction may often be necessary because the child-to-adult ratio in the home or institution prohibits the degree of attention needed to be consistently responsive to individual children. However, if this style of interaction becomes a pervasive feature of children's communicative interactions, it is reasonable to assume that the development of communication skills in mentally retarded children is affected as a result. This style of interaction is imbalanced with respect to opportunities for the child to experience reciprocal turn-taking exchanges in communicative interaction. Exposure to reciprocal turn-taking in communicative interactions is believed to be necessary to the practice and enhancement of ecologically valid communication skills (MacDonald, 1982). Repeated exposure to this imbalanced style of interaction could lead children to develop a negative (i.e., passive) view of their roles as communicators whereby children may become reticient to initiate communicative acts and uncomfortable in the role of initiator when circumstances force the issue. Furthermore, this negative self-image as communicator may lead the child to neglect the use of certain communicative functions such as declarations or questions (Bliss, Allen, & Walker, 1978; Owens & MacDonald, 1982) and may contribute to difficulties in the cognitive monitoring of ongoing speech and comprehension of utterances.

Of course the effect of styles of interaction may be expected to vary with the personality of the retarded child (Beveridge & Hurrell, 1980). Nevertheless the social role adopted by caregivers and parents vis-a-vis the child remains an important consideration for caregivers and professionals who hope to optimize the effects of intervention on mentally retarded children. Particularly where communication skills are concerned, teachers and caregivers should be aware of the need to supplement didactic interactions with situations where the social context maximizes the likelihood that children will experience the role of initiator/speaker as well as listener/responder.

However, those who have worked with handicapped children recognize the caregivers' and interventionists' need for specific and organized training agenda. Therefore, it is very likely that the implementation of this intervention approach will depend upon the availability of simple structured situations for the home and classroom that provide adults with an organized framework for presenting children with nondidactic, reciprocally responsive communication training. Fortunately, models for these types of interactional situations may already be at hand in the form of the measures used to assess communication skills. For example, the procedures used to assess prelinguistic skills present structured situations designed to elicit child-initiated communicative acts while also providing guidelines for the maintenance of a responsive and flexible adult role during the assessment interaction (Seibert & Hogan, 1981). With older children, game playing referential communication situations (Hoy & McKnight, 1977) provide structured interactions that are enjoyable and that allow children to initiate and practice specific functional uses of language with peers and adults (Conant, Budoff, & Hecht, 1983; Hecht, Conant, Budoff, & Morse, 1983).

CONCLUSIONS

A purpose of this chapter has been to argue for the potential of the communication skills literature to contribute to theory and practice concerning developmental deficits in retarded children. This literature, however, is still in its formative period of development. There are many issues remaining that need to be addressed before the potential of this literature reaches fruition. The following presents a brief discussion of some of these issues.

In the beginning of this chapter the distinction between research on speech, language, and communication skills was noted. This distinction reflects the assumption that the capacity to use speech and language as a vehicle for communication emerges somewhat independently from the development of the ability to produce speech and language. Nevertheless, it probably is the case that speech, language, and communication skills interact to produce the overall communicative competence of children. For example, cognitive capacity limits may affect retarded children's ability to monitor ongoing interactions and produce appropriate types of communicative acts. Also, processes involved simply in the production of language may severely tax the cognitive capacity limits of mentally retarded children. Communication skill deficits may emerge in retarded children because these children cannot handle the simultaneous cognitive demands of language production *and* monitoring the context of social interactions. This illustration is intended to underscore the need to integrate speech, language, and communication skills research to better understand the communication problems of the retarded child.

The recurrent theme in this chapter that the communication skills of retarded children are affected by the characteristics or style of interaction of communicative partners reflects another important question for additional study. To what extent are specific communication skill deficits in mentally retarded children the result of perceptions of social context and their own social status, or the result of cognitive retardation per se? A definitive answer to this question will no doubt be difficult to obtain. Nevertheless, information garnered in the attempt to address this complex issue should prove valuable in establishing appropriate methods and goals for communication skills intervention. To begin to answer this question, however, researchers will need to gather better data on the comparative skills of normal and retarded children. All too often studies of communication skills in retarded children have neglected the use of developmentally matched control groups. Although the validity of variables used to developmentally equate normal and retarded children (e.g., MA, MLU) is controversial, continuing to produce research in this area without normal comparison data is less than acceptable.

A third issue of concern involves the question of whether or not there is developmental continuity in communication skill differences found among retarded children. In other words, are individual differences in prelinguistic skills related to differences in linguistic skills in childhood, and are differences in childhood linguistic skills related to adult skill levels. The results of longitudinal research addressing this question would have obvious implications for the validity of attempts to intervene with the development of communication skills. The choice of variables to study in research of this nature may depend on what is learned from comparative studies of retarded and normal children. Also the focus of this research should be guided by a picture of ultimate outcome, that is, the communication skills of retarded adults. At present little is known concerning the skills of retarded adults. However, research on interactive communicative competence (Abbeduto & Rosenberg, 1980; Bedrosian & Prutting, 1978) and referential skills (Kearnan & Sabsay, 1983) of retarded adults have begun to fill this gap in the literature.

Given the context of this volume, perhaps the most important question for study is whether communication skill deficiencies are involved in the development of emotional problems in mentally retarded children. It is plausible that the degree to which children cannot interact effectively with peers and adults is related to the tendency to manifest the symptomology of emotional disturbance (e.g., depression or conduct disorder). Moreover, the research discussed in this chapter (e.g., Beveridge et al., 1979; Gottman et al., 1975) suggests that level of communication skill is directly related to children's ability to interact effectively with others. Thus, it is reasonable to expect that individual differences in communication skills are related to emotional problems in mentally retarded children. Of course, if such a relationship is documented in additional research, it will be necessary to attempt to determine the causal path of association. That is, communication skill deficits may serve as an etiologic agent in the development of emotional problems, or communication skill deficits may be the result of existing emotional disturbance. In addition, a variety of environmental, organic and/or personality factors may to a greater or lesser extent influence the development of emotional disorder in the retarded. Therefore, to address this issue, research will also need to be multivariate in order to determine the relative role of communication skills in the complex network of variables affecting (or affected by) the emotional wellbeing of retarded children.

In summary, we have suggested several issues that would be useful to consider in additional research concerning communication skills in retarded children. These are the need to consider the interaction of speech and language ability with communication skill in understanding communication problems, the question of the relative role of social perception and cognitive deficits in communication skill deficiencies, the need to gather better comparative data on retarded and normal children, the question of developmental continuity in individual differences in communication skills, the need to develop a better picture of outcome, that is, the communication skills of retarded adults, and the question of whether communication skill deficits affect or reflect the development of emotional problems in retarded children.

Acknowledgment

During the preparation of this paper the first author was supported by a National Research Service Award administered through the Clinical Research Center for Childhood Psychosis at the Neuropsychiatric Institute of the University of California at Los Angeles.

REFERENCES

Abbeduto, L, & Rosenberg, S. (1980). The communication competence of mildly retarded adults. *Applied Psycholinguistics, 1,* 405–426

Ammon, P. (1981). Communication skills and communicative competence: A neoPiagetian process—structural view. In WP Dickson (Ed.), *Children's oral communication skills.* New York: Academic Press

Anderson, S, & Messick, S. (1975). Social competency in young children. *Developmental Psychology, 10,* 282–293

Austin, JL. (1962). *How to do things with words.* Cambridge, MA: Harvard University Press

Bates, E. (1976). *Language and context: The acquisition of pragmatics.* New York: Academic Press

Bates, E, Benigni, L, Bretherton, I, Camaioni, L, & Volterra, V. (1979). *The emergence of symbols: Cognition and communication in infancy.* New York: Academic Press

Bayley, N. (1969). *Bayley Scales of Infant Development.* New York: Psychological Corporation

Bedrosian, JL, & Prutting, CA. (1978). Communicative performance of Mentally retarded adults in four conversational settings. *Journal of Speech and Hearing Research, 21,* 79–95

Benedict, H. (1979). Early lexical development: Comprehension and production. *Journal of Child Language, 6,* 183–200

Berger, J, & Cunningham, CC. (1981). The development of eye contact between mothers and normal versus Down's Syndrome infants. *Developmental Psychology, 17,* 678–689

Beveridge, M, & Hurrell, P. (1980). Teachers' responses to severely mentally handicapped children's initiations in the classroom. *Journal of Child Psychology and Psychiatry, 21,* 175–181

Beveridge, M, Spencer, J, & Mittler, P. (1979). Self blame and communication failure in retarded adolescents. *Journal of Child Psychology and Psychiatry, 20,* 129–138

Beveridge, M, & Tatham, A. (1976). Communication in retarded adolescents: Utilization of known language skills. *American Journal of Mental Deficiency, 81,* 96–99

Blacher, J. (1982). Assessing social cognition in young mentally retarded and nonretarded children. *American Journal of Mental Deficiency, 86,* 473–484

Bliss, LS, Allen, DV, & Walter, G. (1978). Sentence structures of trainable and educable mentally retarded subjects. *Journal of Speech and Hearing Research, 21,* 722–731

Blount, WR. (1969). A comment on language, socialization, acceptance and the retarded. *Mental Retardation, 7,* 33–35

Borys, SV. (1979). Factors influencing the interrogative strategies of mentally retarded and nonretarded students. *American Journal of Mental Deficiency, 84,* 280–288

Bricker, D, Dennison, L, & Bricker, W. (1976). A language intervention program for developmentally young children. *Mailman Center for Child Development Monographs, Vol. 1*

Brooks-Gunn, J, & Lewis, M. (1982). Affective exchanges between normal and handicapped infants and their mothers. In T Field & A Fogel (Eds.), *Emotion and interaction: Normal and high-risk infants.* Hillsdale, NJ: Erlbaum

Bruner, JS. (1977). Early social interactions and language acquisition. In HR Schaffer (Ed.), *Studies in mother infant interaction.* New York: Academic Press

Butterworth, G, & Jarrett, N. (1982). *Origins of referential communication in human infancy.* Paper presented at the International Conference on Infant Studies, Austin, TX

Conant, SJ, Budoff, M, & Hecht, BF. (1983). *Teaching language disabled children: A communication games intervention.* Cambridge, MA: The Ware Press

Cunningham, CE, Rueller E, Blackwell, J, & Deck, J. (1981). Behavioral and linguistic developments in the interactions of normal and retarded children with their mothers. *Child Development, 52,* 62–70

Denny, DR. (1974). Recognition, formulation, and integration in the development of interrogative strategies among normal and retarded children. *Child Development, 45,* 1068–1076

Dewart, MH. (1979). Language comprehension processes of mentally retarded children. *American Journal of Mental Deficiency, 84,* 177–183

Dickson, WP. (Ed.) (1981). *Children's oral communication skills.* New York: Academic Press

Dodd, B. (1975). Recognition and reproduction of words by Down's Syndrome and non Down's Syndrome retarded children. *American Journal of Mental Deficiency, 80,* 306–311

Doll, EA. (1965). *Vineland Social Maturity Scale.* Circle Pines, MN: American Guidance Service

Duncham, JF, & Erickson, JG. (1976). Normal and retarded children's understanding of semantic relations in different verbal contexts. *Journal of Speech and Hearing Research, 19,* 749–766

Eheart, BK. (1982). Mother-child interactions with nonretarded and mentally retarded preschoolers. *American Journal of Mental Deficiency, 87,* 20–25

Emde, RN, Katz, EL, & Thorpe, JK. (1978). Emotional expression in infancy: Early deviations in Down's Syndrome. In M Lewis & LA Rosenblum (Eds.), *The development of affect.* New York: Plenum

Fischer, KW. (1980). A theory of cognitive development: The control and construction of hierarchies of skills. *Psychological Review, 87,* 477–531

Flavell, JH. (1981). Cognitive monitoring. In WP Dickson (Ed.), *Children's oral communication skills.* New York: Academic Press

Glucksberg, S, Krauss, RM, & Weisberg, R. (1966). Referential communication in nursery school children: Method and some preliminary findings. *Journal of Experimental Psychology, 3,* 333–342

Gottman, J, Gonso, J, & Rasmussen, B. (1975). Social interaction, social competence, and friendship in children. *Child Development, 46,* 706–718

Greenspan, S. (1979). Social intelligence in the retarded. In NR Ellis (Ed.), *Handbook of mental deficiency, psychological theory & research.* Hillsdale, NJ: Erlbaum

Greenwald, CA, & Leonard, LB. (1979). Communicative and sensorimotor development of Down's syndrome children. *American Journal of Mental Deficiency, 84,* 296–303

Gunn, P, Berry, P, & Andrews, RJ. (1982). Looking behavior of Down's Syndrome infants. *American Journal of Mental Deficiency, 87,* 344–347

Halpern, AS, & Equinozzi, AM. (1969). Verbal expressivity as an index of adaptive behavior. *American Journal of Mental Deficiency, 74,* 180–186

Harding, CG. (1982). Development of the intention to communicate. *Human Development, 25,* 140–151

Hecht, BF, Conant, S, Budoff, M, Morse, R. (1983). *Language intervention: A pragmatic approach.* Manuscript in preparation, University of California, School of Education, Los Angeles, CA

Hoy, EA, & McKnight, JR. (1977). Communication style and effectiveness in homogeneous and heterogeneous dyads of retarded children. *American Journal of Mental Deficiency, 81,* 587–598

Hurtig, R, Ensrud, S, Tomblin, JB. (1982). The communicative function of question production in autistic children. *Journal of Autism and Developmental Disorders, 12,* 57–69

Hymes, D. (1974). *Foundations in sociolinguistics: An ethnographic approach.* Philadelphia, PA: University of Pennsylvania Press

Jones, OMH. (1980). Prelinguitic communication skills in Down's Syndrome and normal infants. In TM Field, S Goldberg, D Stern, & AM Sostek (Eds.). *High-risk infants and children: Adult and peer interactions.* New York: Academic Press

Keane, SP, & Conger, JC. (1981). The implications of communication development for social skills training. *Journal of Pediatric Psychology, 6,* 369–381

Kearnan, K, & Sabsay, S. (1983) *Communication in mildly retarded adults.* Research in progress, University of California, Neuropsychiatric Institute, Los Angeles, CA

Krauss, RM, & Glucksberg, S. (1969). The development of communication: Competence as a function of age. *Child Development, 49,* 255–266

Layton, TL, & Sharifi, H. (1978). Meaning and structure of Down's Syndrome and nonretarded children's spontaneous speech. *American Journal of Mental Deficiency, 83,* 439–445

Leger, HJ, Groff, D, Harris, VW, Finfrock, LR, Weaver, FH, & Kratochwill, TR. (1979). An instrumental package to teach communication behaviors in a classroom setting. *Journal of School Psychology, 17,* 339–346

Lempers, JD, Flavell, ER, & Flavell, JH. (1977). The development in very young children of tacit knowledge concerning visual perception. *Genetic Psychology Monographs, 95,* 3–53

Leonard, LB, Cole, B, & Steckol, KF. (1979). Lexical usage of retarded children: An examination of informativeness. *American Journal of Mental Deficiency, 84,* 49–54

Lobato, D, Barrera, RD, & Feldman, RS. (1981). Sensorimotor functioning and prelinguistic communication of severely and profoundly retarded individuals. *American Journal of Mental Deficiency, 85,* 489–496

Longhurst, TM. (1974). Communication in retarded adolescents: Sex and intelligence level. *American Journal of Mental Deficiency, 78,* 607–618

Longhurst, TM, & Berry, GW. (1975). Communication in retarded adolescents: Response to listener feedback. *American Journal of Mental Deficiency, 80,* 158–164

MacDonald, JD. (1982). Communication strategies for language intervention. In DP McClowerg, AM Guilford, & SO Richardson (Eds.), *Infant communication: Development, assessment, and intervention.* New York: Grune & Stratton

MacMillan, D, Jones, R, & Meyers, CE. (1976). Mainstreaming the mentally retarded: Some questions, cautions, and guidelines. *Mental Retardation, 14,* 3–10

Markman, EM. (1981). Comprehension monitoring. In WP Dickson (Ed.), *Children's oral communication skills.* New York: Academic Press

Masur, EF. (1981). Mothers' responses to infants object-related gestures: Influences on lexical development. *Journal of Child Language, 9,* 23–30

Mayhew, GL, Enyart, P, & Anderson, J. (1978). Social reinforcement and the naturally occurring social responses of severely and profoundly retarded adolescents. *American Journal of Mental Deficiency, 83,* 164–170

McLeavey, BC, Toomey, JF, & Dempsey, PJR. (1981). Nonretarded and MR children's control over syntactic structures. *American Journal of Mental Deficiency, 86,* 485–494

Miller, JF, Chapman, RS, Branstow, MB, & Reichle, J. (1980). Language comprehension in sensorimotor stage V and VI. *Journal of Speech and Hearing Research, 23,* 284–311

Miller, L. (1978). Pragmatics and early childhood language disorders: Communicative interactions in a half-hour sample. *Journal of Speech and Hearing Disorders, 43,* 419–436

Mundy, P, Seibert, J, Hogan, A. (1984). Relationships between sensorimotor and early communication abilities in developmentally delayed children. *Merrill-Palmer Quarterly, 30,* 33–48

Mundy, P, Seibert, J, Hogan, A, & Fagan, J. (1983). Novelty responding and behavioral development in young, developmentally delayed children. *Intelligence, 7,* 163–174

Murphy, CM. (1978). Pointing in the context of a shared activity. *Child Development, 49,* 371–380

Naremore, RC, & Dever, RB. (1975). Language performance of educable mentally retarded and normal children at five age levels. *Journal of Speech and Hearing Research, 18,* 82–95

Nelson, K. (1973). Structure and strategy in learning to talk. *Monograph for Society of Research in Child Development, 3* (149)

Niswander, PS, & Kelley, LW. (1975). Comparison of speech discrimination in nonretarded and retarded listeners. *American Journal of Mental Deficiency, 80,* 217–222

O'Malley, JM. (1977). Research perspective on social competence. *Merrill-Palmer Quarterly, 23,* 29–44

Owens, RE, & MacDonald, JD. (1982). Communicative uses of the early speech of nondelayed and Down Syndrome children. *American Journal of Mental Deficiency, 86,* 503–510

Peterson, CL, Donner, FW, & Flavell, JH. (1972). Developmental changes in children's response to three indications of communicative failure. *Child Development, 43,* 1463–1468

Piaget, J. (1952). *The origins of intelligence in children.* New York: International Universities Press

Prior, M, Minnes, P, Coyne, T, Golding, B, Hendy, J, McGillivary, J. (1979). Verbal interactions between staff residents in an institution for the young mentally retarded. *Mental Retardation, 17,* 65–69

Rheingold, HL, Hay, DF, & West, MJ. (1976). Sharing in the second year of life. *Child Development, 83,* 898–913

Rosenberg, S, & Cohen, BD. (1966). Referential processes of speakers and listeners. *Psychological Review, 73,* 208–231

Rosenberg, S, Spradlin, JE, & Mabel, S. (1961). Interaction among retarded children as a function of their relative language skills. *Journal of Abnormal and Social Psychology, 63,* 402–410

Ross, DM, & Ross, SA. (1972). The efficacy of listening training for educable mentally retarded children. *American Journal of Mental Deficiency, 77,* 137–142

Rubin, KH. (1972). Relationship between egocentric communication and popularity among peers. *Developmental Psychology, 7,* 364

Rueda, R, & Chan, KS. (1980). Referential communication skill levels of moderately mentally retarded adolescents. *American Journal of Mental Deficiency, 85,* 45–52

Sameroff, A. (1975). Transactional models in early social relations. *Human Development, 18,* 65–79

Schiefelbusch, RL. (1981). Development of social competence and incompetence. In MJ Begab, HC Haywood, & HL Garber (Eds.), *Psychological issues in retarded performance* (Vol. 1) Baltimore, MD: University Park Press

Seibert, JM, & Hogan, AE. (1982). *Procedures manual for the Early Social Communication Scales (ESCS).* Mailman Center for Child Development, University of Miami, FL

Seibert, JM, Hogan, AE, & Mundy, PC. (1982). Assessing interactional competencies: The Early Social-Communication Scales. *Infant Mental Health Journal, 3,* 244–258

Seibert, JM, Hogan, AE, & Mundy, PC. (1984). Mental age and cognitive stage in young handicapped and at risk children. *Intelligence, 8,* 11–29

Seibert, JM, & Oller, DK. (1981). Linguistic pragmatics and language intervention strategies. *Journal of Autism and Developmental Disorders, 11,* 75–88

Shatz, M. (1983). Communication. In PH Mussen (Ed.), *Handbook of child psychology. Cognitive development* (Vol. 3). New York: Wiley

Shatz, M, & Gelman, R. (1973). The development of communication skills: Modification in the speech of young children as a function of the listener. *Monographs of the Society for Research in Child Development, 38* (5, Serial No. 152)

Simeonsson, RJ. (1978). Social competence: Dimensions & directions. In J Wortis (Ed.), *Annual review of mental retardation and developmental disabilities* (Vol. 10). New York: Brunner/Mazel

Snyder, L. (1978). Communicative and cognitive abilities and disabilities in the sensorimotor period. *Merrill-Palmer Quarterly, 24,* 161–180

Stevenson, MB, & Lamb, ME. (1982). The effects of social experience and social style on cognitive competence and performance. In ME Lamb & LR Sherrod (Eds.), *Infant social cognition: Empirical and theoretical considerations.* Hillsdale, NJ: Erlbaum

Sugarman-Bell, S. (1978). Some organizational aspects of pre-verbal communication. In I Markova (Ed.), *The social context of language.* New York: Wiley

Trevarthen, C, & Hubley, P. (1978). Secondary intersubjectivity: Confidence confiding and acts of meaning in the first year. In A Lock (Ed.), *Action gesture and symbol: The emergence of language.* New York: Academic Press

Weiss, D, & Weinstein, E. (1968). Interpersonal tactics among mental retardates. *American Journal of Mental Deficiency, 72,* 653–667

West, MJ, & Rheingold, HL. (1978). Infant stimulation of maternal instruction. *Infant Behavior and Development, 1,* 127–140

Veit, SW, Allen, GJ, & Chinsky, JM. (1976). Interpersonal interactions between institutionalized retarded children and their attendants. *American Journal of Mental Deficiency, 80,* 535–542

Yoder, DE, & Reichle, JE. (1977). Some current perspectives on teaching communication functions to mentally retarded children. In P Mittler (Ed.), *Research to practice in mental retardation: Education and training,* (Vol. 2) Baltimore, MD: University Park Press

Zigler, E, & Trickett, PK. (1978). IQ, social competence and evaluation of early childhood intervention programs. *American Psychologist, 37,* 789–797

Douglas C. Smith
Denise Valenti-Hein
Tamar Heller

4

Interpersonal Competence and Community Adjustment of Retarded Adults

With increased emphasis on deinstitutionalization and community placement of mentally retarded adults, concern with the social competence of this group has risen sharply. A substantial body of literature has evolved linking social competence to a number of aspects of successful community adjustment including living independently (Shalock & Harper, 1978; Shalock, Harper, & Carrer, 1981), securing and maintaining competitive employment (Fulton, 1975; Greenspan & Shoultz, 1981), and becoming socially integrated within the community (Reiter & Levi, 1980). Although these relationships appear to be fairly well established across studies, the precise mechanisms by which they exist are far from clear. Part of the difficulty lies in the manner in which social competence is operationalized for research purposes.

Social competence has historically been viewed as a broad construct encompassing a wide variety of personal characteristics and adaptive skills. Anderson and Messick (1974), in their comprehensive review of defining approaches, describe no less than 29 distinct domains of competence. Included among these are such facets as personal maintenance and care, realistic feelings of self-worth, appropriate regulation of antisocial behavior, perceptual and motor skills, and enjoyment of humor, play and fantasy. Simeonsson (1978), in his review of social competence within developmentally disabled populations, organizes his discussion around five prevalent theoretical orientations. These include equating social competence with adaptive behaviors,

CHILDREN WITH EMOTIONAL DISORDERS AND DEVELOPMENTAL DISABILITIES ISBN 0–8089–1700–5

vocational success, personality factors, interpersonal skills, and developmental indices of social maturity.

The descriptions of Anderson and Messick and of Simeonsson illustrate the lack of concensus regarding defining parameters of social competence. Furthermore, many of the skills included appear only tangentially related to "social" competence. Nowhere is this better illustrated than in social skills training programs designed for mentally retarded individuals. Typically, these programs include such skill areas as personal hygiene and grooming, toileting, proper use of eating utensils, money management, use of public transportation, and a number of other essentially "self-help" skills. While training in these areas may be of considerable importance for the adaptive functioning of retarded persons, its relevance for stimulating and enhancing interactions with other people is highly questionable.

In discussing the community adjustment of retarded adults within the present chapter, we wish to focus on a fairly narrow band of social behaviors that we will term "interpersonal competence." A proposed distinction between interpersonal and personal skills as distinct domains of competence has been made elsewhere in the literature, as by Andrasik and Matson (1985) and by Greenspan (1981), and should prove useful in clarifying our discussion.

Interpersonal competence, as we will use the term, refers to a set of behaviors or capabilities that increase the probability of an individual's effectively functioning within a social context (i.e., during interactions with other people). "Effective" functioning stresses the goal-directedness of social behavior and is consistent with prior conceptualizations of competence (Edmonson, 1974; Weinstein, 1969, White, 1959). Inherent here is the prospect of goal attainment as a primary source of competence.

What types of goals then are sought by individuals in interpersonal situations? Typically these include such things as expressing and receiving affection, obtaining information, persuading others to assist with a difficult task, or making positive impressions. Clearly, the more highly skilled individual (e.g., the accomplished conversationalist, the better role-taker, the more adept problem-solver), is likely to be in a better position to reach his or her interpersonal goals.

Our major concern within the present chapter is to emphasize the role that interpersonal competence may play in the successful community adjustment of retarded adults. Our discussion will be organized around three facets that appear to be critical to the quality of life of retarded individuals and have typically been employed as indices of community adjustment. These include peer relationships, job placement and success, and development of satisfactory sexual relationships. Within each area, our intent is to provide information attesting to the current adjustment status of retarded adults. The chapter will conclude with a discussion of two theoretical approaches for improving interpersonal competence and, hence, community adjustment of retarded individuals.

PEER STATUS OF RETARDED ADULTS

With the passage of Public Law 94-142 (Education for All Handicapped Children Act) in 1975, many mildly retarded and a substantial number of moderately retarded school-age children were placed in less restrictive, more "normalized" environments for varying portions of the school day. Whereas many of these children were formerly educated in segregated, self-contained special education classrooms, legislation now encourages and, in some cases, demands integration into the "mainstream" of school activities. Thus, some retarded students, depending on their intellectual and adaptive skills, may now receive instruction within a regular classroom setting. Many other retarded youth participate to some extent in nonacademic activities (i.e., recess, lunch, school programs) with nonretarded peers.

A substantial body of research has accumulated describing the social status of retarded children in mainstreamed school settings. Overwhelmingly the results indicate that retarded students are often the victims of isolation and rejection at the hands of nonhandicapped peers (Gottlieb, 1981, Gottlieb, Semmel, & Veldman, 1978). Apparently, this distressing pattern of social nonacceptance is even more pervasive in the case of mainstreamed students than for those who remain in segregated settings (Goodman, Gottlieb, & Harrison, 1972, Gottlieb & Budoff, 1973).

Mainstreaming of retarded students in educational settings parallels to some extent the "normalization" movement in the field of mental health. Normalization in terms of community placement, independent or supervised living arrangements, and opportunities for gainful employment provide retarded clients with significantly greater opportunities to coexist with nonhandicapped members of society.

If independent living within the community is a goal of normalization efforts for retarded adults, it would appear that an important question for researchers concerns the social status of retarded adults within the community. Our review of the literature, however, revealed little information on the friendship patterns of retarded adults outside institutional or supervised living facilities. One reason for the relative paucity of studies in this area may be that a majority of mildly retarded individuals, identified primarily through the schools, cease to be classified as functionally retarded once they leave the school system (MacMillan, 1982). For all intents and purposes, this group, primarily composed of those diagnosed as retarded due to psychosocial disadvantage (Grossman, 1983), lead normal and productive lives, albeit in the lower socioeconomic strata of society (Goldstein, 1964).

The small number of studies available on the social status of retarded adults living independently within the community have, with few exceptions, been based on client or parent reports. This procedure has yielded descriptive information regarding the social networks of adults who formerly resided in institutional settings or who attended special education classes for the mentally retarded. In the following section, we will review results of these studies.

Studies of Retarded Adults in Independent Living Arrangements

One of the earlier follow-up studies of the social status of retarded adults was conducted in Israel by Katz and Yekutiel (1974). Utilizing parent reports, the study examined the friendship patterns of 128 retarded adults who had "graduated" from sheltered workshops and were, at the time of the study, living in either group homes, with their families, or independently within the community.

Of those clients living independently within the community, lack of social contact appeared to be a major obstacle to this group's successful adjustment. Approximately two-thirds of parents interviewed reported that their retarded offspring had no friends in the community and more than 70 percent reported that these individuals spent no time with members of the opposite sex. In addition, parents maintained that lack of suitable companions was the primary problem facing their retarded offspring in terms of leisure time activities.

Further evidence supporting the limited social networks of retarded adults within the community comes from a follow-up study of 88 young adults who had formerly attended special education classes in the United Kingdom (Richardson, 1978). Based on data obtained from subjects' self-reports and, in some cases, corroborative reports by parents, retarded subjects were compared to a random sample of nonretarded young adults matched on chronological age, sex, and socioeconomic status.

Results indicated that only 58 percent of the retarded group were able to name at least two best friends (as compared to 89 percent of the nonretarded group) and only one-third maintained that they had a special friend of the opposite sex (as opposed to two-thirds of the nonretarded group). Although these figures regarding friendship networks are more optimistic than those reported by Katz and Yekutiel, the fact remains that many retarded adults have considerable difficulty forming intimate social relationships (i.e., friendships with other people in the community).

Studies by Reiter and Levi (1980) and Shalock et al. (1981) provide additional support for the hypothesis that retarded adults have few people whom they can consider friends in community settings. In the Reiter and Levi study, parents of 30 moderately and mildly retarded young adults who had previously attended special education classes were questioned regarding the degree of social integration of their offspring. Only five of the 30 subjects had nonretarded friends, according to parents, and 16 of the 30 were reported to have no friends at all.

Shalock et al. (1981) studied the social networks of retarded adults who were fully integrated into the community (defined here as living in independent housing and engaged in competitive employment). Of the 27 formerly institutionalized adults who met this criterion, one-third reported having no friends, with the remainder reporting only one or two friends, usually a roommate or staff member from a former placement facility.

Although the studies reviewed thus far suffer from the potential inaccuracies inherent in self-report data, several general, albeit tentative, conclusions may be drawn. First, establishing meaningful social contacts within the community is a difficult proposition for many mentally retarded adults. A considerable portion of those interviewed (or their parents) indicated that they had no one in the community whom they could consider as a "friend".

A second conclusion to be drawn is that lack of friendships may constitute a major obstacle to the successful adjustment of retarded adults living independently. A growing body of research with nonretarded populations is indicative of the relationship between lack of friends and concurrent or subsequent emotional and mental health problems (Asher, Oden, & Gottman, 1977; Cowen, Pedersen, Babigian, Izzo, & Trost, 1973). For retarded individuals placed in community settings, lack of friendships, particularly as an aspect of the social support system, may impose an additional burden for adjustment.

As a final point, we might surmise that retarded people who are without friends spend a good deal of their leisure time in solitary activities. In a study of 18 formerly institutionalized retarded adults (most of whom were mildly retarded), McDevitt, Smith, Schmidt, and Rosen (1978) reported that many of their subjects spent considerable amounts of time alone, usually engaged in passive activities, such as watching television. Very few subjects reported participating in community activities, with the exception of church-sponsored socials or activities organized by their former institution's "alumni" club. Thus, it appears that for many retarded adults, social contacts, if they are to be made, are most likely to occur with other retarded people.

Although the evidence reviewed thus far provides some insight into the problems experienced by mentally retarded adults living within the community, many questions remain unanswered. Perhaps the most important concern the characteristics of individuals and of settings that influence peer interactions and friendship formation. What, for example, is the potential of retarded persons for forming meaningful social contacts? Under what circumstances would these most likely occur?

In seeking answers to these complex questions, we turn now to studies of retarded adults living in supervised facilities. Much of the available data is based on direct observation of client social behavior within various facilities. Thus, the information should prove useful in specifying interpersonal competencies that are associated with friendship formation as well as environmental variables that either restrict or enhance opportunities for social interaction among retarded adults.

Studies of Retarded Adults in Community Living Facilities

Extensive investigations of the social behavior of retarded adults in group homes, sheltered workshops, and other community living facilities have been conducted by Landesman-Dwyer and colleagues at the University of Washington (Landesman-Dwyer, Berkson, & Romer, 1979, Landesman-Dwyer, Stein, & Sackett, 1978) and by Berkson, Romer, and colleagues at the University of Illinois, Chicago (Berkson & Romer, 1980, Romer & Berkson, 1980a, 1980b). Both groups of researchers observed the friendship patterns and interactive behaviors of large numbers of mentally retarded adults across placement settings varying on a number of dimensions. Utilizing multiple regression techniques, these studies present evidence regarding the relative contributions of both environmental and client characteristics to social behavior.

Landesman-Dwyer, Berkson, and Romer (1979) observed the interpersonal behavior of 208 mostly mild and moderately retarded adults in 18 community-based group homes. Within these settings, it was observed that clients spent most of their unstructured time engaged in nonaffiliative behaviors (i.e., not in the company of others), considerably less time with one peer, and progressively less time with two and more peers. Almost all of the residents' affiliative behavior occurred in dyads; however, within 8 group homes only 16 pairs of "friends" were observed (defined as pairs who spent more than 10 percent of the observed time together).

Perhaps the most important set of findings from the Landesman-Dwyer et al. study concerns the characteristics of environments and of the residents' themselves that predict affiliative behavior. Interestingly, individual characteristics such as sex and intelligence level were not significant predictors. Group home characteristics including average or collective intelligence level of residents, sex ratio of clients, homogeneity of residents' backgrounds, and size of facility were much more influential in determining the extent and intensity of residents' affiliative behaviors. Specifically, residents from group homes that housed more intelligent clients evidenced more intense social relationships; intense relationships were observed more often in homes that were predominantly female; more intense relationships occurred in homes that were homogeneous in terms of residents' backgrounds; and larger group homes fostered a wider variety of peer contacts.

Berkson and Romer (Berkson & Romer, 1980; Romer & Berkson, 1980a, 1980b, 1981) observed 315 mentally retarded and mentally ill adults within four sheltered workshop settings and a sheltered-care residential facility. Like the Landesman-Dwyer et al. (1979) study, observations of clients' social behaviors took place during informal activities such as coffee breaks, lunch, and recreation periods.

Three dimensions of affiliative behavior were identified. These included extensity—the number of different people an individual associates with; intensity—the amount of time spent interacting with a particular person; and aggregation—proximity of an individual to other people in a noninteractive situation.

Observations indicated that mentally retarded adults spent considerable portions of their time engaged in social activities. Almost 40 percent of observation intervals were coded as affiliative; an additional 40 percent involved clients in close proximity to one another. Consistent with the Landesman-Dwyer et al. (1979) findings, most social interactions occurred in dyads. On the whole, it appeared that retarded clients had social contacts with many different people during a typical day; however, the number of clients with whom frequent interactions occurred was relatively small (2.8 people).

Romer and Berkson (1980a) reported on the characteristics of clients and of settings that were predictive of affiliative behavior. Individual personal characteristics subjected to analysis included sex, age, IQ, diagnosis, physical attractiveness, and desire for affiliation. Context variables corresponded to the settings in which clients were observed. The most striking finding to result from the regression analysis was that from 16 to 63 percent of the variation in affiliative behavior could be accounted for by context as opposed to individual difference predictors.

Context characteristics thus appear to be important determinants of the social behavior of retarded individuals in community facilities. In particular, Romer and Berkson point out that the average IQ of peers within a setting is strongly related to affiliation. Again consistent with the Landesman-Dwyer et al. (1979) findings, it appears that individuals surrounded by others of a higher intelligence level will evidence more sociability, regardless of their own IQ. Such a finding argues against the practice of segregating clients on the basis of IQ in facilities serving the mentally retarded.

The two personal characteristics that best predicted affiliative behavior were age and diagnosis. Older clients and those diagnosed as mentally ill interacted with fewer people on the average and also were seen less in the proximity of other clients. Interestingly, individual IQ was unrelated to any of the dimensions of affiliative behavior. Romer and Berkson (1980a) view this finding as particularly encouraging since it suggests that, "individuals over a broad range of ability can be equally successful in forming and maintaining interpersonal relationships" (p. 241).

Romer and Berkson (1980b) also examined their data for characteristics that helped to describe friendship preferences among mentally retarded adults. One important finding was that clients tended to affiliate most with familiar others. Like many of us, retarded people need time to cultivate friendships; they choose to affiliate with those people with whom they have shared time in the past. The implications of this finding are twofold. First, it appears that retarded adults need opportunities to spend time in each other's company if they are to develop close social ties. Exposure to other individuals on a regular basis may act to encourage affiliation. Second, and perhaps more important, friendship networks among retarded adults should be taken into account in making placement decisions as well as while devising daily activity schedules within institutional or workshop settings (Heller, Berkson, & Romer, 1981). Disruption of friendship patterns may otherwise result in undue physical and/or emotional stress.

Other characteristics of friendships discussed by Romer and Berkson (1980b) include the sex and intelligence levels of partners. Although more intense friendships usually involved same-sex partners, particularly for males, opposite-sex friendships were not uncommon.

Findings for intelligence levels of friendship pairs indicated that most relationships involved pairs differing moderately in IQ. Thus, a limited form of complementarity seemed to exist in which both low and high IQ clients (relative to the group) tended to prefer to affiliate with peers who were different in intellectual ability. It appears that the presence of moderately intelligent clients, since they are more likely to affiliate with both high- and low-level peers, is important for the overall social climate of a particular setting. Romer and Berkson see this as further evidence against the practice of homogeneous grouping of clients in communal living facilities.

Two major conclusions may be drawn from the observational studies summarized in this section. First, mentally retarded adults appear to desire and to benefit from social contacts with peers. Within communal living and work facilities, most of those observed engage in a high percentage of affiliative behaviors. These occurs with a relatively small number of "close" friends, however.

Second, context variables or the characteristics of settings in which retarded adults live are key determinants of the amount of social behavior that occurs within these settings. Overall, context variables appear to be at least as important to the friendship process as individual client competencies per se. Obviously, such a finding has important implications for efforts to improve the social status of retarded individuals in both community living facilities and in more normalized settings. Specifically, interpersonal skills training may be seen as only one component of an effective program for assisting retarded adults in building friendships. This issue will be discussed further in the concluding section of this chapter.

VOCATIONAL ADJUSTMENT OF RETARDED ADULTS

If mentally retarded individuals are to lead satisfying and productive lives in the community, the ability to obtain and hold a job is of vital importance. This section of the chapter will present evidence pertaining to the employability of retarded adults in sheltered and competitive employment situations. In arguing for the importance of interpersonal competence in determining vocational success, we will examine the following factors: attitudes of nonhandicapped coworkers and supervisors toward the retarded, reasons for job termination decisions, and methods for identifying critical interpersonal skills.

Interpersonal competence and social relations of mentally retarded adults play a significant role in their vocational adjustment. This has been documented in several studies that have examined the factors affecting the employability of mentally retarded adults in both competitive and sheltered settings. These studies have operationalized vocational success in terms of the following: job tenure in competitive employment (Brolin, 1972, Brickey, Browning, & Campbell, 1982, Greenspan & Shoultz, 1981; Kolstoe, 1961; Rusch, Martin, & Lagomarcino, 1984; Wehman, Hill, Goodall, Cleveland, Barrett, Brooke, Pentecost, & Bruff, 1982; Windle, Stewart, & Brown, 1961); vocational performance in sheltered workshops (Cunningham & Presnall, 1978; Domino & McGarty, 1972, Melstrom, 1982); and movement into competitive employment (Melstrom, 1982).

Working and earning a living are key hallmarks of competent adulthood in our society. Although progress has been made in demonstrating the ability of mentally retarded people to perform a wide variety of work tasks (Gold, 1980), retarded people still experience considerable problems in finding and maintaining employment. Employers often view retarded people as incapable of learning, needing constant supervision, and causing interaction strain on customers and coworkers (Phelps, 1965). Nonhandicapped coworkers sometimes exhibit negative attitudes toward retarded workers for the following reasons: fears that they will have to absorb extra duties, unreasonable job expectations, hesitation about communicating directly with retarded people, and prejudice towards the disability (Wehman et al., 1982).

From the available data, it is difficult to determine if negative attitudes and stereotypes present more of a problem to the retarded worker in terms of initially securing a job or in performing satisfactorily after having been hired. Statistics on annual employee departures from sheltered workshops range from 12 to 15 percent; of these people, 75 percent are placed in competitive employment within one year after leaving the workshop (Rusch & Mithaug, 1980). The percentage of retarded adults who obtain employment without having been involved in sheltered workshops is unclear.

Figures pertaining to the job tenure of retarded workers in competitive employment situations vary considerably across studies. Job longevity records range from 18 percent of mentally retarded workers in the same job after one year (Margalit & Schuchman, 1978) to 82 percent of former special education students being employed several years after graduation (Crain, 1980). Although some of the variability in these findings may be attributable to job demands and other environmental characteristics, personal characteristics of workers also seem to play an important role.

In order to determine the factors contributing to job failures of retarded adults, studies have identified employees who were involuntarily terminated over several years and the reasons associated with their termination. The two most significant factors emerging from these studies relevant to job failure of retarded adults are inadequate work performance and inadequate interpersonal relations. In one such study, Greenspan and Shoultz (1981) found that the inability to interact effectively with people (57 percent of the cases) was more often cited as a reason for involuntary job terminations than the inability to perform direct job tasks. Using the same coding strategies, Rusch et al. (1984) reported that production problems accounted for approximately 60 percent of termination reasons and interpersonal problems for the remaining 40 percent. In two other studies (Brickey et al., 1982, Wehman et al., 1982), interpersonal difficulties predominated in termination decisions affecting retarded workers.

Interpersonal behavior has also been shown to be a significant predictor of vocational success in sheltered settings. Staff ratings of clients' social adjustment has been positively related to workshop productivity (Cunningham & Presnall, 1978) and to work adjustment ratings (Domino & McGarty, 1972). In one observational study (Melstrom, 1982), clients who demonstrated higher rates of social interaction were more likely to earn more money and to graduate from sheltered workshops to school or competitive employment.

Interpersonal skills also appear to play a significant role in job acquisition. The personnel literature indicates that job qualifications account for only 25 to 50 percent of the variance in influencing interviewer employment decisions (Arvey, 1979). Other important variables include speech intelligibility, degree of responsiveness of an answer to a question, sentence complexity, and verbosity (Elias, Sigelman, & Danker-Brown, 1980).

Additional evidence exists that nonverbal interpersonal skills demonstrated during a job interview influenced the way in which mentally retarded job applicants are evaluated by an interviewer. In particular, the interviewer is influenced by the following: frequency of eye contact, posture (Argyle, Lefebvre, & Cook, 1974), tone of voice (Wexley, Fugiata, & Malone, 1975), attractiveness, and smiling (Elias-Burger, Danley, Sigelman, & Burger, 1981).

Earlier studies of social functioning in relation to job success, such as Brolin (1972) and Kolstoe (1961), used broad descriptors of social adjustment such as arrest records, indicators of cheerfulness, whether an individual was married, and global opinions of others. These studies tended to focus on emotional disturbance or sociopathy as determinants of job placement failure.

More recently, investigators have begun to examine the contributions of specific interpersonal skills to vocational adjustment. Identification of critical social skills can generate necessary information on what to train for improving vocational success. There are two major ways to determine these skills. The first is to examine the social reasons for job termination. The second is to ask vocational counselors, job placement specialists, and employers what skills are critical in vocational settings.

Using the first approach, Greenspan and Shoultz (1981) compared involuntary job terminations of mentally handicapped and nonhandicapped employees. Although both were fired primarily for social reasons, handicapped workers were likely to be fired for lack of "social awareness," whereas nonhandicapped workers were more often fired as a result of "character" deficits. Social awareness referred to understanding social cues, rules, and norms of coworkers, supervisors, and customers. It was manifested in inept and ineffective interpersonal dealings. Character referred to the moral quality of workers' behavior on the job. Character difficulties were associated with antisocial or irresponsible behavior.

Other specific social reasons for termination of mentally retarded workers have included poor relations with peers and supervisors, inappropriate behaviors, poor motivation and attitudes, stealing, noncompliance, inordinate off-task behavior, failure to notify employer of absences, and bizarre or aggressive behaviors (Brickey et al., 1982, Wehman et al., 1982).

The second approach for determining critical interpersonal skills is termed "social validation." It uses significant others to determine the prerequisites for successful placement in sheltered (Johnson & Mithaug, 1978; Mithaug & Hagmeier, 1978) and competitive settings (Rusch, 1983). At least 90 percent of the workshop supervisors surveyed in the above studies agreed that the following basic skills were important for entry into sheltered workshop programs: communicating basic needs, responding to instructions, initiating contacts with supervisors when appropriate, and lack of disruptive, antisocial behavior. Rusch (1983) surveyed the job requisites that employees in service and light industrial settings believed would lead to competitive employment. The following major skills were noted: initiating contacts with supervisors when not able to perform a job, and responding appropriately and immediately after instructions. Similarly, Foss and Peterson (1981) found that job placement specialists rated supervisor–worker relationships, such as following instructions, responding to criticism, or working independently, as the most important determinants of job tenure.

In summarizing the results of studies reviewed in this section, it appears that interpersonal skills play a critical role in determining on-the-job success for mentally retarded workers. These skills are important both for relationships with coworkers and with supervisors. Most of the work reviewed indicates that interpersonal competence, manifested in the ability to positively interact with others, is at least as important as technical job skills in predicting overall vocational success for retarded adults.

SEXUAL RELATIONSHIPS AND INTIMACY AMONG RETARDED ADULTS

A third area in which interpersonal competence may play a critical role in the adjustment of retarded adults is in terms of sexual relations and intimacy. In this section, we will review the major misconceptions about sexuality in retarded individuals, including the manner in which these misconceptions impinge on the legal system, on the attitudes of caretakers, and on the attitudes of retarded people themselves. The section will conclude by addressing the incidence of sexual problems among retarded adults.

Mythology

Interpersonal skills related to sexual behavior is an area that has only recently been systematically addressed. One reason for the delay in recognizing this as an area of need is that a number of widely held myths about retarded people persist in our culture. These are by no means restricted to people who have no experience interacting with retarded individuals. They are also held by those as closely involved as parents and caretakers.

One myth that abounds in our society is that retarded people are "eternal children" and therefore asexual (Szymanski & Jansen, 1980). Since sexual behavior involving children is taboo in our society, the myth has led to the prohibition of sexual relations among retarded individuals. The view that retarded people are asexual may minimize the guilt associated with limiting another individual's freedom. Yet, as these "children" reach their 20s and 30s, it becomes increasingly difficult to deny their adulthood.

Oddly enough, a second myth involves the converse of the first, and regards the retarded as excessively sexual and therefore indiscriminant in their sexual behavior (Szymanski & Jansen, 1980). This myth forms the basis of forced sterilization laws that are still carried on the books of many states. As Szymanski and Jansen point out, the fear of indiscriminant sexual behavior may sometimes result in caretakers overreacting to friendliness and to early signs of sexuality in retarded individuals. Anxiety by parents regarding their retarded offspring's sexuality may be expressed by isolating their retarded children from external social contacts.

A third piece of mythology, closely related to the second, is that negative attributes tend to be correlated within an individual (Blom, 1971). According to this view, retarded people are likely to possess a number of character flaws including tendencies toward violence, craziness, or inappropriate sexual behavior. Such notions are tied to the "just world" hypothesis, i.e., those who have a handicap deserve it in some way. Perpetuation of the myth of negative attributes serves to support the ban on sex education for retarded clients. According to this line of reasoning, if information is provided, the stage would be set for sexual acting-out.

A final half-truth that has served to limit the sexual freedom of retarded adults is the belief that the offspring of retarded persons will themselves be retarded (Schulman, 1980). In actuality, only a small percentage of retardation is genetically determined (Hilliard & Karman, 1965). Moreover, many genetically-linked forms of retardation are more severe and are often accompanied by infertility problems as well. Thus, it appears that education, particularly as it pertains to birth control and value systems, is a better solution to this problem than restriction.

Legislation

Myths regarding the sexuality of retarded adults have been influential in determining legislation pertaining to this topic. At one time, laws required caretakers to sterilize retarded clients who were considering marriage (Vitello, 1978). Such legislation was a direct result of the assumption that retarded couples would beget retarded children.

More recently, as the scientific community began to recognize a number of previously held assumptions as myths, there was resistance to attempts to change the laws. Instead, new reasons for maintaining these laws were identified. It was argued, for example, that retarded parents would not be able to adequately care for their offspring, although this was challenged by some (Krishef, 1972).

One reason for the strong objection by some to sterilization is fear over its indiscriminant use. In an excellent review of legal issues, Vitello (1978) points out that the retarded individual is often denied due process whether involuntary sterilization statutes exist. Most states either have no laws on the topic or allow a third party to decide on sterilization (Krishef, 1972). Where no laws exist, the room for interpretation is great. If decisions are made by a third party, even when the retarded person is under age, this is equivalent to compulsory sterilization.

A related area of legislation pertains to marriage among the retarded. Again, many states have no laws regarding this issue, leaving considerable room for interpretation. A small number of states forbid marriage between retarded people based on the notion that they would not be able to understand the commitment involved. Although it may be true that retarded couples are often beset with the pressures of low income, limited education, and lack of family support, studies of retarded people who have married indicate that the stability of these marriages and the incidence of divorce are comparable to marriages of nonretarded persons (Katz, 1968; Floor, Baxter, Rosen, and Zisfein, 1975). Moreover, compared to unmarried retarded persons who have been discharged from institutions, married couples are more likely to be in financial distress, but also evidence better social adjustment (Floor et al., 1975). This suggests that marriage affords retarded individuals a much needed opportunity for intimacy that is related to later adjustment.

Szymanski and Jansen (1980) points out that laws restricting retarded persons from sexual behavior and marriage are unconstitutional because they are directed at an entire group of people without regard for individual differences. If these laws are meant to limit a particular problem, then they should be applied to all people rather than a subgroup considered to be at-risk. Instead, the laws are applied unevenly in the case of retarded individuals. For example, if a retarded couple cannot demonstrate the ability to support a family, they may be denied the right to marriage. If the purpose of this law is to prevent added Welfare burden or to limit marital discord, it appears that nonretarded people should also bear the burden of proof.

Attitudes of Parents and Caretakers

Attitudes of parents and caretakers play an important role in the sexual adjustment of retarded adults. Misconceptions and adherence to stereotyped attitudes among this group may have serious consequences since these are the people who often exert the greatest amount of control over the lives of retarded individuals.

Studies of caretakers attitudes dramatically reflect the myths we discussed previously. Heshusius (1982) notes that many workers at a residential facility felt that sexual behavior among their clients should be dealt with by segregation, supervision, and rules limiting physical contact to hand-holding and kissing. Furthermore, it was felt that sex education or conversations concerning sex should not be permitted. In another study, Mitchell, Doctor, and Butler (1978) report that a striking 31.2 percent of caretakers felt that no sexual behavior was acceptable among the retarded, including behaviors as innocuous as holding hands. Among the caretakers who believed that some level of sexual behavior was permissible, the general concensus was that the behavior was more acceptable when conducted in privacy rather than in the presence of others. Thus, sexual activity might be considered permissible if retarded people could learn the appropriate time and place to engage in such activity. What is surprising here is that retarded persons are expected to learn this without explicit instruction.

Studies on parental attitudes toward sexual relations among the retarded are far more numerous. In one study (Turchin, 1974), parents were asked about appropriate topics for a sex education curriculum for their moderately retarded offspring. The topics, listed in order of perceived importance, were clean body, menstruation, veneral disease, birth control, and marriage. Parents expressed that they did not want their children to learn about masturbation and premarital sex. Alcorn (1974) found that 80 percent of parents of retarded children felt that the primary responsibility for sex education was in the home; yet 53 percent felt unsure about their ability to convey this information. Sixty percent of those surveyed did not believe in sex education because it "might give the retarded ideas they might not otherwise have" (p. 124).

In a study by Hammar, Wright, and Jensen (1967) parents were asked what they actually taught their retarded daughters regarding sexuality. Most parents reported only discussing menstruation with their daughters. Other topics were addressed only if the child initiated a question.

Although it appears that a sizeable portion of parents and caretakers disagree with the concept of sex education for retarded people, many others feel that it is desirable, particularly if carried out in the home. Unfortunately, it also appears that few retarded persons are taught even the most rudimentary facts, such as basic physical changes that occur with the onset of puberty (Alcorn, 1974). This may be related to the uncertainty regarding this information that many parents feel. Uncertainty among parents and caretakers regarding the sexuality of retarded adults should be addressed in any comprehensive sex education program.

Client Attitudes

Very little direct research has been conducted on the attitudes of retarded people themselves toward sexual behavior. In a recent review of client attitudes, Heshusius (1982) reported a total of five articles that had some reference to sexuality. As he points out, such topics are often actively avoided during interviews with retarded clients. Nevertheless, from client statements reported in these studies, Heshusius organized the material into four major content areas that provide some insight into the sexual concerns of retarded people. The topic areas, from most to least often reported, were enjoyment of or desire for sexual contact, fear or anxiety concerning sex, intimacy and physical contact in marriage, and inaccurate sexual information. Although each individual may have a different set of concerns, it does appear that many retarded persons think independently about sexual issues. When coupled with the limited knowledge of sexual information, this may result in a potentially dangerous situation, increasing the retarded persons risk of unwanted pregnancy, venereal disease, and abuse.

Sociosexual Problems of Retarded Adults

One way to substantiate the need for training sex-related interpersonal skills is to document the incidence rates of problematic sexual behaviors among retarded individuals. Sexual misconduct is a potentially important factor in impeding normalization efforts. Dial (1968), for example, points out that a primary reason for reinstitutionalization of female clients living in a group home and working at jobs in the community was misbehavior in heterosexual relationships.

A number of specific sexual problems have been noted in the literature. Masturbation is one source of concern identified by parents (Goodman, Budner, & Lesh, 1971) as well as caretakers (Mitchell et al., 1978). In the past, treatment consisted of isolation and segregation. In the event that masturbation is prevalent in institutions because of minimal social stimulation, however, isolation would appear to be contraindicated. As mentioned previously, one study of attitudes (Mitchell et al., 1978) indicated that caretakers considered behaviors such as masturbation to be acceptable if done in private. Retarded people in residential and supervised facilities, however, are often so closely monitored that litte privacy is available.

Another problem area among institutionalized retarded adults is homosexuality. This however appears to be a direct function of institutionalization. Since many facilities do not wish to address the heterosexuality of clients, a typical precaution taken is to discourage coeducational activities and to utilize single sex dormitories. As in other facilities where heterosexual activity is prevented (e.g., prisons), homosexuality often becomes prevalent. Like masturbation, it is typically dealt with by aversive means, including isolation and closer supervision (Friedman, 1971).

Heterosexual relations can constitute a third problem area for retarded people. This may be more of a problem in the eyes of caretakers than for clients themselves. Although heterosexual activity may occur in institutional settings, limited exposure of males to females and vice versa, make this possibility fairly remote. In an interesting vignette, Szymanski and Jansen (1980) discuss girls at a residential facility who circumvented the isolation by escaping and returning pregnant. This became a status symbol for the girls because it lent some degree of normalcy to their lives.

Retarded persons living outside residential facilities have more opportunities for opposite-sex relationships. As discussed previously, however, many of these individuals have little knowledge or training in sexual matters. On the one hand, retarded adults find themselves bombarded with sexual stimulation from the media and other sources. On the other hand, they have received very little input as to appropriate means of expressing their needs for sexual contact.

Sexual abuse of retarded people is a final area that has garnered a large amount of public concern. Ironically, the concern is warranted primarily because of the severe limitation placed on the sexual experiences of retarded individuals. Their naivete in sexual matters make them easy targets for exploitation. Szymanski amd Jansen (1980) observe that retarded people may imitate the dress and behavior of their nonretarded peers without being aware of the seductiveness inherent in some styles and mannerisms. Moreover, a desire for closeness and warmth may result in positive evaluations of abusive relationships and reluctance to report abuse.

Sexual relationships of retarded adults are an important aspect of community adjustment. The data reviewed in this section indicate that many parents and caretakers, as well as some professionals, view sexual intimacy among retarded people as something to be discouraged. The prevailing philosophy, particularly in residential facilities, has been to discourage sexual activity by denying information and by isolation and segregation.

Our view is that mentally retarded adults, like most members of society, can benefit from receiving factual information about sexual issues. We further believe that interpersonal competence plays an important role in retarded adults' ability to appropriately initiate and maintain intimate relationships with people of the opposite sex. The final section of this chapter will discuss methods for enhancing interpersonal skills as they apply to social, vocational, and sexual adjustment.

IMPROVING INTERPERSONAL COMPETENCE AND COMMUNITY ADJUSTMENT

Two major approaches for increasing the interpersonal competence of retarded adults include individual or group skills training and social ecological support. Interpersonal skills training assumes that social adaptation primarily depends upon cognitive and behavioral abilities. Since poor adjustment results from skill deficiencies, it is assumed that training can be effective in promoting social adjustment. This approach relies on learning principles and behavior analysis techniques (Bandura, 1969).

The social ecological approach stems from interactionist personality theory (Lewin, 1951) which emphasizes the joint influences of personal and environmental variables on behavior. It assumes that successful adjustment to an environment depends less on personal attributes per se than on the match between the person and the environment. An individual's degree of adjustment within the community would then be determined not only by his or her competencies, but also by the social milieu of the placement environment. Intervention would involve matching the person with the appropriate environment, changing the social milieu, and fostering social support from peers, family, coworkers, supervisors, and significant others.

Interpersonal Skills Training

Easily the most popular approach for increasing the interpersonal competence of retarded persons has been through interpersonal skills training programs. Most training has taken place via operant conditioning procedures and has focused on such skills as cooperative play (McClure, 1968; Paloutzian, Hasazi, Streifel, & Edgar, 1971), social greetings (Stokes, Baer, & Jackson, 1974), question asking (Twardosz & Baer, 1973), and voice tone and volume (Jackson & Wallace, 1974).

More recently, modeling, social reinforcement–feedback, coaching–instructional, roleplaying, and rehearsal techniques have been used separately or in combination to develop and increase various specific behavioral skills of mentally retarded adults. These skills have included assertiveness (Gentile & Jenkins, 1980), appropriate touching (Matson & Martin, 1979), attending (Rusch, 1979), decrease of topic repetition (Rusch, Weithers, Menchetti, & Schutz, 1980), compliance with supervisors (Rusch & Menchetti, 1981), job interview skills (Elias-Burger et al., 1981; Hill, Wehman, & Pentecost, in press), and conversational skills (Matson & Martin, 1979; Rusch, Karlan, Riva, & Rusch, in press). While these studies effectively demonstrate the acquisition of social skills, they have not, for the most part, shown maintenance over a long-term period or generalization to nontraining settings.

In an effort to increase maintenance and generalization of social skills training, researchers have begun to emphasize cognitive components of interpersonal competence. Smith (1983), for example, has included social problem resolution as an integral part of training efforts for retarded children and adolescents. Andrasik and Matson (1985), in their review of interpersonal skills training programs for retarded individuals, emphasize a skills training package that includes instruction involving appropriate ways to respond to interpersonal demands, modeling by trainers of effective social behaviors, roleplays involving modeled behavior, positive and negative feedback on roleplays, and social praise as a reinforcer. Additional research has suggested relatively minor variations in the standard package that may serve to improve maintenance and generalization, such as in-vivo roleplays by clients rather than observation of trainers (Senatore, Matson, & Kazdin, 1982), use of interpersonal problem situations that are familiar to clients (Matson & Zeiss, 1979), and self-monitoring by clients of social behaviors outside the training site (Matson & Andrasik, 1982). Additionally, Rusch and associates, in their work on teaching interpersonal skills to retarded workers, have used coworkers to teach and maintain conversational skills during mealtimes (Rusch et al., in press). Although initial findings are encouraging, the overall effectiveness of these strategies for increasing maintenance and generalization of target behaviors remains questionable.

Social Ecological Approaches

Throughout this chapter, we have emphasized the impact of environmental variables on the interpersonal competence and community adjustment of retarded adults. Results from several long-term follow-ups of retarded adults placed into community living arrangements support the notion that environmental variables play a critical role in subsequent adjustment.

Hull and Thompson (1980), for example, in their follow-up study of 369 retarded adults residing in community facilities, reported that environmental variables such as presence of activities promoting social integration, degree to which staff encouraged independence, and opportunities for freedom and initiative were major determinants of residents' degree of adaptive functioning, more so, in fact, than individual characteristics such as IQ. Hull and Thompson conclude that attention to the social ecology of community facilities may serve as an addendum to skills training in promoting community adjustment among retarded adults.

The impact of the social milieu on interpersonal functioning was demonstrated in a study of the social behaviors of clients who first entered sheltered workshops (Heller et al., 1981). Some clients were assigned to a workshop where the atmosphere was "sociable"; others were assigned to a less sociable workshop. Although the two sets of clients did not differ in sociability prior to assignment, workers assigned to sociable surroundings increased their percentage of affiliative behaviors over time while those assigned to less sociable surroundings actually decreased their extent of affiliation. Apparently, clients tended to adapt their level of sociability to that of the environment. It appears, therefore, that an individual's tendency to develop interpersonal relations depends in part on the sociability of the person's milieu.

In analyzing the social ecology of community placement facilities and its potential for facilitating the interpersonal competence of retarded adults, research indicates a number of factors that should be considered. As suggested earlier in this paper, a major determinant of the degree of affiliation between clients is simply the extent to which clients have opportunities to interact with both same- and opposite-sex peers. Thus, interpersonal competence may be bolstered through structuring or simply providing time for social interaction. Heterogeneous grouping of clients, particularly with regard to IQ, also appears to promote interaction.

In terms of vocational competence, a major environmental factor is the degree of structure and role clarity in the job. Several researchers have suggested that the most successful placements are in jobs with detailed job descriptions (Brickey et al., 1982, Sowers, Thompson, & Connis, 1979). Emphasizing the social validation of training, Rusch (1983) strongly advocates assessing both the behaviors of nonhandicapped employees and the reinforcement contingencies present on the job. This information is then used in setting up training programs that use the same reinforcement contingencies, teach retarded workers to act more like nonhandicapped people, and utilize coworkers to maintain training.

Group placements of retarded individuals into school, vocational, or other community settings may also act to promote friendships and social contacts. Brickey et al. (1982) report that clients placed together in groups were most likely to retain their jobs over a period of 30 months. Since social interactions do not readily occur between retarded and nonretarded individuals, group placements can have the advantage of providing retarded people with peer social support upon entering new settings. Peer networks appear to facilitate adaptation to new settings (Gollay, Freedman, Wyngaarden, & Kurtz, 1978; Heller & Berkson, 1982) and aid in adjustment by providing more secure emotional ties and help with personal difficulties (Wolfensberger, 1967). The strategy of group placement may be particularly relevant to mainstreamed school settings where, as discussed previously, indications are that retarded students face rejection and isolation at the hands of nonhandicapped peers (For a review of other social-ecological adaptations applicable to mainstreaming of retarded students into school settings, see Donaldson, 1980).

The advantages of peer contact as a means of improving community adjustment was further documented in a study of small decision making groups composed of mentally retarded adults (Heller, 1978). Participation in group sessions resulted in subsequent individual decisions that were more socially competent than individual decisions made prior to the group discussion. This improvement apparently resulted from information sharing among members and from the influence of the most able people. This suggests that another means of boosting the interpersonal skills and social supports of retarded adults would be to develop ongoing client groups in sheltered or nonsheltered settings. These groups could be beneficial in terms of teaching many of the same interpersonal skills (basic communication, self-assertion, problem-solving) that are generally taught by professionals in social skills training programs. They may also complement the skills training approach by providing opportunities for generalization and maintenance of learned skills. Advantages of peer-led groups are that they provide clients with decision-making and socialization opportunities frequently denied them while at the same time, freeing-up staff time for other activities. Additionally, these groups could have the effect of increasing clients' self-confidence and independence from staff. Examples of such groups are the job-finding clubs (Azrin & Besalel, 1980) which have been effective in increasing job placements of those seeking competitive employment, and People First, a national movement in the United States toward self-advocacy by developmentally disabled individuals.

Acknowledgment

The authors would like to thank Joseph Szysko for his help with an earlier draft of this paper.

REFERENCES

Alcorn, DA. (1974). Parental views on sexual development and education of the trainable mentally retarded. *The Journal of Special Education, 8,* 119–130

Anderson, S, & Messick, S. (1974). Social competency in young children. *Developmental Psychology, 10,* 282–293

Andrasik, F, & Matson, JL. (1985). Social skills with the mentally retarded. In L L'Abate & MA Milan (Eds.), *Handbook of social skills training and research.* New York: Wiley

Argyle, M, Lefebvre, L, & Cook, M. (1974). The meaning of five patterns of gaze. *European Journal of Social Psychology, 4,* 125–136

Arvey, RC. (1979). Unfair discrimination in the employment interview: Legal and psychological aspects. *Psychological Bulletin, 86,* 736–765

Asher, SR, Oden, SL, & Gottman, JM. (1977). Children's friendships in school settings. In LG Katz (Ed.), *Current topics in early childhood education* (Vol. 1). Norwood, NJ: Ablex

Azrin, NH, & Besalel, VA. (1980). *Job counselor's manual.* Baltimore, MD, University Park Press

Azrin, NH, Philip, RA, Thienes-Hontos, P, & Besalel, VA. (1981). Follow-up on welfare benefits received by Job Club clients. *Journal of Vocational Behavior, 18,* 253–254

Bandura, A. (1969). *Principles of behavior modification.* New York: Holt, Rinehart & Winston

Berkson, G, & Romer, D. (1980). Social ecology of supervised communal facilities for mentally disabled adults: I. Introduction. *American Journal of Mental Deficiency, 85,* 219–228

Blom, GE. (1971). Some considerations about the neglect of sex education in special education. *Journal of Special Education, 5,* 359–361

Brickey, M, Browning, L, & Campbell, K. (1982). Vocational histories of sheltered workshop employees placed in projects with industry and competitive jobs. *Mental Retardation, 20,* 52–57

Brolin, D. (1972). Value of rehabilitation services and correlates of vocational success with the mentally retarded. *American Journal of Mental Deficiency, 76,* 644–651

Cowen, EL, Pederson, A, Babigian, M, Izzo, LD, & Trost, MA. (1973). Long-term follow-up of early detected vulnerable children. *Journal of Consulting and Clinical Psychology, 41,* 438–446

Crain, EJ. (1980). Socioeconomic status of educable mentally retarded graduates of special education. *Education and Training of the Mentally Retarded, 15,* 90–94

Cunningham, T, & Presnall, D. (1978). Relationships between dimensions of adaptive behavior and sheltered workshop productivity. *American Journal of Mental Deficiency, 82,* 386–393

Dial, KB. (1968). A report of group work to increase social skills of females in vocational rehabilitation programs. *Mental Retardation, 6,* 11–14

Domino, G, & McGarty, M. (1972). Personal and work adjustment of young retarded women. *American Journal of Mental Deficiency, 77,* 314–321

Donaldson, J. (1980). Changing attitudes toward handicapped persons: A review and analysis of research. *Exceptional children, 46,* 504–514

Edmonson, B. (1974). Arguing for a concept of competence. *Mental Retardation, 12,* 14–15

Elias, SF, Sigelman, CK, & Danker-Brown, P. (1980). Interview behavior of and impressions made by mentally retarded adults. *American Journal of Mental Deficiency, 85,* 53–60

Elias-Burger, SF, Danley, WE, Sigelman, CK, & Burger, DL. (1981). Teaching interview skills to mentally retarded persons. *American Journal of Mental Deficiency,* 85, 655–657

Floor, L, Baxter, D, Rosen, M, & Zisfein, L. (1975). A survey of marriage among previously institutionalized retardates. *Mental Retardation,* 13, 33–37

Foss, G, & Peterson, SL. (1981). Social interpersonal skills relevant to job tenure for mentally retarded adults. *Mental Retardation, 19,* 103–106

Friedman, E. (1971). Missing in the life of the retarded individual—sex: Reflections on Sol Gordon's paper. *Journal of Special Education, 5,* 365–368

Fulton, RW. (1975). Job retention of the mentally retarded. *Mental Retardation, 13,* 26–27

Gentile, C, & Jenkins, JO. (1980). Assertive training with mild mentally retarded persons. *Mental Retardation, 18,* 315–317

Gold, MT. (1980). *Try another way training manual.* Champaign, IL: Research Press

Goldstein, H. (1964). Social and occupational adjustment. In H Stevens & R Heber (Eds.), *Mental retardation.* Chicago: University of Chicago Press

Gollay, E, Freedman, R, Wyngaarden, M, & Kurtz, NR. (1978). Coming back: The community experiences of institutionalized mentally retarded people. Cambridge, MA: Abt Books

Goodman, H, Gottlieb, J, & Harrison, RH. (1972). Social acceptance of EMR's integrated into a nongraded elementary school. *American Journal of Mental Deficiency, 76,* 412–417

Goodman, L, Budner, S, & Lesh, B. (1971). The parent's role in sex education for the retarded. *Mental Retardation, 9,* 43–45

Gottlieb, J. (1981). Mainstreaming: Fulfilling the promise? *American Journal of Mental Deficiency, 86,* 115–126

Gottlieb, J, & Budoff, M. (1973). Social acceptability of retarded children in non-graded schools differing in architecture. *American Journal of Mental Deficiency, 78,* 15–19

Gottlieb, J, Semmel, MI, & Veldman, DJ. (1978). Correlates of social status among mainstreamed mentally retarded children. *Journal of Educational Psychology, 70,* 396–405

Greenspan, S. (1981). Defining childhood social competence: A proposed working model. In BK Keogh (Ed.), *Advances in special education* (Vol. 3). Greenwich, CN: JAI Press

Greenspan, S, & Schoultz, B. (1981). Why mentally retarded adults lose their jobs: Social competence as a factor in work adjustment. *Applied Research in Mental Retardation, 2,* 23–38

Grossman, HJ. (Ed.). (1983). *Classification in mental retardation.* Washington, DC: American Association of Mental Deficiency

Hammar, SL, Wright, LS, & Jensen, DL. (1967). Sex education for the retarded adolescent: A survey of parental attitudes and methods of management in fifty adolescent retardates. *Clinical Pediatrics, 6,* 621–627

Heller, T. (1978). Group decision-making among mentally retarded adults. *American Journal of Mental Deficiency, 82,* 480–486

Heller, T, & Berkson, G. (1982). *Friendship and residential relocation.* Paper presented at the Gatlinburg Conference on Research in Mental Retardation and Developmental Disabilities. Gatlinburg, TN

Heller, T, Berkson, G, & Romer, D. (1981). Social ecology of supervised communal facilities for mentally disabled adults: VI. Initial social adaptation. *American Journal of Mental Deficiency, 86,* 43–49

Heshusius, L. (1982). Sexuality, intimacy and persons we label mentally retarded: What they think—What we think. *Mental Retardation, 20,* 164–168

Hill, J, Wehman, P, & Pentecost, JH. (in press). Developing job interview skills in mentally retarded adults. *Education and Training of the Mentally Retarded*

Hilliard, LT, & Karman, BH. (1965). *Mental deficiency.* Boston, MA: Little, Brown

Hull, JT, & Thompson, JC. (1980). Predicting adaptive functioning of mentally retarded persons in community settings. *American Journal of Mental Deficiency, 85,* 253–261

Jackson, DA, & Wallace, RF. (1974). The modification and generalization of voice loudness in a fifteen-year-old retarded girl. *Journal of Applied Behavior Analysis, 7,* 461–471

Johnson, JL, & Mithaug, DE. (1978). A replication of sheltered workshop entry requirements. *AAESPH Review, 3,* 116–122

Katz, E. (1968). *The retarded adult in the community.* Springfield, IL: Charles Thomas

Katz, S, & Yekutiel, E. (1974). Leisure time problems and mentally retarded graduates of training programs. *Mental Retardation, 12,* 54–57

Kolstoe, OP. (1961). An examination of some characteristics which discriminate between employed and not-employed mentally retarded males. *American Journal of Mental Deficiency, 66,* 472–482

Krishef, CH. (1972). State law on marriage and sterilization of the mentally retarded. *Mental Retardation, 10,* 36–38

Landesman-Dwyer, S, Berkson, G, & Romer, D. (1979). Affiliation and friendship of mentally retarded residents in group homes. *American Journal of Mental Deficiency,* 83, 571–580

Landesman-Dwyer, S, Stein, JG, & Sackett, GP. (1978). A behavioral and ecological study of group homes. In GP Sackett (Ed.), *Observing behavior: Theory and applications in mental retardation* (Vol. 1). Baltimore, MD: University Park Press

Lewin, K. (1951). *Field theory in social science: Selected theoretical papers.* New York: Harper & Row

MacMillan, DL. (1982). *Mental retardation in school and society* (2nd ed.). Boston: Little, Brown

Margalit, M, & Schuchman, R. (1978). Vocational adjustment of EMR youth in a work-study program and a work program. *American Journal of Mental Deficiency, 82,* 604–607

Matson, JL, & Andrasik, F. (1982). Training leisure-time social-interaction skills to mentally retarded adults. *American Journal of Mental Deficiency, 86,* 533–542

Matson, JL, & Martin, JE. (1979). A social learning approach to vocational training of the severely retarded. *Journal of Mental Deficiency Research, 23,* 9–17

Matson, JL, & Zeiss, RA. (1979). The buddy system: A method for generalized reduction of inappropriate interpersonal behavior of retarded psychiatric patients. *British Journal of Social and Clinical Psychology, 18,* 401–405

McClure, RF. (1968). Reinforcement of verbal social behavior in moderately retarded children. *Psychological Reports, 23,* 371–376

McDevitt, SC, Smith, PM, Schmidt, DW, & Rosen, M. (1978). The deinstitutionalized citizen: Adjustment and quality of life. *Mental Retardation, 16,* 22–24

Melstrom, M. (1982). Social ecology of supervised communal facilties for mentally disabled adults: VII. Productivity and turnover rate in sheltered workshops. *American Journal of Mental Deficiency, 87,* 40–47

Mitchell, L, Doctor, RM, & Butler, DC. (1978). Attitudes of caretakers toward the sexual behavior of mentally retarded persons. *American Journal of Mental Deficiency, 83,* 289–296

Mithaug, DE, & Hagmeier, LD. (1978). The development of procedures to assess prevocational competencies of severely handicapped young adults. *AAESPH Review, 3,* 94–115

Paloutzian, RF, Hasazi, J, Streifel, J, & Edgar, CL. (1971). Promotion of positive social interaction in severely retarded young children. *American Journal of Mental Deficiency, 75,* 519–524

Phelps, WR. (1965). Attitudes related to the employment of the mentally retarded. *American Journal of Mental Deficiency, 69,* 575–585

Reiter, S, & Levi, AM. (1980). Factors affecting social integration of noninstitutionalized mentally retarded adults. *American Journal of Mental Deficiency, 85,* 25–30

Richardson, SA. (1978). Careers of mentally retarded young persons: Services, jobs and interpersonal relations. *American Journal of Mental Deficiency, 82,* 349–358

Romer, D, & Berkson, G. (1980a). Social ecology of supervised communal facilties for mentally disabled adults: II. Predictors of affiliation. *American Journal of Mental Deficiency, 85,* 229–242

Romer, D, & Berkson, G. (1980b). Social ecology of supervised communal facilities for mentally disabled adults: III. Predictors of social choice. *American Journal of Mental Deficiency, 85,* 243 252

Romer, D, & Berkson, G. (1981). Social ecology of supervised communal facilities for mentally disabled adults: IV. Characteristics of social behavior. *American Journal of Mental Deficiency, 86,* 28–38

Rusch, FR. (1979). A functional analysis of the relationship between attending to task and production in an applied restaurant setting. *Journal of Special Education, 13,* 399–411

Rusch, FR. (1983). Competitive vocational training. In ME Snell (Ed.), *Systematic instruction of the moderately and severely handicapped* (2nd ed.). Columbus, OH: Charles E Merrill

Rusch, FR, Martin, JE, & Lagomarcino, T. (1984). *Why mentally retarded workers lose their jobs: A comparison between mentally retarded and their nonhandicapped coworkers.* Unpublished manuscript, University of Illinois, Urbana

Rusch, FR, & Menchetti, BM. (1981). Increasing compliant work behaviors in a non-sheltered work setting. *Mental Retardation, 19,* 107–112

Rusch, FR, & Mithaug, DE. (1980). *Vocational training for mentally retarded adults: A behavior analytic approach.* Champaign, IL: Research Press

Rusch, FR, Weithers, JA, Menchetti, BM, & Schutz, RP. (1980). Social validation of a program to reduce topic repetition in a non-sheltered setting. *Education and Training of the Mentally Retarded, 15,* 208–215

Rusch, JC, Karlan, GR, Riva, MT, & Rusch, FR. (in press). Teaching conversational skills to mentally retarded adults in employment settings. *Mental Retardation*

Schulman, ED. (1980). *Focus on the retarded adult: Programs and services.* St. Louis, C.V. Mosby

Senatore, V, Matson, JL, & Kazdin, AE. (1982). A comparison of behavioral methods to train social skills to mentally retarded adults. *Behavior Therapy, 13,* 313–324

Shalock, RL, & Harper, RS. (1978). Placement from community-based mental retardation programs: How well do clients do? *American Journal of Mental Deficiency, 83,* 240–247

Shalock, RL, Harper, RS, & Carrer, G. (1981). Independent living placement: Five years later. *American Journal of Mental Deficiency, 86,* 170–177

Simeonsson, RJ. (1978). Social competence: Dimensions and directions. In J Wortis (Ed.), *Annual review of mental retardation and developmental disabilities.* New York: Brunner/Mazel

Smith, DC. (1983). *A friendship-building program for mentally retarded adolescents.* Paper presented at the meeting of the American Association on Mental Deficiency, Dallas, TX

Sowers, J, Thompson, LE, & Connis, RT. (1979). The food service vocational training program: A model for training and placement of the mentally retarded. In TG Bellamy, G O'Connor, & OC Karan (Eds.), *Vocational rehabilitation of severely handicapped persons.* Baltimore, MD: University Park Press

Stokes, TF, Baer, DM, & Jackson, RL. (1974). Programming the generalization of a greeting response in four retarded children. *Journal of Applied Behavior Analysis, 7,* 599–610

Szymanski, LS, & Jansen, PE. (1980). Assessment of sexuality and sexual vulnerability of retarded persons. In LS Szymanski & PE Tanguay (Eds.), *Emotional disorders of mentally retarded persons.* Baltimore, MD: University Park Press

Turchin, G. (1974). Sexual attitudes of mothers of retarded children. *Journal of School Health, 44,* 490–492

Twardosz, S, & Baer, DM. (1973). Training two severely retarded adolescents to ask questions. *Journal of Applied Behavior Analysis, 6,* 655–661

Vitello, SJ. (1978). Involuntary sterilization: Recent developments. *Mental Retardation, 16,* 405–409

Wehman, P, Hill, M, Goodall, P, Cleveland, P, Barrett, N, Brooke, V, Pentecost, J, & Bruff, V. (1982). Job placement and follow-up of moderately and severely handicapped individuals: An update after three years. In P Wehman & M Hill (Eds.), *Vocational training and placement of severely disabled persons: Project employability* (Vol. 3). Richmond, VA: Commonwealth University

Weinstein, EA. (1969). The development of interpersonal competence. In D Goslin (Ed.), *Handbook of socialization theory and research.* Chicago: Rand McNally

Wexley, K, Fugiata, S, & Malone, M. (1975). An applicant's nonverbal behavior and student evaluation judgments in a structured interview setting. *Psychological Reports, 36,* 391–394

White, RW. (1959). Motivation reconsidered: The concept of competence. *Psychological Review, 66,* 297–333

Windle, CD, Stewart, E, & Brown, SJ. (1961). Reasons for community failure of released patients. *American Journal of Mental Deficiency, 66,* 213–217

Wolfensberger, W. (1967). Vocational preparation and occupation. In AA Baumeister (Ed.), *Mental retardation: Appraisal, education and rehabilitation.* Chicago: Aldine

SECTION II

Children with Dual Disabilities: Cognitive and Emotional Problems

Dual disability is manifested in a variety of forms and the chapters in this section describe some of these patterns. Chapter 6 provides a general introduction to the disorders often associated with mental retardation while Chapter 7 specifically focuses on emotional disorders of the mentally retarded child and adolescent. The following two chapters analyze the interrelation of cognitive and social disorders in autistic and schizophrenic children. The focus of these chapters is a departure from the overall theme of the book in that the chapters discuss cognitive problems in children with fundamental disturbances of social–emotional development rather than emotional problems in children with delayed cognitive development. These chapters were included in order to view the issue of dual disabilities from both perspectives. The last chapter in this section returns to the theme of emotional problems in the mentally retarded by discussing dual disability adults and presenting assessment and treatment procedures.

Mary J. O'Connor

5

Mental Retardation and Associated Disorders of Childhood

DEFINITION OF MENTAL RETARDATION

The term mental retardation refers to a heterogeneous group of conditions characterized by low scores on intelligence tests and deficits in adaptive behavior. The definition adapted by the American Association of Mental Deficiency (AAMD) is the most currently accepted.

Mental Retardation is defined as significantly subaverage general intellectual functioning with deficits in adaptive behavior manifested during the developmental period (Grossman, 1977). The following three key aspects to the AAMD definition of mental retardation must be considered when evaluating children suspected of being retarded.

Significantly subaverage intelligence. This is defined as a score that is two or more standard deviations below the population mean on a standardized intelligence test. Children scoring in this range theoretically should represent only 3 percent of the general population. In using the AAMD classification system, one must be aware of both the mean and standard deviation scores of the intelligence tests employed. Thus, while most tests utilizing deviation IQs have means of 100, the standard deviation of these tests may vary. For example, the standard deviation of the Wechsler Intelligence Scale for Children—Revised (WISC–R) and the Wechsler Preschool and Primary Scale of Intelligence (WPPSI) is 15, while the standard deviation for the Stanford-Binet—1972 Revision is 16. If the −2SD criterion is used, then a score below −2SD on the

CHILDREN WITH EMOTIONAL DISORDERS AND DEVELOPMENTAL DISABILITIES ISBN 0–8089–1700–5

WISC–R and WPPSI is 69, and is 67 on the Stanford-Binet. Children who are classified as mentally retarded are then identified as functioning in the mild, moderate, severe, and profound ranges based upon levels of intelligence used in concert with adaptive behavior classifications.

Adaptive behavior. This is defined as those behaviors that reflect independence and social responsibility expected of children of the same cultural background and chronological age. Adaptive measures include assessments of self-help skills, physical development, economic and vocational activity, language and academic performance, self-direction, and socialization. Measures of adaptive behavior change in content as a function of the child's chronological age.

Developmental period. This last aspect has been defined as the period between birth and 18 years of age. Thus, the child must be identified as retarded at some point during development prior to reaching the age of 18 years.

An important aspect of the AAMD definition of mental retardation is that the child's performance must reflect deficits in *general* cognitive performance rather than some specific aspect of ability. Therefore, a child manifesting a specific language or learning disability that causes his overall score to fall within the retarded range would not be classified as mentally retarded. Conversely, a child who has superior skill in only one area of ability, causing his score on certain tests to fall in the low average or borderline range of functioning, but whose overall level of functioning in all other areas is much lower, might be classified as retarded. This point is particularly important when evaluating the scores of autistic children who frequently score high on measures of concrete visuospatial skill, but who are functionally retarded.

Thought of in the preceding way, the definition of mental retardation refers to a set of rather specific features that children manifest without regard to etiology. The definition also "*avoids specific differentiations of mental retardation from other childhood disorders* such as childhood schizophrenia or brain damage" (Robinson & Robinson, 1976, p. 31). Mental retardation exists with many forms of childhood disorder, and attempts to determine which is primary or secondary are often frustrating and nonproductive. Nevertheless, it is helpful to delineate various populations of children who manifest mental retardation in order to clarify methods of assessment and treatment with these individuals.

Traditionally, mentally retarded children have been considered to fall into one of two broad categories, familial or organic. Although these classifications are conceptually neat, in practice, both groups often manifest overlapping symptomatology. In general, however, the familial type of mental retardation is characterized by children who are mildly retarded (50 to 69 range of IQ), who come from backgrounds of social or cultural disadvantage, and whose parents may exhibit similar below average intellectual functioning. These children are usually identified later in life (school age) and may show variability in intellectual performance as they grow older. These children also tend to respond to intensive interventive programs designed to facilitate cognitive growth and to provide familial support and education.

Mental retardation in the presence of organic conditions is usually manifested in children showing more severe cognitive delays with IQ's below 50. The etiology of the condition may be known or can be inferred from developmental history and may be associated with genetic, metabolic, or organic brain conditions. Children with organic brain injury usually have diffuse brain dysfunction or malformation and show developmental delays from infancy or following some traumatic environmental insult to the brain. Children with these conditions, while able to learn and develop, do not show dramatic developmental gains with intervention.

Generally, mild and moderate degrees of mental retardation are associated with hereditary, environmental, and/or psychosocial deprivation (familial), and the more severe degrees of mental retardation are related to central nervous system abnormalities and multiple handicaps (organic). Children with known organic etiology, however, represent a small percentage of the retarded population and it has been estimated that about 80 percent of mentally retarded individuals do not fit into a biologic etiological classification (Magrab & Johnston, 1980).

Clinical Disorders Associated With Mental Retardation

Because of the difficulty in classifying children as to the etiology of their general retardation, the following discussion will describe types of children seen in clinical practice, classified according to behavioral manifestations, with a discussion of etiology if it is known. It should become clear in the discussion that, in clinical practice, it is very difficult to determine specific etiologies and to partial out environmental/organic variables in the majority of cases. On rare occasions, we are able to identify a specific event or lesion that can explain the child's behavior, but the probability of this in our experience is so rare as to make it almost unrealistic to hope to do so.

Cerebral Palsy

Children with cerebral palsy represent a heterogeneous group of individuals who manifest a disorganization of motor control as a result of brain injury experienced prenatally or in the first 3 years of life. In addition to neuromuscular dysfunction, children with cerebral palsy may also manifest difficulties in learning, behavior, speech and language, and sensory functioning. Cerebral palsy results from a variety of causes including hypoxia-asphyxia, head trauma, central nervous system infection, and complications of illnesses having a genetic basis.

Denhoff (1976) has suggested four broad categories of cerebral palsy: spasticity, dyskinesia, ataxia, and mixed. This discussion will focus on the more common forms of cerebral palsy, spasticity and dyskinesia.

Children evidencing spasticity represent about two-thirds of all children diagnosed as having cerebral palsy. Within this group are those with congenital spastic hemiplegia and those with acquired or postnatal spastic hemiplegia. About 37 percent of the children with congenital hemiplegia are retarded whereas 46 percent of the children with acquired spastic hemiplegia are retarded (Crothers & Paine, 1959). Children with acquired spastic hemiplegia, who have a seizure disorder and injury prior to 2 years of age, have a poorer cognitive prognosis than those without a seizure disorder and later trauma.

Children with spastic quadriplegia (all four extremities involved) are the most severely cognitively affected of any other group with spasticity, in that 70 percent are retarded. Children with spastic paraplegia have a relatively good prognosis for normal cognitive functioning, since seizure and language disorders are less common in this group.

Dyskinesia or extrapyramidal cerebral palsy is seen in about 25 percent of the cerebral palsied population (Denhoff, 1976) and is characterized by increased tone in the extremities accompanied by choreiform, athetoid, or choreoathetoid movements. Cognitively, about 33 percent of these children function in the retarded range (Crothers & Paine, 1959).

Sensory Disabilities

The two most prominent forms of sensory disabilities seen in children are blindness and deafness. Although the majority of children who are deaf or blind are not retarded, some children do function in the retarded range or show delayed development from very early in life. According to Thompson and O'Quinn (1979) the degree to which functioning is impaired is dependent upon several factors:

> (1) The severity of the disorder of the special sense, (2) the etiology, (3) the time period during which the disorder occurred and became manifest, (4) the reaction of the afflicted person and that of his or her family to the disability, and (5) the availability of appropriate resources to ameliorate the difficulty (pp. 245–246).

Children with sensory deficits who are also retarded usually have a history of experiencing traumatic medical and/or environmental events. In particular, sensory impairment associated with central nervous system damage may result in below-average intelligence. Nevertheless, it is important to remember that often these children are also restricted in their activities, including limited opportunities for social, educational, and cultural stimulation, and that these limitations may also affect intellectual development. Intervention in certain areas, particularly in educational opportunities, may result in dramatic changes in intellectual performance.

Deaf children, as a group, score in the average range of intelligence on nonverbal tests, but their means are somewhat lower than the means of hearing children (Thompson & O'Quinn, 1979). Children with associated neurologic impairment score much lower. Blind children also score in the normal range on intelligence tests but the distribution of their scores is bimodal. That is, there is a high proportion of above average as well as retarded children in this population. According to Lowenfeld (1963), compared to sighted peers, there is a slightly higher percentage of blind children in the superior range and a considerably larger percentage in the below average range.

Genetic and Metabolic Syndromes

In spite of the difficulty in determining an etiologic basis for many forms of mental retardation, there are some common genetic and/or metabolic disorders of which mental retardation is a common symptom. Even in these rare cases, however, the interaction between genetic and environmental factors cannot be ignored. For example, in Down's syndrome children, children who are generally considered to be severely impaired intellectually, it has been shown that intelligence levels are higher as a function of remaining in the home as opposed to being institutionalized (Lodge & Kleinfeld, 1973).

The presence of an extra set of genes of the twenty-first chromosome, manifested as Down's syndrome, has been noted as the most common chromosomal cause of moderate to severe mental retardation. At least 10 percent of children with this degree of retardation exhibit Down's syndrome (Robinson & Robinson, 1976). Other autosomal chromosome aberrations resulting in retardation are trisomy 13 and trisomy 18. Deletion of chromosomal material (other than the Y chromosome) as in *cri-du-chat* syndrome also results in significant mental deficiency. Syndromes associated with aberrations of the sex chromosomes such as Turner's or Klinefelter's syndromes are not characterized by severe mental retardation; nevertheless, mild retardation has been reported in some individuals. Other inherited syndromes that are associated with mental retardation include those where the child manifests neural tube defects (anencephaly and meningomyelocele), tuberous sclerosis, neurofibromatosis, muscular dystrophy, or kernicterus.

A number of genetically determined inborn errors of metabolism, if untreated, result in retardation. Fortunately, if treated vigorously, the child need not suffer severe adverse consequences. Although relatively rare, the more notable metabolic disorders are those involving failure to metabolize carbohydrates, protein and amino acids, lipids, and mucopolysaccharides.

Galactosemia, due to failure to metabolize galactose, can be ameliorated by removal of milk from the diet. Intellectual development in treated children is normal. Disorders of protein and amino acid metabolism resulting in phenylketonuria (PKU) can have profound effects on intellectual development. Untreated children rarely achieve an IQ of over 50 and have considerable behavioral disturbance. If treated at birth, however, development proceeds normally, with some delays relative to family members and other control groups (Dobson, Williamson, Azen, & Koch, 1977).

The cerebral lipidoses, including Niemann-Pick, Gaucher's, Tay-Sachs, and Krabbe's diseases are among the more rare causes of mental retardation (Malone, 1976). In these diseases, children are normal at birth with progressive neurologic deterioration and death in early childhood. The mucopolysaccharidoses are characterized by moderate to severe mental retardation with gradual neurologic deterioration and death in adulthood. Hunter's syndrome, Hurler's syndrome, and Sanfilippo's syndrome are associated with mucopolysaccharide storage problems.

Seizure Disorders

Seizure disorder or epilepsy refers to a paroxysmal and transitory disturbance of cerebral electrical discharge that results in altered states of awareness or consciousness and/or disturbance of sensory/motor activity. Many studies have demonstrated the importance of heredity in seizure disorder, as well as other causes such as traumatic brain injury.

There are many forms of seizure disorder that fall under two broad categories, generalized seizures (grand mal, petit mal, Lennox-Gastaut, and infantile spasms), and partial seizures (focal sensory or motor, psychomotor, and hypothalamic). It is important to note, however, that many people have mixed types of seizures and even manifest different seizure patterns over a lifetime, making classification difficult.

Although there is controversy over the causal relationship of seizures to mental retardation, the majority of evidence suggests that seizures and mental retardation are probably both manifestations of underlying brain pathology. Different types of seizures, however, do have different cognitive outcomes, and it has been suggested that poorer outcomes are associated with more difficult to control and more frequent seizure activity. Recent evidence seems to contradict this notion. Richardson, Koller, Katz and McLaren (1981) in a 22 year longitudinal study of children with seizure disorder found no association between severity of retardation and degree of seizure impairment except that there was greater seizure impairment in the lowest intelligence groups.

Children evidencing secondary generalized seizures such as Lennox-Gastaut or infantile spasms show considerable intellectual impairment with associated neurologic pathology and poor seizure control. Ninety percent or more of children with infantile spasms are seriously retarded (Livingston, 1972; Pincus & Tucker, 1974), and 91 percent of children diagnosed with Lennox-Gastaut score in the below average range (Lugaresi, Pazzaglia, Rogers, & Tassinari, 1974). Forty percent of the 125 children with grand mal seizures studied by Keith (1963) were found to be retarded. In contrast, most children with petit mal seizures are not retarded but do show poor school performance (Thompson & O'Quinn, 1979). Likewise, children with partial or focal seizures generally perform in the average range of intelligence with some school difficulties.

Childhood Psychosis

In this discussion of childhood psychosis, the focus will be on conditions emerging in infancy and early childhood that usually have associated behavioral and cognitive abnormalities and that present difficult diagnostic dilemmas.

According to the Diagnostic and Statistical Manual of Mental Disorders (DSM III) (1980), the current reference on classification of mental illness, psychotic disorders of childhood are now classified as "pervasive developmental disorders." This new classification scheme emphasizes the biologic and developmental aspects of childhood psychosis with less emphasis upon psychogenic variables. These disorders are characterized by distortions in the development of basic psychological functions such as attention, perception, language, cognition, motor movement, reality orientation, and social skill. These disorders bear little relationship to adult psychosis, and children so classified never appear to develop normally. The two common types of pervasive developmental disorder are infantile autism and childhood onset pervasive developmental disorder.

Infantile autism. The hallmark of infantile autism, first discussed by Kanner in 1943, is a disturbance in social relatedness. The symptoms associated with autism appear to reflect an underlying neuropathophysiological process that also affects developmental rate, perception, language and cognition (Ornitz & Ritvo, 1976). The current criteria for a diagnosis of autism are:

1. Onset before 30 months of age.
2. Pervasive lack of responsiveness to other people (autism).
3. Gross deficits in language development.
4. If speech is present, peculiar speech patterns such as immediate and delayed echolalia, metaphorical language, pronominal reversal.
5. Bizarre responses to various aspects of the environment, e.g., resistance to change, peculiar interest in or attachments to animate or inanimate objects.
6. Absence of delusions, hallucinations, loosening of associations, and incoherence as in schizophrenia. (DSM III, 1980, p. 90)

Failure to develop social relatedness is characterized by a general lack of interest in or avoidance of people, with disturbance in attachment behavior. In infancy these deficits may be particularly pronounced but by early childhood, some autistic children develop some form of sociability and relatedness to peers and attachment to parents. This sociability often causes diagnostic confusion when the diagnosis is made retrospectively.

Atypical communication patterns include unusual language patterns (if language develops at all) and often failures in nonverbal expression. For example, autistic youngsters exhibit echolalic and idiosyncratic speech, atypical prosity, and concrete verbal expression. Nonverbally, they often have difficulty with imitation and in using gestures. Unusual responses to the environment include ritualistic behavior, attachment to inanimate objects, insistence upon sameness, perseverative play and over- or under-reactivity to external stimuli.

The recognition and acceptance of mental retardation in autistic children has been slow in coming. Kanner (1943) assumed that because autistic children had behavior problems making them difficult to test on standardized intelligence tests, that they were of normal intelligence. This assumption was supported by the observation that even severely impaired children occasionally did something more advanced than their overall developmental functioning would suggest, causing some examiners to conclude that they were normal or bright. The popular notion that these children were "idiot savants" or had "splinter skills" arose out of these obervations. Although it is now commonly accepted that the majority of autistic children do function in the retarded range, there are still practitioners who hold the view that autistic children are of normal intelligence simply because they appear to function normally in one specific skill area.

In general, autistic children do perform better on measures of visual-spatial and memory abilities. Thus, they are able to complete puzzle and form-board tasks with ease and are sometimes able to recite poems, songs, or jingles verbatim. That is why it is important for examiners testing these children to use a variety of measures to assess many skill areas rather than to rely on a single test that measures only one area of performance.

Research shows that about 75 to 94 percent of autistic children obtain intelligence quotients in the mentally retarded range (Demyer, Barton, Kimberlin, Allen, Yang, & Steele, 1974; Freeman, 1978). About 40 percent score below 50. Intelligence quotients derived at 5 years of age and beyond are predictive of later cognitive and educational attainment. Given the research findings, it is important to recognize that autistic children who function in the retarded range are indeed retarded.

Factors associated with long-term prognosis in autism include intelligence level and the development of language. Those children with higher IQs and some functional expressive language have a better prognosis but fundamental disturbances in behavior as described persist.

Pervasive developmental disorder. Childhood onset pervasive developmental disorder is described as developing after 30 months of age and before puberty. It is characterized by social withdrawal and bizarre or unusual behavior. These children often exhibit a lack of appropriate social or affective responsivity, excessive anxiety, oddities of speech and motor movement, and some self-abusive behavior. There may be preoccupation with morbid thoughts accompanied by bizarre fantasies. The DSM III criteria for childhood onset pervasive developmental disorder are:

A. Gross and sustained impairment in social relationships, e.g., lack of appropriate affective responsivity, inappropriate clinging, asociality, lack of empathy.

B. At least three of the following:
   (1) Sudden excessive anxiety manifested by such symptoms as free-floating anxiety, catastrophic reactions to everyday occurrences, inability to be consoled when upset, unexplained panic attacks
   (2) Constricted or inappropriate affect, including lack of appropriate fear reactions, unexplained rage reactions, and extreme mood lability
   (3) Resistance to change in the environment (e.g., upset if dinner time is changed), or insistence on doing things in the same manner every time (e.g., putting on clothes always in the same order)
   (4) Oddities of motor movement, such as peculiar posturing, peculiar hand or finger movements, or walking on tiptoe
   (5) Abnormalities of speech, such as questionlike melody, monotonous voice
   (6) Hyper- or hypo-sensitivity to sensory stimuli, e.g., hyperacusis
   (7) Self mutilation, e.g., biting or hitting self, head banging

C. Onset of the full syndrome after 30 months of age and before 12 years of age.

D. Absence of delusions, hallucinations, incoherence, or marked loosening of associations. (DSM III, 1980, p. 91)

Because pervasive developmental disorder is a relatively new diagnostic category, there is no published research on the prevalence of mental retardation in these children. Nevertheless, preliminary data from the Clinical Research Center at the University of California at Los Angeles Neuropsychiatric Institute suggests that, as in autism, a substantial percentage of these children function in the retarded range (Tanguay, personal communication).

Schizophrenia. Currently, the diagnosis of schizophrenia in children must be made according to the criteria for adult schizophrenia. Young children who can be diagnosed as schizophrenic rarely exhibit Schneiderian first-rank symptoms such as delusions and hallucinations and are, therefore, diagnosed on the basis of the presence of a formal thought disorder characterized by incoherence, loosening of associations, marked illogical thinking, or poverty of content of speech. Although the symptoms are not part of the DSM III criteria for schizophrenia in childhood, Fish and Ritvo (1979) have described symptoms commonly associated with the diagnosis. These symptoms include autistic withdrawal, fluctuating, incongruous or shallow affect, disruptions in attention and perception, erratic and inconsistent cognitive functioning, variable and erratic development, and possible motility disturbances.

Although mental retardation is more commonly seen in children diagnosed as autistic or as childhood onset pervasive developmental disorder, there is evidence that some schizophrenic children are also retarded. Previous studies of young schizophrenic children have found approximately one-fourth with IQs under 70. Furthermore, investigators have shown that lower intelligence is often associated with more severe early onset psychosis, developmental abnormalities, and disintegration of personality and behavior (Fish & Ritvo, 1979).

As we learn more about psychosis in children and the patterns of cognitive and emotional development manifested by these children, it becomes clear that a diagnostic system like DSM III based solely on symptom description, without regard to developmental issues, is clearly inadequate for understanding young psychotic children. This is particularly true for the diagnosis of schizophrenia. According to Tanguay (1984), "If schizophrenia exists in children, surely one might expect that its symptoms would be altered by emotional and cognitive immaturity, just as one expects to find marked symptomatic differences between adult and juvenile forms of diabetes." Tanguay goes on to point out that, for children "DSM III tells us very little about etiology, treatment, and prognosis . . . This is particularly true for categories in which there are serious disturbances in cognitive and language function, in nonverbal communication, and in social relationships."

In order to better understand psychosis in childhood, Tanguay (1984) proposes a model that considers multiple, fundamental, and independent lines of development. He states that "under normal circumstances the elemental aspects of personality develop in a tightly integrated fashion but under adverse circumstances (be they of a biological or experiental nature) lines of development may fail and become dissociated from each other, leading to clinical features of the pervasive developmental disorders, of non-autistic forms of mental retardation, of specific developmental language or reading disorders, of schizophrenia in children, and of other similar forms of serious psychopathology" (Tanguay, 1984*). When most lines of development fail more or less equally, a picture of mental retardation emerges. When fundamental skills become disassociated in developmental rate, many clinical pictures could emerge, including infantile autism, schizophrenia, or specific language disorder. Tanguay argues that describing children according to arrests or delays in specific developmental lines may be helpful in understanding and in providing interventions for disturbed and handicapped youngsters

Other Disorders Associated With Mental Retardation

There is considerable interest currently in childhood depression, however, research in this area is preliminary and contradictory. The state of the art in diagnosis of childhood depression is such that few studies have examined the incidence of mental retardation in depressed children. However, a review by Reid (1972) documents a prevalence rate of affective illness in retarded adults equal to that of the general population, suggesting that rates might be comparable in retarded and nonretarded children.

---

* Tanguay quotes from: Tanguay, PE. (1984). Toward a new classification of serious psychopathology in children. *Journal of the American Academy of Child Psychiatry, 23,* 373–384; by permission of the Williams & Wilkins Company, © 1984 by the American Academy of Child Psychiatry.

A literature does exist on infants and young children who manifest depressive reactions to separation from a primary caretaker (Call, 1980). This group of children, suffering from "anaclitic depressions," were identified in early studies by Spitz (1946) and Freud and Burlingham (1944). These children characteristically manifest developmental retardation affecting physical, intellectual, and emotional development. The cause of the "depression" is usually attributed to a disruption in the attachment process following a separation from a major attachment figure (Bowlby, 1973).

Literature on infants diagnosed as environmental failure-to-thrive suggests that the continued relationship of a vulnerable child with a caregiver who is insensitive to the child's needs and cues can also result in a clinical picture of depression with concomitant developmental retardation and growth failure (Coleman & Provence, 1967; Ferhalt & Provence, 1976). The importance of a consistent responsive adult in providing appropriately stimulating learning and emotional experiences for reversing these conditions has been noted by several authors (Rutter, 1979). It has been suggested that while cognition is often affected in these children, intellectual growth is more amenable to environmental intervention than is social/emotional development (Rutter, 1979; Sameroff & Chandler, 1975).

Poor parent–child interaction leading to disturbed emotional and intellectual child outcome can also be seen in children of abusing parents. The impact of child abuse on the developmental functioning of very young children is only beginning to be understood. There are suggestions from the literature, however, that abused children exhibit a higher percentage of retardation than nonabused children (Appelbaum, 1977; Sandgrund, Gaines, & Green, 1974). Appelbaum (1977) found the average mental score for 2- to 30-month-olds on the Bayley Mental Scale of Infant Development was 75 (SD, 18.92) for abused children, as opposed to 106 (SD, 18.94) in nonabused controls. Furthermore, on the Revised Denver Developmental Screening Test, 47 percent of the abused children scored in the questionable to abnormal range, whereas all of the control children were in the normal range. Both samples came from lower socioeconomic backgrounds.

Problems in attachment and in mother–infant interaction have been noted in maltreated youngsters (Egeland & Sroufe, 1981). Older abused children also show cognitive impairment, especially in the presence of family instability, parent unemployment, and frequent moves (Martin, Breezley, Conway, & Kempe, 1974). Furthermore, there is evidence that neglect as well as abuse is related to poor cognitive and adaptive outcome (Sandgrund et al., 1974).

A growing number of children that we see are those diagnosed as suffering from "fetal alcohol syndrome" (FAS). More severely affected children manifest facial anomalies, growth deficiency, and mental retardation (Smith, 1979). Although mental retardation is the most striking feature of FAS, a variety of behavioral manifestations often associated with brain dysfunction are also evident. These include fine motor problems such as tremulousness, weak and primitive grasp, poor finger articulation, delay in gross motor development, and delay in establishing hand dominance (Streissguth, 1976). Difficulty with sucking as infants and feeding problems in the preschool years are also noted. These children often appear hyperactive with poor attention and problem solving abilities. While an excellent home environment may offset the effects of alcohol consumption during pregnancy in mild cases, it does not offset brain dysfunction in more severely affected children (Thompson, 1979).

This chapter has delineated the major etiologic factors related to mental retardation and provided a general summary of the association between mental retardation and other psychiatric disorders. I have also tried to describe the complexity of the problem in diagnosis of children with multiple difficulties, with mental retardation as a major underlying substrate. Much remains to be discovered in this area, and new ideas concerning diagnosis and treatment need to replace old prejudices and fatalistic ideas about the mentally retarded. We are now in a position to expose every child to innovative treatment programs so as to meet the child's full social, emotional, and cognitive potential. Many children can benefit from inventions previously untried with the mentally retarded. Chapters in this book include discussions of successful treatment approaches, including individual and group psychotherapy as well as behavioral techniques. In the area of diagnosis, future categorization will need to relate more to the special features of development in the young child in order to guide us in specific interventions.

REFERENCES

Appelbaum, AS. (1977). Developmental retardation in infants as a concomitant of physical child abuse. *Journal of Abnormal Child Psychology, 5,* 417–423

Bowlby, J. (1973). *Attachment and loss: Separation anxiety and anger* (Vol. 2). London: Hogarth

Call, JD. (1980). Other disorders of infancy, childhood and adolescence. In Kaplan, HI, Freeman, AF, & Sadoch, B (Eds.), *Comprehensive textbook of psychiatry* (Vol. 3). Baltimore, MD: Williams and Wilkins

Coleman, RW, & Provence, S. (1967). Environmental retardation (hospitalism) in infants living in families. *Pediatrics, 19,* 285–292

Crothers, B & Paine, RS. (1959). *The natural history of cerebral palsy.* Cambridge, MA: Harvard University Press

Demyer, MK, Barton, S, Kimberlin, C, Allen, J, Yang, E, & Steele, R. (1974). The measured intelligence of autistic children. *Journal of Autism and Childhood Schizophrenia, 4,* 42–60

Denhoff, E. (1976). Medical aspects. In WM Cruickshank (Ed.), *Cerebral palsy: A developmental disability.* Syracuse, NY: Syracuse University Press

Diagnostic and Statistical Manual of Mental Disorders (DSM III). (1980). Washington, DC: American Psychiatric Association

Dobson, JC, Williamson, ML, Azen, C, & Koch, R. (1977). Intellectual assessment of 111 four-year-old children with phenylketonuria. *Pediatrics, 60,* 822–827

Egeland, B, & Sroufe, LA. (1981). Attachment and early maltreatment. *Child Development, 52,* 44–52

Ferholt, J, & Provence, S. (1976). An infant with psychophysiological vomiting. *The Psychoanalytic Study of the Child. 31,* 439–459

Fish, B, & Ritvo, E. (1979). Psychoses of childhood. In I Berlin & J Nospitz (Eds.), *Basic handbook of child psychiatry.* New York, Basic Books

Freeman, BJ, (1978). Appraising children for mental retardation. The usefulness and limitations of I.Q. testing. *Clinical Pediatrics, 17,* 169–173

Freud, A, & Burlingham, D. (1944). *Infants without families.* New York: International Universities Press

Grossman, HJ. (Ed.). (1977). *Manual on terminology and classification in mental retardation* (rev. ed.). Washington, DC: American Association on Mental Deficiency

Kanner, L. (1943). Autistic disturbances of affective contact. *Nervous Child, 2,* 217–250

Keith, HM. (1963). *Convulsive disorders in children.* Boston: Little, Brown

Livingston, S. (1972). *Comprehensive management of epilepsy in infancy, childhood, and adolescence.* Springfield, IL: Charles Thomas

Lodge, A, & Kleinfeld, PB. (1973). Early behavioral development in Down's syndrome. In M Coleman (Ed.), *Serotonin in Down's syndrome,* London: North-Holland

Lowenfeld, B. (1963). Psychological problems of children with impaired vision. In W Cruickshank (Ed.), *Psychology of exceptional children and youth* (2nd ed.). Englewood Cliffs, NJ: Prentice-Hall

Lugaresi, E, Pazzaglia, P, Rogers, J, & Tassinari, CA. (1974). Evolution and prognosis in petit mal. In P Harris & C Maudsley (Eds.), *Epilepsy* (pp. 151–153). Edinburgh: Churchill Livingstone

Magrab, PR, & Johnston, RB (1980). Mental retardation. In S Gobel & MI Erickson (Eds.), *Child development and developmental disabilities.* Boston: Little, Brown

Malone, MJ. (1976). The cerebral lipidoses. *Pediatric Clinics of North America, 23,* 303–326

Martin, HP, Breezley, P, Conway, EF, & Kempe, CH. (1974). The development of abused children. In I Schulman (Ed.), *Advances in pediatrics* (Vol. 21) (pp. 25–73). Chicago: Year Book Medical Publishers

Ornitz, EM, & Ritvo, ER. (1976). Medical assessment. In ER Ritvo (Ed.), *Autism: Diagnosis, current research and management.* New York: Spectrum

Pincus, JG, & Tucker, G. (1974). *Behavioral neurology.* New York: Oxford University Press

Reid, AH. (1972). Psychosis in adult mental defectives: I. Manic-depressive psychosis. *British Journal of Psychiatry, 120,* 205–212

Richardson, SA, Koller, H, Katz, M, & McLaren, J. (1981). A functional classification of seizures and its distribution in a mentally retarded population. *American Journal of Mental Deficiency, 85,* 457–466

Robinson, NM, & Robinson, HB. (1976). *The mentally retarded child.* New York: McGraw-Hill

Rutter, M. (1979). Maternal deprivation, 1972–1979: New findings, new concepts, new approaches. *Child Development, 50,* 283–305

Sameroff, AJ, & Chandler, MJ. (1975). Reproductive risk and the continuum of caretaking casualty. In FD Horowitz (Ed.), *Review of child development research* (Vol. 4). Chicago: University of Chicago Press

Sangrund, A, Gaines, RW, & Green, AH. (1974). Child abuse and mental retardation: A problem of cause and effect. *American Journal of Mental Deficiency, 79,* 327–330

Smith, DW. (1979). The fetal alcohol syndrome. *Hospital Practice,* 121–128

Spitz, RA. (1946). Anaclitic depression. *Psychoanalytic Study of the Child, 2,* 313–342

Streissguth, A. (1976). Psychologic handicaps in children with fetal alcohol syndrome. *Annals New York Academy of Sciences, 273,* 140–145

Tanguay, PE. (1984). Toward a new classification of serious psychopathology in children. *Journal of the American Academy of Child Psychiatry, 23,* 373–384

Thompson, RJ. (1979). Effects of maternal alcohol consumption on offspring: Review, critical assessment, and future directions. *Journal of Pediatric Psychology, 3,* 265–275

Thompson, RJ, & O'Quinn, AN. (1979). *Developmental disabilities: Etiologies, manifestations, diagnosis and treatment.* New York: Grune & Stratton

Andrew T. Russell

6

The Mentally Retarded, Emotionally Disturbed Child and Adolescent

A recent article in a leading psychiatric journal was entitled, "Do the Mentally Retarded Suffer from Affective Illness?" (Sovner & Hurley, 1983). The article was informative but the title was troubling. A professional working with the retarded might answer the title's question with "Of course!" or "Why not?" Yet it is disturbing that the question still needs to be asked some 20 years after the President's Panel on Mental Retardation set in motion a national effort to study and combat the problems of mental retardation. Such a title should remind us how little we actually know and how much we have to learn about the relationship between mental retardation and psychiatric disorder.

In the last decade it has become clear that we do not know enough. With the trends toward deinstitutionalization and mainstreaming of the retarded, along with the development of separate service delivery systems for the mentally ill and the developmentally disabled, a serious problem has been brought into clearer perspective. What has been found is that a large proportion of mentally retarded children and adolescents are also emotionally and behaviorally disturbed. These so called "dual-diagnosis" children have tended to fall between the cracks of the two health care delivery systems and have also exposed serious gaps in training and research in the two fields. Many mental health professionals are poorly trained in mental retardation and many care providers in mental retardation often do not have sufficient knowledge or resources to provide needed psychiatric and psychological care for their clients (Cushna, Szymanski, & Tanguay, 1980). One need look no further than the

CHILDREN WITH EMOTIONAL DISORDERS AND DEVELOPMENTAL DISABILITIES ISBN 0–8089–1700–5

misuse of psychotropic medication in some institutions for the retarded to observe the consequences of such ignorance. Of equal concern has been a serious lack of research into the special problems of the emotionally disturbed and mentally retarded individual (Gualtieri, 1979). It is hoped that this volume and other recent reviews reflect a long overdue but growing interest in clinical research in this area (Matson and Barrett, 1982; Szymanski and Tanguay, 1980).

The goals of this chapter will be first to review what we do know about the epidemiology of retardation in children and adolescents. This will provide a perspective to examine the nature of the association between retardation and psychiatric disorder in this age group. Finally, implications for clinical assessment and treatment will be briefly discussed.

DEFINITIONS

Unless otherwise noted, the definition of mental retardation used in this chapter will be that employed by the American Association of Mental Deficiency and discussed in Chapter 1. The definition has two basic components, cognitive functioning and adaptive behavior. Although widely accepted in this county and elsewhere, this definition is not immune from criticism. "Subaverage" intellectual functioning depends on psychometric testing, which itself has been criticized from many viewpoints. Particularly problematic is the definition and reliability of the concept of adaptive behavior (Rutter, 1970). It is beyond the scope of this chapter to debate these issues here but it will be seen that what definitions are employed may dramatically affect such basic questions as, "What is the prevalence of mental retardation?" and "Do certain psychiatric disorders occur more commonly in the retarded child and adolescent?"

The definition and reliable diagnosis of mental disorder, emotional disturbance, or psychiatric disorder is another major problem for research in this field. Although no entirely satisfactory definition for mental disorder exists, the general definition used by the authors parallels the statement used in the *Diagnostic and Statistical Manual of Mental Disorders,* Third Edition (DSM-III) (American Psychiatric Association, 1980, p. 6).

> In DSM-III each of the mental disorders is conceptualized as a clinically significant behavioral or psychological syndrome or pattern that occurs in an individual and that is typically associated with either a painful symptom (distress) or impairment in one or more important areas of functioning (disability). In addition, there is an inference that there is a behavioral, psychological, or biological dysfunction, and that the disturbance is not only in the relationship between the individual and society. (When the disturbance is limited to a conflict between an individual and society, this may represent social deviance, which may or may not be commendable, but is not by itself a mental disorder.)

How researchers have defined and diagnosed psychiatric disorder in the retarded has varied greatly and has led to different empirical results and conclusions. Some symptoms considered pathological in cognitively normal individuals may be within the normal range of behavior in the retarded (Chess, 1970). As the literature in this area is reviewed, we will try to point out the definitions and diagnostic criteria employed by the authors and how they may have affected the results. We will also emphasize the need for the use of similar diagnostic criteria of increased diagnostic reliability to allow useful comparisons between future studies in this field.

EPIDEMIOLOGY OF MENTAL RETARDATION

An important and sometimes overlooked variable in the study of children with dual disabilities is the prevalence of mental retardation itself. It is often assumed that there is a relatively stable population of individuals who can be classified as retarded. Such an assumption is probably erroneous. If one uses the definition of mental retardation given above, both predictive estimates and empirical data confirm that the measured prevalence of mental retardation varies dramatically depending on a variety of factors. Important variables that influence the differing prevalence rates include the definition of mental retardation, age, the degree of intellectual handicap, socioeconomic factors, and the mutability of tested intelligence.

If one uses measured intelligence (IQ scores) as the sole definition of mental retardation it can be predicted that around 3 percent of the population would test two standard deviations below the mean. In a study (to which we will refer frequently) of the entire population of 9-, 10- and 11-year-olds on the Isle of Wight, Rutter and his colleagues found that 2.5 percent of the children were intellectually retarded, a finding consistent with the above prediction (Rutter, Tizard & Whitmore, 1970). However, if different age groups are studied, and definitions of retardation include the concept of adaptive behavior, prevalence figures vary considerably from the 3 percent figure. For example, Richardson and colleagues are now publishing data from a longitudinal study of all children born between 1951–1955 in a city in Britain (Birch, Richardson, Baird, Horobin, & Allsley, 1970; Richardson, 1980). They used an administrative rather than a psychometric definition of mental retardation (i.e., all those children who received special services for the retarded at any time up to the age of 15 years). They found an overall prevalence rate of 16/1000, approximately one-half the 3 percent rate. They point out that if they had used IQ testing as their sole criteria the overall prevalence rate would have approached 3 percent (Richardson, Koller, Katz, & McLaren, unpublished manuscript).

In an important predictive study, Tarjan, Wright, Eyman, and Keeran (1973) argued that the general assumption that 3 percent of the population is retarded is overly simplistic and inaccurate. They pointed out that the 3 percent estimate is based on a definition of mental retardation based primarily on measured intelligence (IQ below 70), the diagnosis is made in infancy, the diagnosis does not change over time, and mortality statistics for the retarded are similar to those of the general population. Each of these assumptions do not reflect clinical experience or empirical research. By using a definition of retardation that includes the concept of adaptive behavior, and takes into consideration the above factors, the authors predicted an overall prevalence rate of 1 percent.

At least one community-based epidemiological study using similar definitions, has confirmed their prediction (Mercer, 1973). This study utilized a representative sample of 7000 children and adults who were then tested and screened. Measures of adaptive behavior were developed and norms established. Mercer then examined how applying different classification criteria affects who was labelled as retarded and who was not. Using traditional criteria (IQ below 70, adaptive behavior scores within the lower 3 percent), she found an overall prevalence rate of 9.7/1000 or just under 1 percent. If IQ alone was used as a criteria, the prevalence rate was 21.4/1000. If standards for retardation were broadened, i.e., IQ below 80, the prevalence rates correspondingly increased. One interesting finding was that the inclusion of adaptive behavior criteria lowered prevalence rates among lower socioeconomic groups and ethnic minorities much more significantly than among white or middleclass groups. These findings obviously have important implications for public policy but also emphasize the importance of selection criteria for research that depends on the identification of a representative sample of mentally retarded individuals.

It is clear from the above examples that in any study that uses a two-dimensional definition of mental retardation, what constitutes adaptive behavior assumes great importance. Rutter has argued that the inclusion of adaptive behavior as a diagnostic criteria leads to spuriously high estimates of psychopathology in children with intellectual deficits (Rutter, 1970). Quantifying adaptive behavior is at best a difficult process and may vary dramatically with developmental level and cultural expectations. Given these difficulties of assessment and measurement, a great deal of additional research is required. One example of important research in this area has been a useful scale to assess a variety of behaviors taking into consideration developmental level developed by Nihira and his colleagues (Nihira, Foster, Shellhaas, & Leland, 1974). Although it is a carefully constructed instrument, the author has found it to be less useful for older children and adolescents who fall into the mild ranges of mental retardation. Additional assessment techniques for this population are sorely needed.

In addition to problems of definition, age and degree of intellectual impairment are important interrelated variables that influence prevalence statistics. Research studies looking at emotional disturbance in retarded children and adolescents must be particularly careful to define which subpopulations are being examined. Severely retarded preschoolers and mildly retarded adolescents are certainly more different than they are alike even though both groups fall into the general class of the retarded.

In the Tarjan study cited previously it was estimated that prevalence rates for retardation in the preschool group were about 0.7/1000 (Tarjan, et al., 1973). A proportionally large number of these children would have IQs below 50 and also have diagnosable organic impairments. This simply reflects that the more severe forms of retardation are often associated with neurologic and physical handicaps and are identified the earliest. In contrast, the prevalence and incidence of retardation rises dramatically in the school-age years with the vast majority of children identified falling in the mild range (IQ 50–70) of retardation. These children make up a very distinct population from their younger, more handicapped peers. The limitations of the school-age children often only become apparent with the increased developmental and cognitive demands of having to learn and function in a classroom, and the majority of these children and adolescents have no clear organic etiology for their retardation. Children from lower socioeconomic backgrounds are overrepresented in this group (Stein & Susser, 1970; Zigler, 1967). Statistics from the Richardson longitudinal study are illustrative of this pattern (Richardson, et al., unpublished manuscript). In their study, based on how many children were identified as requiring special services, the prevalence rate rose rapidly from 3.5/1000 at age 5 years to 14/1000 at age 10 years. It then leveled off until age 15 years, where it again dropped rapidly to approximately 6.5/1000. This drop in prevalence from adolescence to adulthood was explained by the fact that by age 22 years two-thirds of the index cases were not receiving any special mental retardation services. Within this population 89 percent of the males were employed in fulltime jobs, although at a somewhat lower skill level than a comparison group of nonretarded subjects (Richardson, 1978). In summary, many mildly retarded adolescents, identified as such during their school years, make a relatively successful transition to adulthood and are no longer identified as retarded.

Incidence statistics reveal similar patterns. "New" cases of children with more severe forms of retardation are identified at an early age and almost all cases are identified by the early school years. In contrast, fewer new cases of mild mental retardation are identified in the preschool years and the majority are diagnosed during the school years. By late adolescence both prevalence and incidence rates drop sharply.

Two other factors significantly affect epidemiological patterns of mental retardation; the mutability of tested intelligence over time and socioeconomic status. The factors are closely related because there is considerable evidence that environmental disadvantage contributes to progressive deficits in tested intelligence both for individuals and groups and some evidence that a reversal of environmental conditions may lead to an improvement in tested intelligence (Clarke & Clarke, 1975; Stein & Susser, 1970). In addition to the fact that tested intelligence may change, it is a striking phenomenon that children and adolescents classified as mildly mentally retarded and without organic disease, predominantly come from disadvantaged backgrounds (Zigler, 1967). This population has been referred to as the familial retarded or the sociocultural retarded. It is beyond the scope of this chapter to review the evidence supporting these findings (see Baumeister & MacLean, 1979, for an alternative conceptualization) but it is evident that research in this area must take into account the impact of environmental deprivation. For example, in a study of psychopathology in the mildly mentally retarded, comparison groups must be matched for socioeconomic status to avoid spuriously high correlations between mental retardation and psychiatric disorder.

The purpose of this brief overview of the epidemiology of mental retardation has been to put the research on psychiatric disorder in retarded children and adolescents into perspective. As will be seen, the immense variability among subpopulations of the retarded, the differing criteria for classification and diagnosis, the study of institutionalized as opposed to community-based populations, and the lack of consideration of socioeconomic factors are just some of the issues that face research in this area.

MENTAL RETARDATION AND PSYCHIATRIC DISORDER

There is a general consensus amongst researchers and clinicians that a significant number of retarded children and adolescents exhibit symptoms of behavioral and emotional disturbance (Beier, 1964; Webster, 1970). To review the nature of this association several basic questions must be asked. How prevalent is psychiatric disorder in retarded children? What is the relationship between differing levels of IQ and psychiatric disorder? What types of emotional and behavioral disorder are commonly seen in retarded children and adolescents? What are the mechanisms that may underlie the association between retardation and psychiatric disorder? Although these questions appear fundamental, finding clear answers in the scientific literature is difficult. As has already been suggested, there are several reasons for this. There is a relative lack of well-constructed research in this area. The majority of research populations have consisted of institutionalized or referred subjects, samples that are hardly representative of the general population of mentally retarded children and adolescents. Few studies have used matched control groups of nonretarded children. There is a tremendous heterogeneity within the general population of mentally retarded children and adolescents, which is often not accounted for in research designs. Different researchers use different definitions of mental retardation. Last, until recently, there has been a lack of standardized and reliable diagnostic criteria for various psychiatric disorders. The extent to which studies we will review have overcome these methodological difficulties determines to a large extent how useful they are in answering the basic questions posed above.

PREVALENCE OF PSYCHIATRIC DISORDER IN MENTALLY RETARDED CHILDREN AND ADOLESCENTS

Two major epidemiological studies published within the last 15 years provide our best information about the prevalence of psychiatric disorder in retarded children and adolescents. Both are particularly significant in that they more or less overcome the problem of selecting a representative sample and both allow comparisons between a retarded population and children of normal intelligence. The differing methodologies of these two studies will be described and their findings compared. Results from other studies with prevalence data will then be more briefly presented.

In the 1960s Rutter and colleagues conducted an epidemiological study of all 9-, 10-, and 11-year-old children on the Isle of Wight (Rutter, Graham, & Yule, 1970; Rutter, Tizard, & Whitmore, 1970). This study has served as a model for investigations of this type and is a major source of information concerning the relationship between mental retardation and emotional disturbance in children.

Several characteristics of the Isle of Wight study need to be highlighted. First it screened an entire age cohort (ages 9–11 years and again at age 14 years) and did not depend on a referred or selected sample. Such a sample is by definition representative (for the age group and geographical area studied) and more importantly allows direct comparisons between groups of children at all IQ levels.

Secondly, the measures employed were carefully tested for reliability and validity and used in a standardized fashion. Children were classified on the basis of intellectual functioning as measured by IQ tests. Thus the results from the Isle of Wight must not be automatically interpreted as applying to mentally retarded children as defined by AAMD or DSM-III criteria, which include a dimension of adaptive behavior in the diagnosis.

A third notable feature of the Isle of Wight study was the comprehensive range of assessments that were obtained (IQ testing, educational testing, behavioral ratings, neurologic assessment, etc.). In addition, ratings were often obtained from a variety of sources. For example, in selecting children with psychiatric disorder, rating scales were completed by both teachers and parents. These screening instruments were then followed by direct interviews of parent and child. Thus a child's behavior was assessed in several environments and by several different methods.

Results from a second major epidemiological study from Britain have recently been published (Koller, Richardson, Katz & McLaren, 1982, 1983; Richardson, 1978, 1980). This study, cited earlier, differs from the Isle of Wight survey in several important respects. It is similar in that the problem of a representative sample was avoided by studying an entire population, in this case every child born between 1951–1955 in a city in Britain. It differs in that it is a longitudinal study and that behavior disturbance was assessed retrospectively at age 22 years. Another important difference was in the criteria used for sample selection. Rutter used a psychometric definition of mental subnormality while the Richardson and Koller study defined their sample in an administrative way; their sample consisted of those individuals who had received special services for the retarded at some time before the age of 16 years. Keeping these important methodological differences in mind, it is now possible to compare the results from both studies.

The Isle of Wight studies found that emotional disturbance is indeed significantly more common in children with low IQs. The prevalence rate for psychiatric disorder in children with IQs less than 70 was 30.4 percent, using the parental questionnaire and 41.8 percent using the teacher questions. Rates for a representative sample of the total age cohort were 7.7 percent and 9.5 percent respectively. Thus psychiatric disorder was found to be 4–5 times more prevalent in intellectually retarded children. Similar findings were obtained using direct psychiatric interviews.

Koller et al. (1983) have just reported data on behavioral disturbances from the British longitudinal birth cohort study. They found that 61 percent of the mentally retarded population showed evidence of behavioral disturbance in childhood, and 59 percent in the postschool period. The rates for moderate or more severe disturbance were 36 percent in childhood and 30 percent in the postschool period. To compare these rates of disturbance with those of the general population, the authors selected a comparison group from a one-in-five random sample of all children born in the same years as the retarded subjects (Koller et al., 1982). These subjects were then matched with the retarded group on age, sex, and social class. Using the same retrospective methodology, they found evidence of behavioral disturbance in 24 percent of the comparison sample during childhood. The rate for moderate or more severe disturbance was only 5 percent. Thus behavioral disturbance was approximately 2.5 times more common in the retarded group (similar to the Isle of Wight results) and the more serious behavioral problems were 7 times more frequent.

The higher overall rates for behavioral disturbance (as compared to the Isle of Wight studies) may be the result of the different definitions and methodologies employed. Just one of the many differences was the fact that information was gathered in retrospective fashion (at age 22 years) and covered the entire range of childhood rather than focusing on current functioning.

Another recent study, notable for the size of the population surveyed, also provides some information concerning the prevalence of psychiatric disturbance in a mentally retarded population (Jacobson, 1982). This study reports on data from 30,000 individuals receiving developmental disability services in New York State. In spite of the size of the sample, the author points out the population is not entirely representative and is skewed toward greater disability, with underrepresentation of persons with mild mental retardation and overrepresentation of the more severely handicapped groups. On the other hand,

Jacobson (1982) feels that problem behaviors and psychiatric disorder may be overestimated in their sample of mildly or moderately retarded individuals because without such difficulties they might not be recipients of specialized services. The results are based on the *New York Developmental Disabilities Information Survey* (DDIS) (Janicki & Jacobson, 1979, 1982), in which raters are able to code a maximum of 3 problem behaviors from a list of 29, as well as the frequency that they occur. The absence of problem behaviors must also be indicated. After correcting the sample for a normal distribution of mental retardation, Jacobsen estimates that 13.7 percent of children and 17.1 percent of adult developmentally disabled (DD) population would be classified as psychiatrically impaired. These figures are considerably lower than those from the Isle of Wight or the British birth cohort study. When problem behaviors are examined (as opposed to being classified as psychiatrically impaired), a somewhat different picture emerges. When sample results are adjusted to the general population, Jacobson estimates that 47.7 percent of the DD population displays some type of problem behavior. These results are not directly comparable with the previous studies but serve to underline the magnitude of psychiatric problems among the retarded.

A number of other studies, which will be discussed briefly here and more extensively later, also provide some information regarding the prevalence of emotional disturbance among mentally retarded children. All these studies use a referred or selected sample, which may not be representative of the general population of mentally retarded children. Only rarely are nonretarded comparison groups employed. Menolascino (1969) described 256 emotionally disturbed and mentally retarded children out of a total sample of 1025 children referred with suspicion of mental retardation for a prevalence rate of 25 percent. Ten years later, Eaton and Menolascino (1982) reported on an additional sample of 798 retarded individuals referred to their community-based program in Nebraska. Of these children 168 were referred for psychiatric evaluation and 114 were found to exhibit both mental retardation and emotional disturbance, for a prevalence rate of 14.3 percent.

Chess and Hassibi (1970) conducted a follow-up study on 52 children, aged 5 to 11 years. The study is interesting in that the patients in effect were *not* a representative sample in that each was living at home as part of a middleclass family and all were in the mildly retarded range. Of this group, 60 percent were felt to have some type of psychiatric disturbance in association with mild retardation. Six years later (Chess, 1977), 40 percent of the sample still exhibited behavioral disturbance. Phillips and Williams reported on 100 consecutive referrals to a clinic at the Langley Porter Institute. Eighty percent of the referrals were diagnosed as exhibiting emotional disturbance. Szymanski (1977) found 54 percent of 132 children referred to a developmental disabilities clinic in a pediatric hospital setting to be emotionally disturbed.

A rather different approach to the assessment of behavioral disorders in mentally retarded as opposed to cognitively normal children has been taken by

Curry and Thompson (1979, 1982). The study is important in that it applies the same methodology to three different groups of children. In these studies the mother completed the Missouri Children's Behavior Checklist. The results were then subjected to cluster analysis. The three samples consisted of children referred to a developmental disabilities clinic (DEC), a comparison group from a psychiatric clinic, and a third group, which was nonreferred. Cluster membership in the normal cluster was found to be 39 percent for the DEC population, 12 percent for the psychiatric clinical population, and 70 percent for the non-referred population.

Two major conclusions concerning the prevalence of psychiatric disturbance in the mentally retarded can be made on the basis of the above selective review. First, prevalence rates in the studies cited have varied from 14 to 80 percent, depending on definitional criteria and the representativeness of the sample. However, most of the studies report prevalence rates ranging from approximately 14 to 40 percent and these figures perhaps can serve as a rough approximation of the importance of the problem of psychiatric disturbance in mentally retarded children. A second conclusion is that the few studies that compare a mentally retarded sample with a representative sample of the general population consistently report that emotional disturbances are more common in the retarded than they are in the nonretarded. Perhaps the best information in this area comes from the Isle of Wight studies, which reported a 4–5 times greater rate of behavioral disturbance in an intellectually retarded population.

PREVALENCE OF PSYCHIATRIC DISORDER AT VARYING LEVELS OF IQ

Given the fact that psychiatric disorder is more common in the general population of children with intellectual deficits, it is necessary to examine whether the relationship holds for all levels of IQ. A related question is whether certain types of abnormal behavior are more common at certain IQ levels. To answer these questions large sample sizes are required, and we again turn to the large scale epidemiological studies cited previously.

One of the more interesting findings of the Isle of Wight studies was the fact that associations between behavioral disturbance (almost all types) and intellectual functioning held for all levels of IQ and was not limited to the retarded group. For example, Table 6-1 summarizes teacher ratings for the items "miserable," fighting, and poor concentration for boys at five different IQ levels (Rutter, 1970). In summary, the Isle of Wight survey found that the frequency of behavioral deviance of almost all types is inversely related to IQ and this relationship holds at the upper as well as the lower ranges of intelligence in an almost linear fashion.

Table 6-1
Relationship of Behavior to IQ in Boys
(Teacher Ratings—% of Sample)

	IQ			
Symptom	<79	80–99	100–119	>120
"Miserable"	20	11	6	3
Fighting	26	17	11	5
Poor Concentration	76	50	30	11

Data from Rutter, M. (1970). Psychiatry. In J Wortis (Ed.), *Mental retardation, An annual review* (Vol. 3).

The British birth cohort study also examined the relationship of level of IQ to behavioral disturbance (Koller et al., 1982). The results differed considerably from the Isle of Wight study, perhaps for some of the methodological differences already mentioned. The IQ subsets examined were less than 50, 50–59, 60–69 and 70 and greater. The rates for behavioral disturbance were 58, 62, 49, and 81 percent respectively. The lack of any kind of linear relationship with IQ and a high percentage of behavioral disturbance in the mildly impaired children may in part be explained by the selection criteria for the mentally retarded population. As discussed previously, children were included in the study only if they had received some type of services for the developmentally disabled. Children with milder cognitive impairment tend to be identified and referred for services if they have associated behavioral disturbance and may not be identified if they do not. Interestingly, Birch et al. (1970) had earlier examined a subsample of the same birth cohort (at age 10 years), using methodology more similar to that of Isle of Wight studies (parent and teacher questionnaires and psychiatric interviews with the children). Birch found 45, 48, 21, and 7 percent of children exhibited behavioral disturbance for the same IQ subsets mentioned above. These results more closely parallel conclusions of the Isle of Wight survey.

The large size of the population in the New York developmental disabilities survey also allowed the examination of the relationship between problem behavior and the IQ level (Jacobson, 1982). As in the Isle of Wight studies, it was found that the frequency of most problem behaviors increased as IQ levels decreased. However, not all 29 problem behaviors surveyed followed that pattern. For example, in the population from 0–21 years of age, perseveration, echolalia, extreme mood changes, lack of interpersonal responsiveness, physical assault upon others, property destruction, self-injurious behavior, hyperactivity, stereotyped movements, crying and temper tantrums, and wandering/running away were more frequent as IQ decreased. In contrast, delusions and hallucinations, suicide threats/attempts, depression, fire-setting, coercive sexual behavior, verbal abusiveness, and substance abuse were more common in the less handicapped individuals.

The relationship between individual behavioral items and IQ reported in the New York study confirmed results of another large community study, which reported on the frequency of certain behavioral items taken from the Adaptive Behavior Scale (Eyman & Call, 1977). That study also found a clear relationship between a variety of problem behaviors (e.g., threatens or does physical violence, damages property, physical violence to self) and level of IQ. However, some behaviors requiring verbal ability (e.g., using profane or hostile language) were more common in the mildly retarded group. Unfortunately, the more aggressive behaviors were more common in the more severely handicapped individuals, making successful community placement doubly difficult.

All the above studies are relatively consistant in their findings that the frequency of behavioral disturbance is inversely related to IQ. This relationship holds across the entire spectrum of intelligence. Although some individual items of behavior may not follow this pattern, most indeed do, and it can be concluded that children with low IQs are significantly at risk for a variety of behavioral and psychiatric disturbances during their developmental years.

TYPES OF PSYCHIATRIC DISORDER

Given the fact that psychiatric disturbance is relatively common in retarded children and adolescents, the next question that must be asked is whether certain types of psychiatric disorder are more prevalent in the retarded as opposed to children with normal intelligence. In other words, are mentally retarded children subject to the same spectrum of psychopathological disorders as other children or does the presence of cognitive handicap lead to specific types of disturbance? The preponderance of the evidence suggests that the types of psychiatric disorder seen in retarded children do not differ in kind from those seen in the general population. While evaluating the research in this area, however, several cautions must be noted. First, it is difficult to compare different epidemiological studies that have addressed this question because of the lack of consistency in diagnostic criteria between studies. In the United States, earlier studies used DSM-I or DSM-II criteria and only recently have the more specific criteria of DSM-III been applied. In Great Britain, research has tended to use other diagnostic criteria, most recently, that developed by Rutter and colleagues for the World Health Organization (Rutter, Shaffer, & Shepherd, 1975). Other researchers have developed their own diagnostic categories. In summary, varying diagnostic criteria make it extremely difficult to generalize about what specific types of psychiatric disorder are most commonly seen in the retarded and whether the patterns of disorders seen differs significantly from that of children and adolescents without intellectual impairment. Another important consideration in reviewing research in this area is, once again, the heterogeneity of the retarded population. As will be seen, there is considerable evidence that more severely handicapped children (IQs less than 50) may exhibit somewhat different types of psychiatric disorder than children in the mild ranges of mental retardation. The presence or absence of clear-cut neurologic disorders may also influence the type of psychiatric disturbances seen. A final question concerns the reliability of the diagnostic process in retarded individuals. Reiss and colleagues have demonstrated the phenomena of diagnostic overshadowing in which the presence of obvious mental retardation can lead diagnosticians to overlook other psychiatric diagnoses (Reiss, Levitan, & Szysko, 1982., Reiss & Szysko, 1983). The converse is also probably true. When patients present with major psychiatric disturbance, the presence of mild forms of mental retardation may be overlooked. Field trials that were conducted by the World Health Organization demonstrated that in complex clinical cases (i.e., mental retardation, neurologic disorder, and psychiatric disturbance in the same child), the clinician would often diagnose only one of the disorders that was present (Tarjan, Tizard, Rutter, Begab, Brooke, De La Cruze, Lin, Montenegro, Strotzka, & Sartorius, 1972). The DSM-III field trials also showed that when a child required multiple diagnoses on one axis, the second and third diagnoses tended to be made with less reliability (Russell, Cantwell, & Mattison, 1979). For this reason, the inclusion of mental retardation as one of many Axis I diagnoses in DSM-III has been criticized and it has been suggested that mental retardation and/or intellectual functioning based on IQ testing be allocated a separate axis in future multiaxial diagnostic schemes (Rutter & Shaffer, 1980). To these methodological problems must be added the clinical reality that delineating psychiatric syndromes in a retarded population is often a difficult task (Menolascino, 1970; Szymanski, 1980). This is particularly true when diagnostic criteria have been developed for use in cognitively normal populations (Corbett, 1977a; 1977b).

Keeping these methological and clinical problems in mind, some of the studies focusing on "dual-diagnosis" children and adolescents will be briefly reviewed. Many of these studies have already been cited in the discussion of the prevalence of psychiatric disorder in mentally retarded children.

Using nomenclature from DSM-I, Menolascino (1969) diagnosed 256 children who had been evaluated at a psychiatric clinic in Nebraska. Menolascino saw the majority of these children as suffering from a chronic brain syndrome with either behavioral or psychotic reactions. The distinctions between the behavioral and psychotic group were made "primarily on the basis of the degree of the emotional disturbance noted and associated family interaction dynamic." Of the sample, 68 percent was diagnosed in these categories, while an additional 23 percent were felt to have an adjustment reaction, 3 percent functional psychoses, 2 percent personality disorders, and 6 percent unspecified. In a more recent study, diagnostic categories "based primarily on DSM-III criteria" were used (Eaton and Menolascino, 1982). Of a subsample aged 6–20 years, 48 percent received a diagnosis of organic brain syndrome with either transient psychotic reaction or transient behavioral reaction. Of this age group, 29 percent was classified as suffering from adjustment reactions, 9 percent personality disorders, and 15 percent schizophrenia. Of the 8 children or adolescents who received a diagnosis of schizophrenia, 3 were diagnosed as having childhood schizophrenia, symptoms of which had developed between 4 to 6 years of age in previously retarded children; and 5 had chronic undifferentiated schizophrenia.

Chess and Hassibi (1970) studied and followed up a group of 52 mildly retarded children. These children ranged in age from 5–11 years and were all living at home in middle class families. Eleven of the 52 children (21 percent) were diagnosed as having cerebral dysfunction. Assignment to this category was based on neurologic findings (two or more soft signs and/or focal findings) "beyond the cognitive disability plus behavior symptoms which are not explained in terms of reactive or neurotic behavior disorders." These children would probably be similar to those diagnosed by Menolascino as having organic brain syndromes with behavioral reactions. Of the sample, 35 percent were diagnosed as having a reactive behavior disorder reflecting environmental stress. These children exhibited such symptoms as fear of going outside, tantrums and aggressive behavior. One child was classified as having a neurotic behavior disorder and one as psychotic. Twenty-one children (40 percent) were felt to have no psychiatric disorders. Chess and Hassibi emphasize that many of the observed behaviors (e.g., stereotyped and repetitive movements, speech, and play activities) usually considered "pathological," were not correlated with psychiatric disturbance in these retarded children and more parsimoniously, could be seen as related to their cognitive handicaps. More recently Chess (1977) has reported follow-up data on the original sample. One important finding from this study was that the prognosis for the children without significant neurologic findings was relatively good, while none of the children in the cerebral dysfunction group had improved.

Phillips and Williams (1975) studied 100 mentally retarded children referred to a psychiatric clinic. They found that 38 of the children had disorders of "psychotic proportions." This group included children with infantile autism, childhood schizophrenia, and chronic brain syndromes. Out of the remaining 62 children, 26 were diagnosed as having behavior disorders, 16 were diagnosed as having personality disorders, 5 neuroses, 2 transient situational disorders, and 13 had no psychiatric disorder. In contrast to Menolascino, Phillips and Williams assessed organicity independently and did not categorize all children with organic findings as exhibiting chronic brain syndromes. Forty-eight children showed evidence of definite neurologic findings, while 52 did not. Of the 38 children, 21 in the psychotic group had neurologic findings and 27 of the 62 other children had neurologic findings. One virtue of the Phillips and Williams study was that it compared the retarded group with a group of nonretarded children also referred to the psychiatric clinic. They found similar symptoms in both groups and concluded that psychopathology in mentally retarded children is no different in kind from that of children of normal intelligence. These findings were interpreted as supporting the view that emotional disturbance in the retarded is not so much the result of cognitive handicaps but rather is related to "delayed disordered personality functions," and "disturbed interpersonal relationships with meaningful people in the environment" (Phillips, 1967, p. 29).

Similar to the Phillips and Williams study, the Isle of Wight study found that intellectual retardation was associated with a wide range of disorders in children (Corbett, 1977b; Rutter, 1970). Although psychiatric disorder was more common in retarded children, it was felt that there was nothing particularly distinctive about the types of disorders seen. Exceptions to the generalization were the syndromes of infantile autism, severe hyperkinetic disorder, and certain types of abnormal behavior such as stereotyped movements and pica, which were strongly associated with cognitive handicaps. The relationship of mental retardation and infantile autism is discussed at length elsewhere in this volume.

Although the pattern of psychiatric disorders seen in retarded children is similar to that seen in nonretarded children, there is some evidence that more severely handicapped children may exhibit a somewhat different spectrum of psychopathology. Corbett, Harris, and Robinson (1975) examined 140 children with IQs below 50 out of a Southeast London population of 175,000. Using a methodology similar to that employed on the Isle of Wight, it was found that 43 percent of the children exhibited behavioral disturbance. In their sample, psychosis (including autism) was diagnosed in 13 percent of the children, hyperkinetic disorders 12 percent, and severe stereotypies 5 percent. Only 3 percent of the sample were diagnosed as having a neurotic disorder and only 9 percent as having a conduct disorder. This pattern of disorder is considerably different than found in most studies of children predominantly in the mildly retarded range and in the general population. Of particular note are the high prevalence rates of childhood psychosis, hyperkinetic disorders, and severe stereotypies in the severely retarded children.

Reid (1980) has reviewed the psychiatric diagnoses of 60 children and adolescents referred to a psychiatric clinic and followed for an average of almost 5 years. Reid used the diagnostic scheme developed by Rutter, et al. (1975) for the World Health Organization. Like DSM-III, this classification system is multiaxial. Although the sample was referred and biased toward psychopathology, the use of a multiaxial classification scheme helped to identify the wide variety of disorders seen in children who are both mentally retarded and psychiatrically disturbed. The most common diagnosis on Axis I (clinical psychiatric syndrome) was conduct disorders, which occurred in 45 percent of the sample. This was followed by neurotic disorders (42 percent), hyperkinetic syndrome (15 percent), childhood psychosis (8 percent), and adjustment reaction (4 percent). One child was suffering from manic depressive psychosis and one child was unclassified. Fourteen children received a secondary diagnosis on Axis I and 6 children required 3 diagnoses on Axis I to appropriately capture the variety of disorders seen in these children. This finding simply underlines the clinical experience that these children often present with a complex variety of disorders. One of six of the children received a diagnosis on Axis II (specific delays in development). These children in general had speech and language delays more severe than could be accounted for by their level of retardation. Axis III recorded the intellectual level of the children and on Axis IV (accompanying medical conditions) almost one-half the children in the study had associated medical disorders. One of five of the children had epilepsy and there was a tendency for children with hyperkinetic syndromes to have clear-cut structural brain damage.

In the British birth cohort study cited earlier (Koller et al., 1982, 1983) the authors classified the subjects into four broad groups: emotional disturbance, which included anxiety disorders and symptoms of psychosis and depression; hyperactive behavior; aggressive conduct disorder including fighting, bullying and unsocialized aggression; and antisocial behavior focusing primarily on delinquent and illegal acts where aggression was not the primary component. They found that 29 percent of the sample exhibited emotional disturbance, 12 percent hyperactive behavior, 33 percent aggressive conduct disorder, 27 percent antisocial behavior, and 39 percent no behavior disturbance. The results were then analyzed in terms of sex and IQ subsets. In comparison with age and sex matched controls, emotional disturbance was more common at higher IQ levels, hyperactivity more common in males with lower IQs, aggression more common in males and females with IQs less than 50 and in males with IQs 70 or greater, and antisocial behavior more common in males with IQs over 70.

Several tentative conclusions can be drawn from the somewhat confusing picture presented by such a wide variety of studies using different methodologies and different diagnostic criteria.

Although psychiatric disorder is more common in a retarded population, the types of disorder are quite heterogenous and there seem to be no dramatic differences in the types of disorder seen in retarded children and nonretarded children. An exception to this generalization is the more severe forms of retardation in which neurologic disorder, severe forms of hyperkinesis, stereotypic movements, and childhood psychoses are relatively more common. Given the fact that psychiatric disturbance does not differ in kind in most retarded children, it is extremely important to make careful psychiatric assessments and evaluations in children who present with mental retardation. As has been pointed out by several authors, diagnosis is more difficult in mentally retarded children and significant emotional disturbance may be overlooked. As a consequence, many retarded children may not receive appropriate treatment interventions. Multi-axial diagnostic schemes may be particularly useful in making comprehensive diagnoses in these children who often present with a complex combination of psychiatric disturbances, intellectual handicaps, other learning disorders, and neurologic disorders.

THE BASIS OF THE ASSOCIATION BETWEEN MENTAL RETARDATION AND PSYCHIATRIC DISORDER

Having established that psychiatric disorder is more common in mentally retarded children and adolescents, and that a wide variety of nonspecific disorders is seen in this population, the final basic question that must be asked is what mechanisms underlie the strong association. The answer to this question is complex and at best the evidence is incomplete. As may be expected from the fact that such a broad spectrum of psychiatric disorders is seen in the retarded and that the retarded themselves are such a heterogenous group, it is clear that there are multiple factors involved. This topic has been reviewed by Rutter (1970), Corbett (1977b), and Matson and Barrett (1982). These reviews suggest that several probable and potential mechanisms must be considered.

Brain Damage and Neurologic Disorder

Baumeister and Maclean (1979) have reviewed the evidence linking brain damage with mental retardation. It is well known that the great majority of individuals with IQs less than 50 have diagnosable organic brain disease. This is also true for a significant number of children with milder degrees of retardation. There is also considerable evidence that the presence of neurological disorder is associated with higher rates of psychiatric disturbance at all IQ levels (Rutter, Graham, & Yule, 1970). The most useful information in this area comes from the Isle of Wight study. Using identical assessment techniques, the Isle of Wight study looked at children without physical or neurologic disorders, children with chronic physical disorders not involving the brain, and children with neuroepileptic disorders directly involving the central nervous system. Rates for psychiatric disorder within these populations were 7 percent, 12 percent, and 34 percent respectively. Psychiatric disorder was also found to be somewhat more common in mentally retarded children with associated neurologic damage as compared to mentally retarded children without evidence of neurologic dysfunction. The importance of intellectual retardation as an independent factor was demonstrated by the fact that psychiatric disorder was much more common in children with neuroleptic conditions whose IQ was less than 85 than in those whose IQ was in the higher ranges (Rutter, 1970). Corbett, Harris, and Robinson (1975) summarized the relationship between mental retardation, epilepsy, and behavioral disturbance in the severely retarded. They found that the association between seizure disorders and behavioral disturbance was much stronger in children with normal intelligence than in severely retarded individuals. They felt that the behavior disturbance in the more severely retarded group might be more strongly associated with other factors that tended to overshadow the presence or absence of epileptic disorder.

Temperament

Both Chess (1970) and Rutter (1970) have emphasized the importance of temperament in the genesis of behavior disorders in the mentally retarded. Temperamental factors such as general activity level, quality of mood, intensity of reactions to new situations, distractability, and attention span all influence how well and how smoothly a child adapts to his or her environment. Temperamental qualities of many mentally retarded children may seriously affect how well he or she can adjust to his environment, with lack of adjustment making a child more susceptible to a variety of behavioral disorders. Particularly striking was how often poor concentration was cited by both parents and teachers in retarded children as well as children with a wide variety of behavioral disorders (Rutter, Tizard, & Whitmore, 1970).

Interpersonal Relationships

Reiss (1982 and this volume) have emphasized the importance of social rejection of mentally retarded children and adults. It is clear that one of the many stresses in a retarded child's environment is his or her lack of acceptability to peers, at times accompanied by outright ridicule. How important social rejection is in the actual genesis of behavioral disorder in these children is a complex question and a difficult one to research adequately. The problem is compounded by the fact that presence of a behavioral disturbance in children in itself leads to rejection by peers. It is often difficult to tell which preceded the other.

Education and Reading Retardation

There is ample evidence from the work of Rutter and colleagues (Berger, Yule, & Rutter, 1975, Rutter, Tizard, Yule, Graham, & Whitmore, 1976) that specific reading retardation and other educational handicaps, over and above the effects of measured intelligence, are strongly associated with behavioral disorders, particularly of the antisocial type. On the Isle of Wight, psychiatric disorder was approximately three times more common in children with educational retardation compared to the normal population. Many retarded children have specific developmental and educational handicaps disproportionate to their level of retardation (Reid, 1980). Both intellectually and educationally retarded children may experience multiple failures and many difficulties in the school environment. It can be assumed that similar mechanisms may be at work in the genesis of psychiatric disorders in both of these groups. These concerns are particularly true for mildly retarded children and perhaps of less importance in more severely retarded children (Corbett, 1977b).

Speech and Language Disorders

Children with speech and language disorders are vulnerable to a wide variety of psychiatric disorders (Cantwell & Baker, 1980). In the cited study, 53 out of 100 children aged 2 to 13 years referred to a community speech and hearing clinic were found to suffer from emotional disorders. As with specific reading retardation, one can hypothesize that language disorders, common in the retarded, may be a contributing factor to the high rates of emotional disturbance in retarded children.

Family Pathology and Socioeconomic Factors

Family psychopathology, environmental deprivation, and stressful environments are of course important factors in the genesis of emotional disorders in all types of children. There is no clear-cut evidence that mentally retarded children are more susceptible to such factors than other children, but it can be assumed that the presence of cognitive handicaps may make it more difficult for retarded children to cope with a wide variety of environmental stresses (Phillips, 1967). It is also true that the presence of a mentally retarded child is in itself a stress on many family systems. In the sample of 60 mentally retarded and psychiatrically disturbed children described by Reid (1980), 61 of the family members of the 60 children were found to be suffering from mental disturbance. For almost one-third of the children there was a background of "scapegoating, ambivalent attitudes, gross disharmony and rejection by parents and siblings," (p. 289). On the other hand, Rutter concludes that the high rates of psychiatric disorder in retarded children cannot be explained by the fact they come from more disturbed homes than children of normal intelligence (Rutter, 1970). For example, mentally retarded children are not more likely to come from broken homes than children in the general population (Rutter, Tizard, & Whitmore, 1970). It is also probably true that the effects of a disturbed family situation may be overshadowed by the wide variety of other handicaps and stresses that face the retarded child during his or her development. In terms of intervention, of course, it is vital to carefully evaluate the family environment of a retarded child who is exhibiting emotional disturbance. Major interventions may be directed at the family situation with considerable improvement in the behavior of the child.

In summary, a variety of factors may and probably do influence the high rates of emotional disturbance among retarded children. Some of the different types of handicap and their influences on the genesis of psychiatric disorder are summarized in Figure 6-1. It should be noted that all the factors that are associated with psychiatric disorder also interact and overlap with each other. In other words, a child with mental retardation may also have a neuroepileptic condition, and/or language and educational handicaps making him or her even

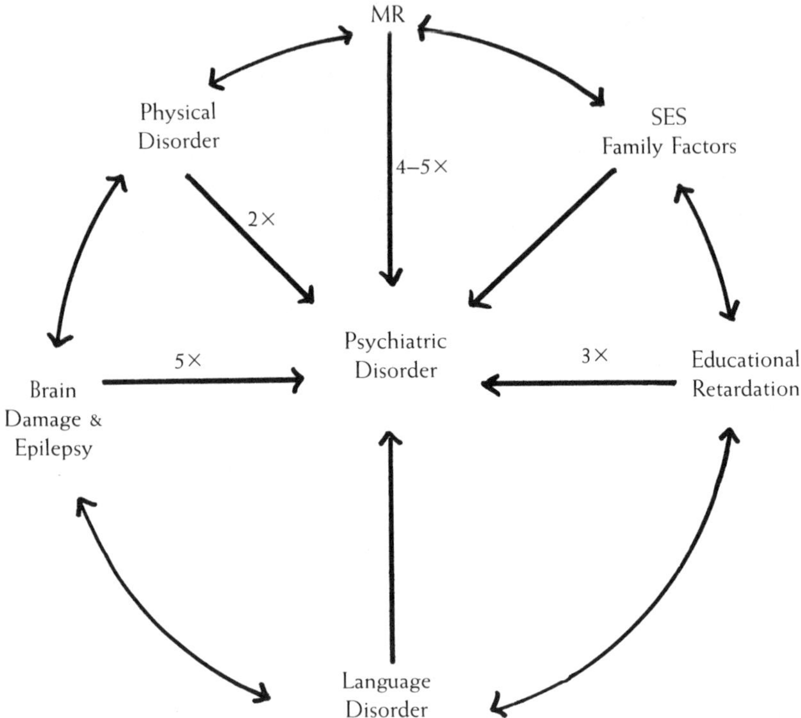

Fig. 6-1. Association of psychiatric disorder in children with other handicaps. Rates of psychiatric disorder shown as multiples of prevalence figures for normal or comparison population. [Data from Rutter, M, Graham, P, & Yule, W. (1970). *A neuropsychiatric study in childhood.* London: Spastics International Medical Publications and Heinmann; and from Rutter, M, Tizard, J, & Whitmore, K. (1970). *Education, health, and behavior.* London: Longmans.] Approximately 50 percent of language disordered children have associated psychiatric and behavioral disorders. [Data from Cantwell, DP, & Baker, L. (1980). Psychiatric and behavioral characteristics of children with communication disorders. *Journal of Pediatric Psychology, 5,* 161–178.]

more vulnerable to the emergence of a psychiatric disorder. Corbett has summarized the information in this area succinctly:

> There is ... a complex interaction between intellectual retardation and psychiatric disorder and only limited evidence of the relative importance of different mechanisms (Rutter, 1971). However, it seems that in the severely retarded child organic brain dysfunction and deviant temperamental attributes are the two most important factors. These also play a part in the mildly retarded child, but the adverse social consequences of educational failure, social rejection, general immaturity and language retardation are equally important. Institutional care and the side effects of drugs, for example, anticonvulsants, may be contributory factors and, as in any child, family and social pathology may be important. (Corbett, 1977b, p. 835)

CONCLUSIONS

This review of the association between mental retardation and psychiatric disorder has several implications for both the clinician and the researcher concerned with the mental health of retarded children.

Every mentally retarded child and adolescent undergoing a clinical evaluation should be carefully assessed for emotional and psychiatric disturbance. This review of epidemiological studies suggests that between 14 and 40 percent of the general population of the retarded may suffer from emotional disturbance. In spite of this high prevalence rate, screening for behavioral and emotional problems is often given insufficient emphasis by clinicians with primary care responsibility for the retarded. This may be particularly true for the "quietly disturbed" child or adolescent who exhibits a gradual decline in adaptation (as a result of depression, for example) without flagrant behavioral problems.

To facilitate the evaluation of psychiatric disturbance in the retarded, screening and diagnostic tools must be developed. Existing instruments must be tested on retarded populations and modified as needed. A significant amount of clinical research is now under way to develop more reliable diagnostic instruments for children and adolescents. One example is the development of structured and semistructured psychiatric interviews (Herjanic & Campbell, 1977; Orvaschel, Puig-Antich, Chambers, Tabrizi, & Johnson 1982). Research is needed to test the applicability of these interviews to retarded populations. Clinical rating scales and similar instruments should also prove to be very useful in the assessment of emotional disturbance in the retarded. Kazdin, Matson, and Senatore (1983) are now developing a screening instrument to be used with retarded adults. As mentioned previously, Nihira and colleagues have developed and extensively researched a scale to assess adaptive behavior in the retarded (Nihira et al., 1974). Rating scales developed for the general population may also be applicable to retarded populations (Kazdin et al., 1983). Beck, Carlson, Russell, and Brownfield (1982) found the Beck depression inventory to be useful and reliable in detecting depression in a group of adolescents, some of whom were mildly retarded. The unfortunate fact is that most research in this area excludes retarded children and adolescents from experimental samples, making it difficult to determine the clinical utility of these diagnostic instruments in retarded populations. Assessment research with children and adolescents must be expanded to include carefully described populations of the intellectually handicapped.

The use of standard and reliable diagnostic criteria should be encouraged in clinical practice and required by extramural funding agencies supporting research with retarded populations. This review emphasizes that the use of widely discrepant diagnostic criteria has made it very difficult to compare findings from different research projects. An important step towards greater diagnostic reliability has been the publication of DSM-III (APA, 1980). Although the diagnostic criteria have been criticized, they have at least provided a framework for research that can be applied across different projects. An important strength of DSM-III is its multiaxial structure. As discussed previously, retarded children often present with multiple behavioral and medical problems, which can be best diagnosed using a multiaxial framework. Discussions are now underway with the goal of revising DSM-III. One consideration has been to move the Mental Retardation category from Axis I to Axis II (Spitzer, 1983). This should encourage clinicians to more carefully consider the presence of more acute syndromes (Axis I) in children with developmental disorders (Axis II).

Effective treatment methods for the "dual diagnosis" child must be developed. As is true with diagnostic research, retarded populations tend to be excluded from treatment research. As a result, clinicians have very few guidelines in applying treatment strategies to retarded children and adolescents who are also psychiatrically disturbed. On the other hand, if a psychiatric disorder has been clearly identified in a retarded child, there is little reason not to apply the treatment regimens that have been proven effective in the general population of children. Yet, this is often not done. For example, mildly retarded children and adolescents may not be offered psychotherapy because it is felt they are not "verbal" enough. Hyperactive retarded children, particularly in institutions, are often treated with antipsychotic medications such as Mellaril® (Sandoz) and Thorazine® (Smith Kline & French), and relatively infrequently with stimulants (Lipman, DiMascio, Reatig, & Kirson, 1978). This occurs in spite of some evidence that the antipsychotics may impair cognitive performance in these children (Aman, 1978). If we do not have research that suggests we should treat retarded children differently, we should at least apply the diagnostic and treatment methodologies proven effective with nonhandicapped children.

Finally, it is clear from this review that mentally retarded persons are at risk for a wide variety of emotional and behavioral disorders. The artificial categorization of individuals as mentally retarded or mentally ill all too often leads to inadequate and incomplete care. Improved training of primary care providers as well as specialists in both fields is a necessity. This must be coupled with expanded clinical research programs that cross disciplinary lines. With an improved knowledge base from these efforts we may be better able to meet the many needs of these underserved and understudied young people.

REFERENCES

Aman, MD. (1978). Drugs, learning and the psychotherapies. In JS Werry (Ed.), *Pediatric psychopharmacology: The use of behavior modifying drugs in children* (pp. 79–108). New York: Brunner/Mazel

American Psychiatric Association. (1980). *Diagnostic and statistical manual of mental disorders* (3rd ed.). Washington, DC: American Psychiatric Association

Baumeister, AA, & MacLean, WE, Jr. (1979). Brain damage and mental retardation. In NR Ellis (Ed.), *Handbook of mental deficiency* (2nd ed.). Hillsdale, NJ: Erlbaum

Beck, D, Carlson, G, Russell, A, & Brownfield, F. (1982, October 22nd). *Use of the Beck Depression Inventory in developmentally disabled adolescents.* Paper presented at the American Academy of Child Psychiatry, Washington, DC

Beier, DC. (1964). Behavioral disturbances in the mentally retarded. In HA Stevens, & R Heber (Eds.), *Mental retardation.* Chicago: University of Chicago Press

Berger, M, Yule, W, & Rutter, M. (1975). Attainment and adjustment in two geographical areas: II. The prevalence of specific reading retardation. *British Journal of Psychiatry, 126,* 510–519

Birch, HG, Richardson, SA, Baird, D, Horobin, G, & Allsley, R. (1970). *Mental subnormality in the community: A clinical and epidemiological study.* Baltimore, MD: Williams and Wilkins

Cantwell, DP, & Baker, L. (1980). Psychiatric and behavioral characteristics of children with communication disorders. *Journal of Pediatric Psychology, 5,* 161–178

Chess, S. (1977). Evolution of behavior disorder in a group of mentally retarded children. *Journal of the American Academy of Child Psychiatry, 16,* 5–18

Chess, S. (1970). Emotional problems in mentally retarded children. In FJ Menolascino (Ed.), *Psychiatric approaches to mental retardation.* New York: Basic Books

Chess, S, & Hassibi, M. (1970). Behavior deviations in mentally retarded children. *Journal of the American Academy of Child Psychiatry, 9,* 282–297

Clarke, AM, & Clarke, AD. (1975). *Mental deficiency: The changing outlook* (3rd ed.). New York: The Free Press

Corbett, JA. (1977b). Mental retardation—psychiatric aspects. In M Rutter, & L Hersov (Eds.), *Child psychiatry: Modern approaches.* Oxford: Blackwell Scientific Publications

Corbett, JA. (1977a). Populations studies of mental retardation. In PJ Graham (Ed.), *Epidemiological approaches in child psychiatry.* London: Academic Press

Corbett, JA, Harris, E, & Robinson, R. (1975). Epilepsy. In J Wortis (Ed.), *Mental retardation and developmental disabilities.* (Vol. 7). New York: Brunner/Mazel

Curry, JF, & Thompson, RJ. (1979). The utility of behavior checklist ratings in differentiating developmentally disabled from psychiatrically referred children. *Journal of Pediatric Psychology, 4,* 345–352

Curry, JF, & Thompson, RJ. (1982). Patterns of behavioral disturbance in developmentally disabled children: A replicated cluster analysis. *Journal of Pediatric Psychology, 7,* 61–73

Cushna, B, Szymanski, LS, & Tanguay, PE. (1980). Professional roles and unmet manpower needs. In LS Szymanski, & PE Tanguay, (Eds.), *Emotional disorders of mentally retarded persons.* Baltimore, MD: University Park Press

Eaton, LF, & Menolascino, FJ. (1982). Psychiatric disorders in the mentally retarded: Types, problems and challenges. *American Journal of Psychiatry, 139,* 1297–1303

Eyman, RK, & Call, T. (1977). Maladaptive behavior and community placement of mentally retarded persons. *American Journal of Mental Deficiency, 82,* 137–144

Gualtieri, CT. (1979). Psychiatry's disinterest in mental retardation. *Psychiatric Opinion, May,* 26–30

Herjanic, B, & Campbell, W. (1977). Differentiating psychiatrically disturbed children on the basis of a structured interview. *Journal of Abnormal Child Psychology, 5,* 127–134

Jacobson, JW. (1982). Problem behavior and psychiatric impairment within a developmentally disabled population: Behavior frequency. *Applied Research in Mental Retardation, 3,* 121–139

Janicki, MP, & Jacobson, JW. (1979). *New York's Needs Assessment and developmental disabilities: Preliminary report* (technical monograph #78-10). Albany, NY: OMRDD

Janicki, MP, & Jacobson, JW. (1982). The character of developmental disabilities in New York State. *International Journal of Rehabilitation Research, 5,*

Kazdin, AE, Matson, JL, & Senatore, V. (1983). Assessment of depression in mentally retarded adults. *American Journal of Psychiatry, 140,* 1040–1043

Koller, H, Richardson, SA, Katz, M, & McLaren, J. (1982). Behavior disturbance in childhood and the early adult years in populations who were and were not mentally retarded. *Journal of Preventive Psychiatry, 1,* 453–468

Koller, H, Richardson, SW, Katz, M, & McLaren, J. (1983). Behavior disturbance since childhood among a 5-year birth cohort of all mentally retarded young adults in a city. *American Journal of Mental Deficiency, 87,* 386–395

Lipman, RS, DiMascio, A, Reatig, N, & Kirson, T. (1978). Psychotropic drugs and mentally retarded children. In MA Lipton, A DiMascio, & KF Killam (Eds.), *Psychopharmacology: A generation of progress.* New York: Raven Press

Matson, JL, & Barrett, RP. (1982). *Psychopathology in the mentally retarded.* New York: Grune & Stratton

Menolascino, FJ. (1969). Emotional disturbances in mentally retarded children. *American Journal of Psychiatry, 126,* 168–179

Menolascino, FJ. (1970). The research challenge of delineating psychiatric syndromes in mental retardation. In FJ Menolascino (Ed.), *Psychiatric approaches to mental retardation.* New York: Basic Books

Mercer, JR. (1973). *Labeling the mentally retarded: Clinical and social systems perspectives on mental retardation.* Berkeley, CA: University of California

Nihira, K, Foster, R, Shellhass, M, & Leland, H. (1974). *Adaptive Behavior Scale.* Washington, DC: American Association on Mental Deficiency

Orvaschel, H, Puig-Antich, J, Chambers, W, Tabrizi, M, & Johnson, R. (1982). Retrospective assessment of prepubertal major depression with the kiddie-SADS-E. *Journal of the American Academy of Child Psychiatry, 21,* 392–397

Phillips, I. (1967). Psychopathology and mental retardation. *American Journal of Psychiatry, 124,* 29–35

Phillips, I, & Williams, N. (1975). Psychopathology and mental retardation: A study of 100 mentally retarded children: I. Psychopathology. *American Journal of Psychiatry, 132,* 1265–1271

Reid, AH. (1980). Psychiatric disorders in mentally handicapped children: A clinical and follow-up study. *Journal of Mental Deficiency Research, 24,* 287–298

Reiss, S. (1982). Psychopathology and mental retardation: Survey of a developmental disabilities mental health program. *Mental Retardation, 20,* 128–132

Reiss, S, Levitan, GW, & Szyszko, J. (1982). Emotional disturbance and mental retardation: Diagnostic overshadowing. *American Journal of Mental Deficiency, 86,* 567–574

Reiss, S, & Szyszko, J. (1983). Diagnostic overshadowing and professional experience with retarded people. *American Journal of Mental Dificiency, 87,* 396-402

Richardson, SA. (1978). Careers of mentally retarded young persons: Services, jobs, and interpersonal relations. *American Journal of Mental Deficiency, 82,* 349–358

Richardson, SA. (1980). Growing up as a mentally subnormal young person: A follow-up study. In SA Mednick, & AE Baert (Eds.), *An empirical basis for primary prevention: Prospective longitudinal research in Europe.* Oxford: Oxford University Press

Richardson, SA, Koller, H, Katz, J, & McLaren, J. (unpublished manuscript). *Adolescents with mental handicaps: An epidemiological perspective*

Russell, AT, Cantwell, DP, & Mattison, R. (1979). A comparison of DSM II and DSM III in the diagnosis of childhood psychiatric disorders: III. Multiaxial features. *Archives of General Psychiatry, 36,* 1223–1226

Rutter, M. (1970). Psychiatry. In J Wortis (Ed.), *Mental retardation: An annual review* (Vol. 3). New York: Grune & Stratton

Rutter, M, Graham P, & Yule, W. (1970) *A neuropsychiatric study in childhood.* London: Spastics International Medical Publications and Heinemann

Rutter, M, & Shaffer, D. (1980). DSM III: A step forward or back in terms of the classification of child psychiatric disorders. *Journal of the American Academy of Child Psychiatry, 19,* 371–394

Rutter, M, Shaffer, D, & Shepherd, M. (1975). *A multiaxial classification of child psychiatric disorders*. Geneva: WHO; London: Blackwell Scientific Publications

Rutter, M, Tizard, J, & Whitmore, K. (Eds.). (1970). *Education health and behavior.* London: Longmans

Rutter, M, Tizard, J, Yule, W, Graham, P, & Whitmore, K. (1976). Research report: Isle of Wight studies, 1964–74. *Psychological Medicine, 6,* 313–332

Sovner, R, & Hurley, AD. (1983). Do the mentally retarded suffer from affective illness? *Archives of General Psychiatry, 40,* 61–67

Spitzer, RL, Chairperson. (1983). Work group to revise DSM III (personal communication)

Stein, Z, & Susser, M. (1970). Mutability of intelligence and epidemiology of mild mental retardation. *Review of Educational Research, 40* (1)

Szymanski, LS. (1977). Psychiatric diagnostic evaluation of mentally retarded individuals. *Journal of the American Academy of Child Psychiatry, 16,* 67–87

Szymanski, LS. (1980). Psychiatric diagnosis of retarded persons. In LS Szymanski, & PE Tanguay, (Eds.), *Emotional disorders of mentally retarded persons.* Baltimore, MD: University Park Press

Szymanski, LS, & Tanguay, PE. (Eds.). (1980). *Emotional disorders of mentally retarded persons.* Baltimore, MD: University Park Press

Tarjan, G, Tizard, J, Rutter, M, Begab, M, Brooke, EM, De La Cruz, F, Lin, T-Y, Montenegro, H, Strotzka, H, & Sartorius, W. (1972). Classification and mental retardation: Issues arising in the fifth W.H.O. seminar on psychiatric diagnosis, classification, and statistics. *American Journal of Psychiatry, 128*(Suppl.), 34–45

Tarjan, G, Wright, SW, Eyman, RK, & Keeran, CV. (1973). Natural history of mental retardation: Some aspects of epidemiology. *American Journal of Mental Deficiency, 77,* 369–379

Webster, TG. (1970). Unique aspects of emotional development in mentally retarded individuals. In FJ Menolascino (Ed.), *Psychiatric approaches to mental retardation.* New York: Basic Books

Zigler, E. (1967). Familial mental retardation: A continuing dilemma. *Science, 155,* 292–298

Judy A. Ungerer

7

The Autistic Child

Mental retardation in children often coexists with other developmental disabilities. Among the most severe of the associated disorders is infantile autism, a form of psychosis appearing in children before 30 months of age. The incidence of infantile autism is approximately 4.9 per 10,000 (Wing & Gould, 1979), and the majority of autistic children are also mentally retarded. About 70 to 80 percent of autistic children achieve IQ scores on standardized tests in the mentally retarded range (DeMyer, Barton, Alpern, Kimberlin, Allen, Yang, & Steele, 1974; Wing & Gould, 1979). The frequent association of infantile autism and mental retardation often leads to diagnostic confusion between the groups, particularly at the younger ages. However, infantile autism is considered to be a unique disorder (APA, 1980), and characteristics can be identified which differentiate autistic children from their mentally retarded peers. In general, autistic children show different patterns of dysfunction across skills than mentally retarded children, and the severity of their disabilities is usually greater. Nevertheless, considerable overlap in symptomatology between autistic and mentally retarded children does occur, and differential diagnosis is sometimes difficult.

Several attempts have been made to identify the primary behavioral characteristics of infantile autism since Kanner first described the syndrome in 1943 (Kanner, 1943; Ritvo & Freeman, 1978; Rutter, 1978; Schopler, Reichler, DeVellis, & Daly, 1980). Although consensus among the approaches is not complete, two features have emerged consistently as critical for differentiating infantile autism from other related conditions. These are profound impairments

CHILDREN WITH EMOTIONAL DISORDERS AND DEVELOPMENTAL DISABILITIES ISBN 0–8089–1700–5

of social relatedness and communicative speech (De-Myer, Hingtgen, & Jackson, 1981). Autistic children have always been considered socially aloof and incapable of forming normal attachments and social relationships. Originally, this deficiency was attributed to inadequate parenting (Bettelheim, 1967), but research has failed to support this relation. The parents of autistic children do not demonstrate more psychopathology than parents of children having clear organic disorders with or without psychosis, and their parenting skills have not been shown to be deficient (McAdoo & DeMyer, 1978). With respect to communicative speech, the language development of autistic children has been shown to be deviant, with specific deficits in comprehension and the social usage of language (Tager-Flusberg, 1981). More recent work has emphasized that the language disorder may be only one aspect of a more general cognitive deficit that also incorporates sequencing, abstraction, and coding skills (Rutter, 1978).

Most descriptions of infantile autism include impaired social and language development as primary features in conjunction with a third characteristic, atypical responses to objects. Onset of symptoms must occur before 30 months of age in order to differentiate infantile autism from the later occurring psychoses of childhood, like schizophrenia. Stated formally in the third edition of the *Diagnostic and Statistical Manual* (DSM-III) of the American Psychiatric Association (1980), the criteria for infantile autism are onset before 30 months of age; pervasive lack of responsiveness to other people; gross deficits in language development; if speech is present, peculiar speech patterns such as immediate and delayed echolalia, metaphorical language, or pronominal reversal; bizarre responses to various aspects of the environment such as resistance to change, peculiar interest in or attachments to animate or inanimate objects; and no evidence of delusions, hallucinations, loosening of associations, and incoherence as in schizophrenia.

The DSM-III criteria identify the primary deficits in infantile autism, but they are stated too generally to reflect the current level of knowledge of the autistic child's disorders. More detailed information is essential, particularly because autistic children are a heterogeneous group and share symptoms with other childhood disorders, like mental retardation and aphasia. To understand the uniqueness of infantile autism, it is necessary to specify how autistic children differ from these other diagnostic groups. To understand the diversity of the disorder, it is essential to have an appreciation of the range of symptom expression within the autistic group.

In this chapter literature will be surveyed contrasting the cognitive, language, and social functioning of autistic children with that of mentally retarded and aphasic children. These comparison groups were selected because their symptoms overlap with those of the autistic child, and diagnostic confusion among these groups is not uncommon. Only studies in which a reasonable attempt has been made to match autistic and comparison groups on both mental and chronological age will be cited, because these variables are known to influence symptom expression in all three groups. The symptoms manifested by young autistic children are often very different from those seen in older age groups, although the underlying pathology remains unchanged. The interrelationship between social and cognitive/language functioning within the autistic group also will be explored. Although social and cognitive/language dysfunctions have long been recognized as essential features of the autistic syndrome, there is little understanding of the relation between these different aspects of the disorder. An understanding of the relation between these functions may help identify the primary etiology of the disorder and clarify the role of social and cognitive development in the genesis of autistic symptoms. Finally, the diversity of symptom expression within the autistic group will be discussed with particular emphasis on the effects of differences in mental age. The majority of autistic children are also mentally retarded, and the degree of retardation has a clear influence on both the type and severity of presenting symptoms.

DEFICIENCIES IN COGNITION AND LANGUAGE

Performance on Standardized Tests

The cognitive and language skills of autistic children have frequently been assessed using standardized IQ tests like the Stanford-Binet, Merrill-Palmer, and Wechsler scales. IQ scores have been shown to be reliable indices of current functioning in autistic children as well as good predictors of later social and intellectual status. Lockyer and Rutter (1969, 1970) conducted a longitudinal followup of 63 children with a diagnosis of infantile psychosis seen at the Maudsley Hospital between 1950 and 1958. The stability in IQ of this group from the initial to the follow-up assessment 5 to 15 years later was comparable to that of 63 control children with nonpsychotic disorders matched for age, sex, IQ, and year of attendance at the same clinic. The correlation in these groups between initial IQ and the Wechsler Full Scale IQ at follow-up was .63 for the psychotic children and .77 for the controls. However, the relation between verbal and nonverbal performance skills was different within each group. For the psychotic children, verbal skills assessed by the Peabody Picture Vocabulary Test (PPVT) were inferior to nonverbal skills measured by the Wechsler Performance IQ. In the control group, scores on verbal and nonverbal assessments were not significantly different. Gillies (1965) reported similar findings using the Seguin Formboard as a measure of nonverbal performance IQ. For both psychotic children and a mentally subnormal control group, verbal scores were lower than nonverbal scores, but the differences in performance were greater in the psychotic group.

The pattern of subscale scores within the Wechsler Verbal and Performance scales also has been shown to differentiate psychotic and control groups matched on mental and chronological age. On the Verbal scales, psychotic children in the Lockyer and Rutter (1970) study performed significantly better on the Digit Span scale, which assesses attention and short-term memory, while the performance of the control children across scales showed little variation. In addition, while Digit Span was the highest scale in the psychotic group, it was the second lowest scale for the controls. Performance on the Comprehension scale, which assesses verbal reasoning, was highest for the control group but lowest for the psychotic children.

The psychotic and control children also showed different patterns of scores on the Wechsler Performance subscales (Lockyer & Rutter, 1970). The psychotic children were characterized by relatively good performance on the Object Assembly and Block Design scales, which measure perceptual organization. In contrast, the most notable feature of the control group's performance was relatively poor scores on the Digit Symbol/Coding and Block Design scales. Results consistent with these findings have been reported by Wolf, Wenar, and Ruttenberg (1972) and Tymchuk, Simmons, and Neafsey (1977). These studies also emphasized the greater variability in scale scores found among psychotic children. Significant differences between scale scores were consistently found in the psychotic groups, while the performance of mental and chronological age-matched control groups was more uniform. The skills of the psychotic children appeared fragmented and compartmentalized when compared to the more even functioning of the nonpsychotic control groups.

The standardized test performance of autistic children also has been compared to that of children with developmental receptive language disorders (Bartak, Rutter, & Cox, 1975) to determine which aspects of the autistic child's deviant functioning are unique to autism and cannot be accounted for solely by impaired language skills. These comparisons showed that the differences between autistic and language-disordered groups were similar to those found with predominantly subnormal children matched for mental and chronological age. The autistic children demonstrated a greater disparity between their Wechsler Verbal and Performance IQs and greater variability in scores on the Verbal scales than the children with developmental receptive language disorders. The language-disordered children performed better than the autistic group on three of the Verbal scales: Comprehension, Similarities, and Vocabulary. On the Performance subscales, there were no significant differences between the groups in individual scale scores and in the pattern of performance across scales. Both groups performed best on the Block Design, Picture Completion, and Object Assembly scales, and for the autistic children only, scores on the Block Design scale were significantly better than on all other Performance scales.

The pattern of Wechsler scale scores found among autistic children indicates that they have very poor verbal skills and relatively good spatial–performance, perceptual organization, and attention/short-term memory skills. Compared to mentally retarded children of similar chronological and mental age, autistic children have superior perceptual organization skills but inferior verbal skills. Their performance skills are similar to those found in children with developmental language disorders, but their verbal skills are inferior even to this severely language-delayed group.

The relatively good performance skills of autistic children have also been observed in tests of sensorimotor development. Sigman and Ungerer (1984b) used the Casati-Lezine Scales (1968) to compare the sensorimotor performance of autistic and mentally retarded children matched on mental and chronological age. No significant differences between the groups were found on any of the sensorimotor scales, which included tasks assessing object permanence, the use of objects as tools for manipulating other objects, and the ability to separate and integrate components of an object. However, the language skills of the autistic children were significantly poorer than those of the mentally retarded group, a finding consistent with the pattern of verbal and performance scores found on the Wechsler Scales.

Language Development

The significance of the verbal dysfunction in autistic children has prompted considerable investigation of language development in this group. Of interest was determining which aspects of language were uniquely disordered in autistic children and whether the autistic child's primary dysfunction was limited to language or included more general cognitive skills. When the language development of autistic children was compared to that of mentally retarded children, both groups appeared delayed, but the nature of the delay was different in each group. In mentally retarded children, all language functions were delayed to a similar extent, and they tended to follow the same developmental sequence observed in normal children, albeit at a slower rate. In contrast, language development in autistic children was more uneven, and deviant rather than merely delayed language functions were commonly observed even in the older, most linguistically sophisticated children. However, not all language functions were considered deviant or delayed beyond what would be expected from the autistic child's generally retarded development.

The phonologic development of autistic and mentally retarded children was similar, showing the same frequency distribution of phonemes and phonologic errors (Tager-Flusberg, 1981). Syntactic or grammatical development also was similar in autistic and mentally retarded groups. Pierce and Bartolucci (1977) compared the syntactic competence of autistic and mentally retarded children matched on chronological age and on a nonverbal measure of mental age, the Leiter Scales. The two groups showed comparable development when the grammatical complexity of their speech was assessed using Lee's Developmental Sentence Scoring and a Chomskian transformational grammar analysis of speech. The only difference between the groups was in the lower frequency with which a single, complex transformation was used by the autistic children. An alternate means of assessing grammatical competence yielded results that were interpreted to be consistent with these findings. Bartolucci, Pierce, and Steiner (1980) compared the use of 14 grammatical morphemes in autistic and mentally retarded children matched on nonverbal mental age and IQ. Although the facility with which different morphemes were used varied between the groups, they concluded that the results were attributable not to differences in grammatical competence but rather to the inability of autistic children to comprehend the meaning conveyed by certain grammatical forms. The autistic children had difficulty using verb tense markers and articles, which suggested a deficiency in the understanding of deictic categories. Deictic terms like *this* and *that*, *here* and *there*, or *yesterday* and *tomorrow* may be difficult for autistic children because their meanings shift as a function of space, time, or person, and often depend on the relationship between the speaker and listener. Thus, their meanings are abstract concepts that often entail the understanding of social relationships.

The grammatical development of autistic children also has been shown to be comparable to that of children with a developmental receptive language disorder, or dysphasia (Bartak et al., 1975). Autistic children with a nonverbal IQ in the borderline or normal range (IQ $\geq$ 70) showed syntactic development similar to dysphasic children in a comparable mental age and IQ range. The groups did not differ in grammatical complexity, mean length of utterance, or in age of acquisition of both single word and phrase speech. A follow-up analysis of the same children two years later continued to show no significant differences between the autistic and dysphasic groups. The children were comparable in their use of morphologic, phrase structure, and transformational rules (Cantwell, Baker, & Rutter, 1978).

In contrast to the finding of similarities in syntactic and phonologic development, several studies have reported differences in the semantic competence of autistic and mentally retarded children. As noted above, autistic children have difficulty using deictic terms because their meanings are abstract and depend, for example, on understanding the relationship of the speaker and listener to each other and to points in time and space. The autistic children's difficulty with deixis suggests an underlying cognitive deficiency, since their failure to use specific language terms derives from a difficulty in understanding the concepts they represent. Other evidence supporting semantic deficiencies in autistic children comes from the experimental work of Hermelin and O'Connor (1970). These researchers noted that when autistic children were given lists of words to remember from different categories, they failed to use the meaning of the words to assist recall. Autistic children reordered words into related clusters in recall significantly less often than mentally retarded children of comparable mental age. The semantic deficiencies reported for autistic children appear to be associated with cognitive impairments in the ability to form higher level abstractions and to appreciate complex relationships among objects and people. Thus, the autistic child's language deficits may derive from impairments that extend beyond language to more general cognitive skills.

The final aspect of language that has been investigated in autistic children is pragmatics, the development of the communicative use of language. In this domain, as in semantic development, autistic children show deficiencies when compared to mentally retarded children of comparable mental and chronological age. Cunningham (1968) compared language samples from autistic and mentally retarded children matched on mental and chronological age. The groups were comparable in terms of the number of complete grammatical sentences produced and the mean number of words per sentence, but differed in their pragmatic use of language. The autistic children used more egocentric or noncommunicative speech (echolalia, repetition of self, thinking aloud) and more inappropriate or purposeless remarks than the mentally retarded children. The autistic children also volunteered information less and used less socialized speech. Similar results were reported when autistic children were compared to children with developmental receptive language disorders (Bartak et al., 1975; Cantwell et al., 1978). These studies also noted that autistics were less able than dysphasics to use complex gestures to communicate, for example, to use gestures to describe the functions of objects (Bartak et al., 1975; Tubbs, 1966). The autistic child's impoverished use of communicative gestures extends to the production of functional and symbolic play gestures in noncommunicative contexts (Riguet, Taylor, Benaroya, & Klein, 1981; Wing, Gould, Yeates, & Brierley, 1977). Autistic children typically show less spontaneous functional and symbolic object use in play than mentally retarded children of comparable mental and chronological age (Sigman & Ungerer, 1984b).

In summary, comparisons of language skills in autistic, mentally retarded, and dysphasic children are consistent in showing similar developmental achievements in the domains of syntax and phonology. However, for those language skills that depend on general cognitive achievements for their acquisition, autistic children are clearly inferior. Specifically, they show impairments in semantic and pragmatic development, and these deficiencies extend to the use of gesture in both communicative and play contexts. These results imply that the language impairment in autistic children derives from a more general cognitive deficit affecting abstraction and symbolization skills. In addition, it is important to note that many of the cognitive/language skills that are impaired in autistic children involve a social component. The use of deictic categories requires an understanding of speaker–listener relationships and of the relations among people, objects, and events in time and space. The pragmatic use of language entails communicative interaction that is necessarily social, while functional and symbolic play gestures are defined by social conventions and learned by observation and interaction with others. Thus, the language deficiencies of autistic children reflect impairments in both cognitive and social development that are more severe than those found in mentally retarded or dysphasic groups.

DEFICIENCIES IN SOCIAL DEVELOPMENT

Impaired social development has always been a primary characteristic of autistic children, who typically are described as socially aloof and incapable of forming normal attachments and social relationships. Although disturbances of social functioning are found in many clinical groups, the severity and pervasiveness of social impairment is generally greater in autistic children. Rutter and Lockyer (1967) compared the social functioning of psychotic children with a nonpsychotic control group matched on mental and chronological age, sex, and year of attendance at the same clinic. Although nearly all children in both groups showed disturbed interpersonal relationships, the nature of the disturbance was different in the psychotic group. Most of the psychotic children, but only a very few of the control children showed "autism," which was defined as appearing markedly aloof and distant, showing an apparent lack of interest in other people, having little variation in facial expression, rarely exhibiting feelings or appreciating humor, and failing to show sympathy or empathy for other people. Wing (1978) also noted differences in social behavior between psychotic and nonpsychotic children of comparable mental age. She conducted an epidemiological survey in the London borough of Camberwell of all children under 15 years of age with a diagnosis of psychosis or severe mental retardation. Comparing groups of children with mental ages less than 20 months, she found that the psychotic children were less likely to use facial gestures, pointing, and vocalizations to communicate with others than the mentally retarded children. In addition, elaborate routines were observed only in the psychotic group and were generally restricted to those children with mental ages greater than 20 months.

RELATION BETWEEN SOCIAL AND COGNITIVE/LANGUAGE FUNCTIONS

Social and cognitive/language dysfunctions are essential features of the autistic syndrome, but there is little understanding of the relation between these two aspects of the disorder. When autism was originally described, its etiology was considered psychogenic, and deviant social development was emphasized as the primary deficit. Problems in language development were considered to be one result of the autistic child's inability to form normal social relationships. As the popularity of the psychogenic theory waned, however, the emphasis switched. Cognitive/language problems became the primary focus of research, and deviant social development was considered secondary to the cognitive and communicative problems. Rutter (1968), in particular, has presented evidence supporting this latter approach. For example, he noted that the social behavior of autistic children tended to be more malleable than their level of cognitive functioning. Social withdrawal in autistic children generally lessened considerably with age, while cognitive functioning as measured by IQ was as stable as in any other group. In addition, although social withdrawal and language impairment tended to improve or deteriorate together, there were cases in the Maudsley Hospital follow-up study demonstrating marked improvements in social relatedness with no change in speech (Rutter & Bartak, 1971). Finally, IQ and degree of language impairment were the best predictors of the autistic child's intellectual, social, and behavioral adjustment in adolescence and adult life, while social withdrawal was only weakly associated with outcome.

Although Rutter's evidence supporting the primacy of the cognitive/language dysfunction in autistic children appears strong, there are two issues that need to be addressed. First, the social relatedness of autistic children may improve with age, but their social adjustment is in many ways still profoundly impaired. As adolescents and adults they have been described as lacking empathy for other people and as failing to perceive social cues. Even the most intellectually competent autistic children fail to establish normal social relationships (Eisenberg, 1956; Kanner, Rodriguez, & Ashenden, 1972). Given the changes in social behavior observed in autistic children and their marked social impairment even in adulthood, it is possible that the degree of social dysfunction in autism remains constant, while the specific manifestations of the dysfunction vary with age. However, until measures of social functioning are developed that, like the IQ, have validity across a broad age range, meaningful comparisons of the degree of impairment of cognitive and social development cannot be made.

The second issue to be addressed concerns the poor ability of early social behavior to predict later development. Rutter (1968) found social withdrawal to be a poor predictor of outcome, and it is known that the occurrence of actual physical withdrawal does not differentiate psychotic and retarded children of matched mental and chronological age (Rutter & Lockyer, 1967). However, other forms of social behavior, like attachment to the caregiver, may be more closely linked to outcome in psychotic groups. Further research is necessary to establish the predictive significance of these alternate social behaviors.

Rutter's own work suggests a role for social behavior in the prediction of outcome since social skills are necessarily involved in the communicative use of language. Rutter and Bartak (1971) identified language as one of the best predictors of outcome in psychotic children, and several other investigators have shown specifically that the *communicative* use of language is related to the later development of cognitive, language, and social skills (DeMyer, Barton, DeMyer, Norton, Allen, & Steele, 1973; Eisenberg, 1956; Lotter, 1974). Thus, social behavior as it relates to the communicative use of language may be a useful predictor of outcome in psychotic children.

Studies directly assessing the relation between social and cognitive/language development in autistic children are scarce, but the results of those available do suggest an interdependence between the domains. A few training studies have noted changes in social behavior occurring in conjunction with improvements in specifically trained cognitive and language skills. Casey (1978) attempted to teach manual signs and verbalizations to four children in classroom and home-based teaching programs. The clearest results of the intervention were an increase in the number of solicited verbal responses produced by the children and in the appropriateness of their interaction with teachers and other pupils, for example, following directions and cooperative play. In addition, decreases in inappropriate behaviors like self-stimulatory and ritualistic body movements, social withdrawal, and disruptive behavior were noted. Similarly, Churchill (1969) reported improved social relatedness in autistic children participating in behavior modification skill training programs. The children were observed to become more affectionate and attached to the adults working with them. It is probably inaccurrate to assume that the changes in social behavior observed in these studies were completely fortuitous, since some training of social behaviors certainly occurs as a function of maintaining attention and cooperation in teaching interactions. In addition, language training by necessity strengthens social relatedness since any use of language entails communication and interaction with others. However, the changes in social behavior appeared to generalize beyond the specific training tasks and seemed to reflect a substantive change in social functioning, which was associated with improved cognitive and language skills.

Relations between social and cognitive/language functioning in psychotic children have also been reported by Wing and Gould (1979). Comparing high- and low-functioning psychotic children, they found that the degree of social withdrawal was less in children with better intellectual skills. However, even the most competent children showed some social impairment. They initiated social contact less and had more inappropriate eye contact like staring at others and making eye contact at unusual times than did nonpsychotic children of comparable mental age. Finally, McHale, Simeonsson, Marcus, and Oller (1980) found positive correlations between social and symbolic levels of communication and standardized tests of social and cognitive functioning for 11 autistic children attending special education classes. In this group, high scores on the Vineland Scale were associated with the ability to use words symbolically and to communicate with another person within the context of a social interaction. IQ scores also were significantly correlated with these same skills.

The studies reported above indicate that social and cognitive/language functions are related in autistic children, but the nature of this relationship may be different from that found in mentally retarded or normal children of comparable mental age. Sigman and Ungerer (1984a) reported a positive association in autistic children between attachment to the primary caregiver and symbolic play skills. Specifically, autistic children who sought to be close to their mothers following a brief separation were able to treat dolls in play as if they were the agents of their own actions, for example, putting a spoon in a doll's hand as if it could feed itself. In contrast, mentally retarded and normal children do not require this sophisticated level of representation to form attachments. Literature on the development of attachments in normal children indicates that the most intense responses to separation from the primary caregiver occur at 12 months of age, several months before the emergence of symbolic play.

Standardized tests also reveal differences in the relation between social and cognitive/language skills in autistic and retarded groups. Lockyer and Rutter (1970) reported that the Vineland Social Maturity Scale scores of psychotic children were higher than their Peabody Picture Vocabulary Test scores but lower than their Wechsler Performance IQs. In contrast, mentally retarded children had their highest scores on the Vineland Scale. Wechsler Performance IQs for the retarded children were significantly lower than the Vineland Social Quotients but no different from scores on the PPVT.

In summary, attempts to establish either social or cognitive/language dysfunctions as the primary disability in infantile autism are open to question. Progress in this area has been hindered by the absence of well-standardized measures of social development that have validity across a broad age range. The available research does not provide strong support for the primacy of either function, but rather suggests a significant degree of interdependence between the social and cognitive/language domains. Furthermore, the relation between social and cognitive/language development in autistic children appears to differ from that found in either normal or mentally retarded children of comparable mental age.

EFFECTS OF MENTAL RETARDATION ON SYMPTOMATOLOGY AND PROGNOSIS IN AUTISTIC CHILDREN

Infantile autism is considered to be a unique psychiatric disorder. However, there is considerable variability among autistic children in the type and severity of their presenting symptoms. One of the strongest influences on symptom expression within the autistic group is the degree of associated mental retardation. Psychological testing indicates that 70 to 80 percent of autistic children are mentally retarded (DeMyer et al., 1974), with the majority scoring in the moderate to severe ranges of mental retardation (IQ 20 to 50). Despite the frequency with which mental retardation is associated with autism, it is not a defining characteristic of the disorder. However, mental retardation does influence both symptom expression and prognosis in autistic children.

Bartak and Rutter (1976) compared 8.5-year-old normally intelligent (IQ $\geq$ 70) and mentally retarded autistic children on several measures of social, language, ritualistic, stereotyped, and self-injurious behavior. They found that the two groups were very similar on most behaviors characteristically associated with autism. However, the extent of behavioral deviance was frequently greater in the mentally retarded group. Children in both groups lacked personal friendships and functioned poorly in play groups, but the mentally retarded autistic children were more likely to cause disturbances in public places and to show deviant social responses like smelling and touching strange adults. Both groups showed delays in language development, but these were significantly greater in the mentally retarded group. In terms of ritualistic and compulsive behaviors, the mentally retarded autistics showed more resistance to change while the normally intelligent children demonstrated more rituals. In addition, both groups showed some stereotyped behaviors during a test situation, but the mentally retarded children demonstrated more hand stereotypies, and they were more likely to have a history of self-injurious behavior. Wing (1978) reported similar results from her comparisons of high- and low-functioning autistic children. Low-functioning autistics with mental ages below 20 months showed lower sociability, poorer eye contact, and simpler stereotypies than autistic children with mental ages above 20 months. In addition, elaborate routines were found predominantly in the higher-functioning group.

Degree of mental retardation clearly influences current functioning in autistic children, and it is significantly related to outcome in both cognitive and social domains. Early IQ has been shown to be a good predictor of later IQ and school achievement. As noted earlier, Lockyer and Rutter (1969) found a correlation of .63 between initial IQ and Wechsler Full Scale IQ at follow-up 5–15 years later. In addition, 75 percent of children rated as having an overall poor outcome and 83 percent rated as having a very poor outcome had initial IQs below 60 (Rutter, Greenfield, & Lockyer, 1967). Only one child with a fair outcome and no child with a good outcome had an IQ in the same low range. The relation between initial IQ and later school achievement is very similar. DeMyer et al. (1974) found that Performance IQ predicted school placement in their group of 115 autistic children. Children in classes with normal peers at follow-up had mean Performance IQs at initial evaluation in the 70s, while those in classes for the educable retarded had early IQs in the 60–70 range. Children in classes for the trainable retarded had initial IQs in the 50–60 range and those in classes below the trainable level or not attending school had early IQs below 50. Treatment effects also were found to be related to IQ in the DeMyer et al. (1974) study. Children with IQs greater than 50 who were in treatment programs showed greater increases in IQ scores at follow-up than untreated children in the same IQ range. In contrast, treatment had no effect on IQ at follow-up for children with initial IQs below 40. The effects of treatment, particularly improvements in verbal skills, were likely to be maintained and even incremented in the higher-functioning group but were likely to show no change or to deteriorate in the lower-functioning group.

Level of mental retardation also has been shown to relate to later social functioning in autistic children. DeMyer et al. (1973) reported that 30 percent of their high-functioning autistic children were able to achieve "normal" interfamily relationships in later years. However, only a few of these children also were considered to relate normally with peers. Among the lower-functioning autistic children, many were found to demonstrate some affection toward their parents, but most of the children in this group were considered to prefer to be alone. Fifteen percent of the lower-functioning children were oblivious socially to others. Lockyer and Rutter (1969) noted relationships between the presence versus absence of useful speech at 5 years and later scores on the Vineland Social Maturity Scale. For those children without useful speech at 5 years, Vineland Social Quotients were an average of 23 points lower than earlier assessed IQ scores. These low-functioning children also showed decreases in intellectual functioning with age. In contrast, autistic children with useful speech at 5 years had more stable skills. Initial IQ scores and followup Vineland SQs were not significantly different in this higher-functioning group.

Finally, level of intellectual functioning has been related to neurologic status in autistic children. High functioning autistics tend to manifest few neurologic abnormalities, while lower functioning autistics have a much higher frequency of impairment (Lotter, 1974; Kolvin, Humphrey, & McNay, 1971). These neurologic problems are not always evident when the children are first diagnosed in the early years, but may appear during adolescence or later. Seizure disorders are particularly common in mentally retarded autistic children (Bartak & Rutter, 1976).

SUMMARY

Infantile autism is a unique psychiatric disorder that frequently coexists with mental retardation. As a consequence, there is considerable overlap in symptoms between autistic and mentally retarded children, but characteristics differentiating the groups can be identified. Specifically, autistic children show greater disparities in their verbal and performance skills on standardized tests than do mentally retarded children. Their perceptual organization skills are superior to those found in mental age-matched retarded children, while their verbal skills are more delayed. However, not all verbal skills in autistics are equally depressed. Phonologic and syntactic development are comparable in autistic and mental age-matched retarded children, while semantic and pragmatic development in autistic children are significantly less mature. The use of gesture for communication and in play also is markedly delayed in autistic groups. Similar deficits in semantic, pragmatic, and gestural skills are found when comparisons between autistics and children with developmental receptive language disorders are made.

The pattern of impairments found in autistic children indicates that their deficits extend beyond language to incorporate more general symbolic skills. Symbolization in both verbal and gestural domains is deficient, and these impairments are associated with the autistic child's deviant social development. The specific aspects of language that are most delayed in autistic children involve the learning of socially defined meanings (semantics) and rules for using language to communicate with others (pragmatics). Autistic children also are deficient in gestural communication and in the functional use of objects in play, for example, using a cup and spoon for eating, which must be learned from social observation. The autistic child's impairments are not only cognitive deficiencies, but also involve difficulties in understanding social relationships and in learning from social interactions. Neither the cognitive nor social deficits are clearly primary, but rather development in both domains appears to be closely interrelated.

Wing (1981) has suggested that the autistic child's impaired social interaction, verbal and nonverbal communication, and imaginative activities result from the abnormal development of specific brain areas or functions. In normally intelligent autistic children, the impairment is specific and limited to the triad of social, imaginative, and language dysfunction. In mentally retarded autistic children, the brain damage is more widespread and other functions are affected as well. Wing (1981) reported a high incidence of the triad of autistic symptoms in profoundly retarded children, indicating that the more severe and widespread the brain damage, the more likely that the brain areas controlling social interaction, communication, and imagination will be affected. Children who are mentally retarded without these autistic symptoms have brain damage that excludes specific impairment of the areas responsible for these social and language functions. At present there is little physiological data to support or refute Wing's etiologic speculations. However, Wing's approach does provide a model for representing the qualitative differences in behavior between autistic and mentally retarded children as well as the overlap in symptoms that occurs when the disorders coexist to varying degrees within the same child.

Acknowledgments

This work was supported by NIMH Grant MH33815. I thank Holly Hackman and Luisa Castillo for their help in preparing the manuscript. Marian Sigman, Ph.D., Peter Mundy, Ph.D., and Tracy Sherman, Ph.D. provided thoughtful and stimulating comments.

REFERENCES

American Psychiatric Association. (1980). *Diagnostic and statistical manual of mental disorders* (DSM-III) (3rd ed.). Washington, DC: American Psychiatric Association

Bartak, L, & Rutter, M. (1976). Differences between mentally retarded and normally intelligent autistic children. *Journal of Autism and Childhood Schizophrenia, 6,* 109–120

Bartak, L, Rutter, M, & Cox, A. (1975). A comparative study of infantile autism and specific developmental receptive language disorder: I. The children. *British Journal of Psychiatry, 126,* 127–145

Bartolucci, G, Pierce, S, & Steiner, D. (1980). Cross-sectional studies of grammatical morphemes in autistic and mentally retarded children. *Journal of Autism and Developmental Disorders, 10,* 39–50

Bettelheim, B. (1967). *The empty fortress.* New York: The Free Press

Cantwell, D, Baker, L, & Rutter, M. (1978). A comparative study of infantile autism and specific developmental receptive language disorder: IV. Analysis of syntax and language function. *Journal of Child Psychology and Psychiatry, 19,* 351–362

Casati, I, & Lezine, I. (1968). *Les etapes de l'intelligence sensorimotrice.* Paris: Les Editions de Centre de Psychologie Appliquee

Casey, L. (1978). Development of communicative behavior in autistic children: A parent program using manual signs. *Journal of Autism and Childhood Schizophrenia, 8,* 45–59

Churchill, D. (1969). Psychotic children and behavior modification. *American Journal of Psychiatry, 125,* 1585–1590

Cunningham, M. (1968). A comparison of the language of psychotic and non-psychotic children who are mentally retarded. *Journal of Child Psychology and Psychiatry, 9,* 229–244

DeMyer, M, Barton, S, Alpern, G, Kimberlin, C, Allen, J, Yang, E, & Steele, R. (1974). The measured intelligence of autistic children. *Journal of Autism and Childhood Schizophrenia, 4,* 42–60

DeMyer, M, Barton, S, DeMyer, W, Norton, J, Allen, J, & Steele, R. (1973). Prognosis in autism: A follow-up study. *Journal of Autism and Childhood Schizophrenia, 3,* 199–246

DeMyer, M, Hingtgen, J, & Jackson, R. (1981). Infantile autism reviewed: A decade of research. *Schizophrenia Bulletin, 7,* 388–451

Eisenberg, L. (1956). The autistic child in adolescence. *American Journal of Psychiatry, 112,* 607–613

Gillies, S. (1965). Some abilities of psychotic children and subnormal controls. *Journal of Mental Deficiency Research, 9,* 89–101

Hermelin, B, & O'Connor, N. (1970). *Psychological experiments with autistic children.* New York: Pergamon Press

Kanner, L. (1943). Autistic disturbances of affective contact. *Nervous Child, 2,* 217–250

Kanner, L, Rodriguez, A, & Ashenden, B. (1972). How far can autistic children go in matters of social adaptation. *Journal of Autism and Childhood Schizophrenia, 2,* 9–33

Kolvin, I, Humphrey, M, & McNay, A, VI. (1971). Cognitive factors in childhood psychoses. *British Journal of Psychiatry, 118,* 415–419

Lockyer, L, & Rutter, M. (1969). A five- to fifteen-year follow-up study of infantile psychosis: III. Psychological aspects. *British Journal of Psychiatry, 115,* 865–882

Lockyer, L, & Rutter, M. (1970). A five- to fifteen-year follow-up study of infantile psychosis: IV. Patterns of cognitive ability. *British Journal of Social and Clinical Psychology, 9,* 152–163

Lotter, V. (1974). Factors related to outcome in autistic children. *Journal of Autism and Childhood Schizophrenia, 4,* 263–277

McAdoo, W, & DeMyer M. (1978). Personality characteristics of parents. In M Rutter & E Schopler (Eds.), *Autism: A reappraisal of concepts and treatment* (pp. 251–267). New York: Plenum

McHale, S, Simeonsson, R, Marcus, L, & Oller, J. (1980). The social and symbolic quality of autistic children's communication. *Journal of Autism and Developmental Disorders, 10,* 299–310

Pierce, S, & Bartolucci, G. (1977). A syntactic investigation of verbal autistic, mentally retarded, and normal children. *Journal of Autism and Childhood Schizophrenia, 7,* 121–134

Riguet, G, Taylor, N, Benaroya, S, & Klein, L. (1981). Symbolic play in autistic, Down's, and normal children of equivalent mental age. *Journal of Autism and Developmental Disorders, 11,* 439–448

Ritvo, E, & Freeman, BJ. (1978). National Society for Autistic Children definition of the syndrome of autism. *Journal of Autism and Childhood Schizophrenia, 8,* 162–169

Rutter, M. (1968). Concepts of autism: A review of research. *Journal of Child Psychology and Psychiatry, 9,* 1–25

Rutter, M. (1978). Diagnosis and definition of childhood autism. *Journal of Autism and Childhood Schizophrenia, 8,* 139–161

Rutter, M, & Bartak, L. (1971). Cause of infantile autism: Some considerations from recent research. *Journal of Autism and Childhood Schizophrenia, 1,* 20–32

Rutter, M, Greenfield, D, & Lockyer, L. (1967). A five- to fifteen-year follow-up study of infantile psychosis: II. Social and behavioral outcome. *British Journal of Psychiatry, 113,* 1183–1199

Rutter, M, & Lockyer, L. (1967). A five- to fifteen-year follow-up study of infantile psychosis: I. Description of sample. *British Journal of Psychiatry, 113,* 1169–1182

Schopler, E, Reichler, R, DeVellis, R, & Daly, K. (1980). Toward objective classification of childhood autism: Childhood Autism Rating Scale (CARS). *Journal of Autism and Developmental Disorders, 10,* 91–103

Sigman, M, & Ungerer, JA. (1984a). Attachment behavior in autistic children. *Journal of Autism and Developmental Disorders, 14,* 231–244

Sigman, M, & Ungerer, JA. (1984b). Cognitive and language skills in autistic, mentally retarded, and normal children. *Developmental Psychology, 20,* 239–302

Tager-Flusberg, H. (1981). On the nature of linguistic functioning in early infantile autism. *Journal of Autism and Developmental Disorders, 11,* 45–56

Tubbs, V. (1966). Types of linguistic disability in psychotic children. *Journal of Mental Deficiency Research, 10,* 230–240

Tymchuk, A, Simmons, J, & Neafsey, S. (1977). Intellectual characteristics of adolescent childhood psychotics with high verbal ability. *Journal of Mental Deficiency Research, 21,* 133–138

Wing, L. (1978). Social, behavioral, and cognitive characteristics: An epidemiological approach. In M Rutter & E Schopler (Eds.), *Autism: A reappraisal of concepts and treatment* (pp. 27–45). New York: Plenum

Wing, L. (1981). Language, social, and cognitive impairments in autism and severe mental retardation. *Journal of Autism and Developmental Disorders, 11,* 31–44

Wing, L, & Gould, J. (1979). Severe impairments of social interaction and associated abnormalities in children: Epidemiology and classification. *Journal of Autism and Developmental Disorders, 9,* 11–29

Wing, L, Gould, J, Yeates, S, & Brierley, L. (1977). Symbolic play in mentally retarded and in autistic children. *Journal of Child Psychology and Psychiatry, 18,* 167–178

Wolf, E, Wenar, C, & Ruttenberg, B. (1972). A comparison of personality variables in autistic and mentally retarded children. *Journal of Autism and Childhood Schizophrenia, 2,* 92–108

Tracy Sherman
Robert Asarnow

8

The Cognitive Disabilities of the Schizophrenic Child

Traditionally the diagnosis, treatment, and study of psychiatric disorders and mental retardation have been separate fields. As noted previously in this book, different professionals with sometimes quite divergent theoretical orientations have purview over the respective fields of mental retardation and mental illness. This situation is now changing. A major factor for this change is the recognition that psychiatric disorders and mental retardation coexist. The developmentally-disabled child is at increased risk for developing a wide range of psychiatric disorders (Szymanski, 1980). Another factor is the recognition that in some psychiatric disorders, notably schizophrenia, which will be the topic of this chapter, there is some generalized cognitive deficit. There has been some disagreement over the extent of this generalized impairment and whether this mild general impairment is a consequence of the schizophrenic disorder or might be observed prior to the onset of frank schizophrenic symptoms. There is little doubt, however, that schizophrenic individuals as a group suffer from some degree of generalized cognitive deficit (Lane & Albee, 1968; Offord & Cross, 1969). What distinguishes them from nonschizophrenic mentally retarded individuals is not only the degree of general deficit but, more importantly, the presence of specific cognitive impairments that transcend their general deficits. This chapter will review attempts at understanding the nature of these specific cognitive impairments and will examine the relation between these specific cognitive impairments and aspects of social and emotional functioning.

As with the individual who develops a schizophrenic disorder during adulthood, the schizophrenic child suffers from multiple disabilities. These include impairment in the ability to develop and maintain adequate social relationships (particularly with peers), distortions in affective experiences, inability to monitor reality adequately, and the presence of intense and sometimes chronic anxiety. One of the issues confronting the clinicians and educators working with these children is whether this panoply of impairments results from diverse causes or has a common origin. The contention of the present paper will be that a case can be made for considering a wide range of these disabilities as resulting from impairments in certain cognitive functions. The framework that will be adopted for understanding these impairments is provided by modern theories of information processing.

Over the past 10–15 years, theoreticians attempting to summarize the current work on cognitive and perceptual processing in adult schizophrenics have returned again and again to the conclusion that something is wrong with the schizophrenic's ability to deploy attention efficiently and effectively. We shall review the conclusions of a few of these seminal papers in order to benefit from both the ideas put forth in these early reviews as well as the criteria by which they were later evaluated.

ATTENTION AND SCHIZOPHRENIA

Venables (1964) integrated data from a number of seemingly disparate research areas (e.g., incidental learning, stimulus generalization) in order to support his contention that the pattern of deviant performance evidenced by chronic, process schizophrenics was different from the deviant pattern of performance shown by the acute, paranoid schizophrenics. He tied both patterns of performance to inappropriate levels of arousal. Chronic schizophrenic patients were hypothesized to have elevated states of sympathetic and cortical activation. As a result, they suffer from a restriction in their attentional field that is reflected in their inability to use the contextual constraints of language, their poor incidental learning, and their problems with size constancy tasks. In contrast, the acute patient was thought to display a low level of cortical activation and, therefore, an inability to restrict the range of his attention. The acute patients shifted their judgement of an object's weight more than normal controls did following the experience of lifting a heavy weight. They also were more affected than normal controls, or chronic schizophrenic patients, by the presence of anchor stimuli when making judgements of length. Finally, the acute patient showed his inability to restrict his range of attention in studies of conceptual overinclusion. These conclusions seemed very promising because they summarized a wide body of literature by suggesting a reasonably elegant set of hypotheses to explain why chronic patients differed from the acute, paranoid patients.

Neale and Cromwell (1970) pointed out that Venables' conclusions rested on three assumptions: the validity of the hypothesized relationship between attention and arousal (i.e., that heightened cortical arousal results in an overly restricted range of attention, while reduced cortical arousal results in an overly broad field of attention); that chronic and process patients have supernormal arousal, while acute and reactive patients have subnormal levels of arousal; and that arousal differences relate to performance differences in appropriate experimental tasks. Neale and Cromwell concluded that while Venables' overall point of view might have some merit, the theory has limited utility because the terms and concepts of the theory did not have enough specificity. Venables did not have a significantly precise definition of attention to differentiate between tasks that were highly demanding of attention and those that were only minimally demanding. For example, size estimation tasks require judgements about the relative size of target and standard stimuli. The stimuli, however, are not presented simultaneously. Therefore, the task makes demands on the subject's ability to maintain and access information in working memory. Overall, many of the tasks Venables used to derive his theory are open to alternative descriptions, thus raising questions about this particular conceptualization.

Before advancing still another theory of schizophrenia that relies on the concepts of arousal and attention, we must heed Neale and Cromwell's critique of Venables' work. First, we must use a model of attention that provides a clear, operational definition of attention, such that testable hypotheses may be derived. Second, we should use multiple, converging measures of a particular set of cognitive abilities so that we can be confident that any identified limitation is not merely tied to a specific task.

Recent work published after Venables' (1964) and Neale and Cromwell's (1970) papers does seem to provide converging evidence that schizophrenics have trouble with tasks that demand controlled, cognitive processes. These processes make extensive demands on attentional capacity. Cognitive processes that can be described as automatized (i.e., processes that do not seem to draw on our limited attentional capacity; Gjerde, 1983; Neale & Oltmans, 1980; Schneider & Shiffrin, 1977) do not seem to be impaired in schizophrenics. Schizophrenics, for example, do well in tasks involving recognition, but not as well in tasks requiring recall. The claim made is that recall differs from recognition in that it requires some additional processing, such as organization of information at the time of original learning. It is in this structured process that schizophrenics are believed to be impaired.

However, if the studies are examined carefully, it does not appear that we have been able to identify a specific process that is consistently impaired in the schizophrenic individual. Rather, it seems that under certain conditions, controlled processes are not executed. Impaired performance is often revealed in tasks that involve a time pressure such as tachistocopic presentations of materials (Cromwell, 1984). Kahneman (1973) has shown that putting the cognitive system under time pressure places greater demands on the capacity of the system. This can be seen in studies of the subjective organizational structure that is necessary for effective recall. Schizophrenic patients typically fail to show the clustering or other structured behaviors that enhance recall. This is true even when the stimulus materials afford easy category organization (Koh, Kayton, & Berry, 1973). By contrast, normal adults show greater recall when a list of words contains clusterable sublists. Findings such as these might lead to the suggestion that schizophrenics do not have available in long-term memory categories similar to normal adults, or that the category information is not retrievable or otherwise available to aid in current information processing. Yet, if the task is changed from a recall task, where the demand to sort the items is only implicit, to a sorting task, where the demand to sort the items into categories is explicit, schizophrenics are shown to have the necessary category information and to be able to employ it effectively in a task situation (Koh, Kayton, & Schwartz, 1974).

A second example of a cognitive ability that is seen to be available only in certain task situations is illustrated in Neale's work (Neale, 1971) using the span of apprehension task. He derived estimates of the number of items schizophrenics and normals can process from a tachistoscopically presented array of letters. Conditions varied according to the number of distractor letters presented along with the target letter. For a given display size, the schizophrenics consistently processed fewer items than the normals. Moreover, as the number of distractor letters increased, the schizophrenic's performance fell further behind the level of performance achieved by the normals. Yet, interestingly, *both* groups actually process increasing numbers of letters as the number of distractors increased. What this means is that both the schizophrenic subjects and the normal subjects are able to enhance their performance as more distractors are added to the display. This indicates that both schizophrenic and normal individuals have greater processing abilities than are always employed. What is the crucial change that allows the schizophrenic as well as the normal to process more items as the number of distractors is increased?

One further direct example that the schizophrenic has abilities that are employed under one set of conditions and not under others is found in Larsen and Fromholt's (1976) study. They showed that making sorting an explicit task requirement raised the recall performance of schizophrenics to the level of normals. In addition, the self-paced sorting of study items into self-determined categories led to schizophrenic recall at the same level as normal (Koh, 1978; Koh, Kayton, & Streicker, 1976).

When limits are probed, what seems to emerge is that schizophrenics perform necessary processes but fail to do so under certain task situations. Psychologists typically use this type of data to identify or isolate specific impairments in a processing system. There are two reasons, however, that suggest that schizophrenic individuals might not have isolated or *specific* impairments in their information processing system. First, the range of deficits seen in schizophrenic subjects seems very widespread. In recent years, schizophrenic individuals have been variously characterized as suffering from impairments in smooth pursuit eye movements, sensory integration, iconic, short-term and long-term memory, cross-modal integration of information, selective attention, flexibility of cognitive set, and visual persistance. This ubiquity of dysfunction suggests to us that the impairment is more systemic, rather than contained within a small set of isolable information processing functions. Second, our review of the extant literature suggests that the schizophrenic's impairment seems to be related to broad task requirements involving demands for speeded performance and/or controlled processes in general.

Tasks that appear to tap common psychological processes or structures (e.g., organization of long-term memory, clustering strategies, sorting, recall) do not result in a consistent set of findings, i.e., that schizophrenics always do less well than normals. Attempts at converging operations have not isolated specific impairments; rather, questions about general modes of processing, such as automatic versus controlled deployment of attentional capacity, must be raised. The common characteristic of tasks on which schizophrenics show impaired performance is that controlled, effortful information processing is required. Thus, in the span of apprehension task, schizophrenics perform as well as do normals when there are only 0 or 3 distractors. Their performance deviates markedly from that of the normal controls, though, when the number of distracting items goes up to 5 or 10. These are conditions that require the speeded scanning of many letters before the target letters will be detected.

One profitable way to understand aspects of information processing in schizophrenics can be derived from Kahneman's model of effort and attention. Kahneman's model of attention (1973) shifted the focus from structural limitations (bottlenecks and filters) on perceptual processing and cognitive work to capacity limitations on what information processing can occur in a given moment in time. Capacity, or effort, is the measure of cognitive resources that are available to do specific cognitive tasks. The major assumption of Kahneman's model is that the total amount of attention that can be deployed at any time is limited. Two constructs that are central to this model are the rules by which the total pool of capacity is made available or *recruited* to do cognitive work, the governor system; and the rules by which resources are directed to specific tasks, the system by which resources are *allocated*. We shall argue that the functioning of each of these rule-bound systems is impaired in schizophrenics. In this chapter, though, the major emphasis will be on impairments of the functioning of the governor system.

Kahneman argues that the governor system is controlled by two importantly different sets of influence. The first factor that determines the amount of capacity available for cognitive work is the effort required by the currently ongoing or immediately upcoming cognitive activity that the individual is engaged in. Interestingly, Kahneman postulates that while available capacity rises with task demand, it does not increase proportionally. Rather, with increasing task difficulty, the discrepancy between the effort required for successful completion of the task and the effort supplied seem to increase steadily. Thus the tasks that make the greatest demand on capacity are the occasions where there is the greatest discrepancy between available capacity and task demand. The second set of factors affecting the size of the pool of available capacity are what Kahneman terms miscellaneous determinants. These include physiological effects of drugs or drive states and the current level of ambient stimulation. In order to have a chance of successfully completing a task the governor system must adequately evaluate the demands of the task and make available a sufficient pool of processing resources.

Once the necessary capacity is available for cognitive work, these processing resources must still be effectively allocated if task completion is to be successful. Kahneman offers four rules that describe how available capacity will be channelled.

The first rule is that capacity will be involuntarily channelled to certain classes of events. For example, attention is involuntarily drawn to stimulus novelty and to motion. The second rule is that attention may be voluntarily allocated in accordance with current intentions. Adults can intentionally attend, for example, to the words they hear through a right earphone of a headset. The third rule applies when two activities demand more capacity that can be made available. Priorities are applied and one of the tasks will be successfully completed.

The fourth rule refers to the fact that the overall allocation policy will change when the system is either in a high state of arousal or a very low state of arousal. When the system is in a very low state of arousal, the subject may fail to adopt a task set or may fail to evaluate his own level of performance. Lack of attention to feedback on the adequacy of performance will in turn result in insufficient adjustments in the recruitment of capacity in accordance with the demands of the task. Just as very low levels of arousal may result in an overall poor level of performance, so too will extremely high levels of arousal. However, the reasons for impoverished performance will be different. As arousal increases, subjects become more selective in the cues to which they attend. At moderate levels of arousal, this selectivity may facilitate performance. If arousal becomes too great though, the subject's ability to determine which are the most relevant cues is reduced. Thus while attention is focused, it may be focused on aspects of the environment that are irrelevant for successful performance. Moreover, as arousal level rises, the focus of attention appears to become more labile. Thus under conditions of high arousal, subjects become more distractible.

Kahneman's fourth rule captures the phenomenon summarized by the Yerkes-Dodson law. Performance is an inverted U-shaped function of arousal. Performance will suffer if arousal is either too high or too low. Moreover, task difficulty interacts with optimal arousal level. For difficult tasks there is a narrow range of arousal level over which performance will be adequate and a relatively low level of arousal is required for maximal performance. In this way, Kahneman's model adds to our understanding of why performance deteriorates at both very high and very low levels of arousal, and why performance level is a function of both arousal level and task difficulty.

In the terms of Kahneman's model, the pattern of information processing failures seen in schizophrenic subjects may result because the governor system does not or cannot supply sufficient cognitive resources in the time frame required for successful task completion, or because the allocation policy fails to award sufficient resources for the task, for example, by squandering resources on alternative functions.

We will now review work from our laboratory that supports the hypothesis that the information processing dysfunction found in schizophrenic children is due to the governor system's inability to provide the necessary capacity. The reason that controlled processing appears to be impaired in schizophrenics is that this mode of information processing tends to be most resource-demanding. When the governor system fails to allocate sufficient cognitive resources, the first systems that will show failure will be these highly resource-demanding processes.

STUDIES OF VISUAL INFORMATION PROCESSING IN SCHIZOPHRENIC CHILDREN

In our laboratory, we have examined the performance of schizophrenic children on both the full and partial report versions of the span of apprehension (see Asarnow & Sherman, 1984, for a more detailed account of these studies). The partial report span of apprehension task requires subjects to report which of two predesignated target letters are present in arrays of tachistoscopically (50 ms) presented stimuli varying in the number of nontarget items. In the full report version of the span task the identical stimulus arrays and presentation time are used. However, the subject is required to report verbally all the letters he or she can remember seeing. These tasks were chosen because previous work with schizophrenic adults in various phases of the disorder (acutely disturbed and partially recovered) has shown that across wide variations in clinical state, schizophrenic individuals manifest impairments on a partial-report version of the span of apprehension task (Asarnow & MacCrimmon, 1978, 1981, 1982). Also children at-risk for schizophrenia, by virtue of having a schizophrenic parent, also show impairment on a partial-report version of the span of apprehension task (Asarnow, Steffy, MacCrimmon, & Cleghorn, 1977). Thus, like the disorder itself, which seems to entail an enduring vulnerability, the schizophrenic subject's performance on the span of apprehension task seems to continue at a depressed level regardless of clinical state.

In contrast to their performance on the partial-report version of the span, schizophrenic adults do not seem to show impaired performance on the full-report version of the span (Cash, Neale, & Cromwell, 1972). The pairing of success and failure on these two tasks allows one to begin to delimit the source of impairment tapped by the partial-report task. Specifically, the schizophrenic individuals seem to be impaired in the controlled attentive processes that are needed to scan quickly the stimulus array for the presence of one of the target letters.

We studied the performance of schizophrenic children on partial- and full-report versions of the span of apprehension to determine if the same patterns of success and failure found in schizophrenic adults and children at-risk for schizophrenia would be observed. The schizophrenic children performed in a manner equivalent to their MA-matched peers on the full-report version of the span of apprehension, but at a significantly poorer level on the partial-report version of the span (when five or more distractors were presented along with the target stimulus). The performance of the schizophrenic children on a partial-report version of the span was equivalent to that of normal children who were on the average 4 years younger in mental age than the schizophrenic children.

The schizophrenic children's performance paralleled that of the adult schizophrenics. We hypothesized that the schizophrenic children and adults have impairments in the early attentional processes required to identify the presence of one of the target letters in the fading stimulus array before its representation in iconic memory fades.

Given that the schizophrenic children performed at the same level as the younger normals, we were curious to see if these two groups of children were performing the task using the same strategies. If this were true, then we could deem it tenable that the schizophrenic children were merely delayed in the development of the strategies required for successful performance on the partial report version of the span of apprehension. We examined the accuracy of detecting the target letter as a function of its location in the display for both groups of children. Both the older normals and the schizophrenic children made more correct target identifications in the upper half of the display than when the target appeared in the lower half of the display. Target location did not affect the performance of the younger normals. Thus, it appears that the schizophrenic children were using a scanning strategy similar to that of the older normals but not of the younger normals. Interestingly, though, it is only when the target is in one of the upper quadrants that the older normals perform better than the schizophrenics and younger normals. Thus, we concluded that while the overall level of performance of the schizophrenic children is equivalent to that of the younger normals, the schizophrenics are not performing the task as the younger children do. Rather, they are employing the same strategy as their MA-matched peers, but they are less efficient and effective in the implementation of that strategy.

We hypothesize that the schizophrenics perform the search strategy less well than do the MA-matched normals either because the normals, unlike the schizophrenics, have found a better set of critical features to search for and therefore their search is more efficient, or because the schizophrenic and normal children are essentially using the same search strategy, but the schizophrenics are either slower in initiating or in moving through the steps of the search strategy. If the first explanation were the case, then the performance of the schizophrenics would rise to the level of the MA-matched normals with a very simple intervention. We would merely tell the children which features to search for. If the second explanation were true, the remediation of the schizophrenic's deficit would be much more difficult.

From this study alone, we cannot confirm or disconfirm either of these explanations. We think, however, that the schizophrenic's difficulty is less task and modality specific and more ubiquitous than that suggested by the first explanation. It seems likely that schizophrenic individuals have trouble with the partial report version of the span of apprehension because their governor system fails to provide sufficient cognitive resources for the effective and rapid execution of the scanning strategy.

EVENT-RELATED POTENTIAL CONCOMITANTS OF INFORMATION PROCESSING DYSFUNCTION

Cromwell and Neale's critique of Venables, and of "attention" explanations in general, underscores the need to specify precisely what aspect of attention is hypothesized to be impaired and how it might be measured. The results of both of our own set of studies and of the extant literature examining cognitive deficits in schizophrenic subjects suggest that schizophrenic individuals show impairment in cognitive performance when the capacity or effort demanded by the task is greater than their governor system is capable of recruiting. Why the governor system fails to provide sufficient capacity is a question to be addressed as well. But first we would like to establish the plausibility of our hypothesis: that the schizophrenic's governor system chronically fails to provide adequate capacity for cognitive work.

We tested this hypothesis by determining if physiologic measures of capacity recruitment provide evidence that confirms that obtained from our behavioral measures. A collaborating research team (James Marsh, Robert Strandburg, Warren Brown, and Donald Guthrie of the UCLA Department of Psychiatry) measured evoked potentials from multiple electrodes while schizophrenic and normal children were performing the partial-report version of the span of apprehension. Their results (see Strandburg, Marsh, Brown, Asarnow, & Guthrie, 1984, for a more detailed presentation of this study) speak directly to the hypothesized deficit in the governor system's ability to recruit the necessary processing resources. These researchers focused on four components in the event related potential (ERP)—a contingent negative variation (CNV) elicited in response to a warning tone; and an N1, a P300, and a slow wave that followed presentation of the visual span stimuli.

The CNV to the warning tone reflects a variety of different cognitive operations: attention, arousal, anticipated energy output, preparation for decision making or action (Donchin, Ritter, & McCallum, 1978; Syndulko & Lindsley, 1977). The significantly lower amplitudes of the CNV in the schizophrenic children suggested that they were less prepared for, and have mobilized fewer cognitive resources for processing the upcoming visual span stimuli.

The N1 component reflects task difficulty (Naatanen & Michie, 1979). It increases with the complexity of the stimulus discrimination demanded by the task. The schizophrenic children showed the same, relatively small N1 for all array difficulty levels. In contrast, the normal children showed the expected pattern where increasing task difficulty over the various conditions of the experiment was tracked by an increase in N1 amplitude.

The P300 component is believed to reflect the allocation of perceptual resources to higher-level processing of stimulus material. P300 has been hypothesized to reflect the activity of the limited capacity central processor (Donchin et al., 1978; Posner, 1978). Larger P300s are associated with successful task completion. As task demands outstrip the subject's processing capacity, the P300 latency is extended in time and the amplitude is diminished. The normal children generated significantly larger P300 amplitudes than did the schizophrenic children. Diminished amplitude of the P300 has been observed in adult schizophrenics (Roth, Horvath, Pfefferbaum, & Kopell, 1980) and in children at-risk for schizophrenia (Friedman, Vaughan, & Erlenmeyer-Kimling, 1982). This reduced positivity in schizophrenic individuals implies less activation of the physiological substrate underlying the process of allocating attentional resources for perceptual processing.

The slow wave is believed to reflect further processing following the P300 component, which is necessitated by increased task difficulty (Ruchkin, Munson, & Sutton, 1982). Here again, the normal children show an orderly increase of the slow wave with increasing task difficulty, while the schizophrenic children produce slow waves with constant and intermediate amplitudes for all array types.

Schizophrenic children are impaired both in the initial mobilization of resources (auditory component, CNV) and in the specific processsing of the visual stimuli (N1, P300, slow wave). Across a number of ERP components, the schizophrenic children showed diminished response amplitude that was little effected by increases in task difficulty. Amplitude differences may reflect lack of activation of necessary physiological substrates, overinhibition of necessary subcomponents, or a lack of appropriate synchrony. The overall effect, however, is to provide less of the necessary processing resources required for successful task completion.

In summary, schizophrenic children have been shown to have difficulty in a task requiring speeded functioning of the early attentive processes. This pattern of performance is analogous to that seen in adult schizophrenics and children at-risk for schizophrenia.

We have argued that the literature on information processing deficits in adult schizophrenics has failed to isolate a specific memory store or cognitive process that is consistently impaired. Rather, the schizophrenics' deficits seems to be observed across of wide variety of tasks that tap diverse aspects of information processing, but that share the common characteristic of making extensive demands on information processing capacity. One way to account for these findings is to attribute the information processing impairment associated with schizophrenia to a malfunctioning of the governor system described by Kahneman. Both the behavioral data and the electrophysiological findings cited above in studies of schizophrenic adults and children, and in children at-risk for schizophrenia, support the plausibility of this hypothesis.

CAPACITY MODELS OF HUMAN INFORMATION PROCESSING

In this section we will explore the implications of the hypothesized deficit in the governor system for the cognitive functioning of schizophrenic individuals. We will use the model of human information processing proposed by Norman and Bobrow (1975) as the framework for this discussion.

Norman and Bobrow (1975) describe two factors that limit the quality of human information processing. These are data limitations and resource limitations. Clearly, incomplete data will make high quality task performance impossible, just as insufficient cognitive resources will. Norman and Bobrow (1975) argue that to understand how behavior deviates from optimal we need to describe the human information processing system as a stagelike processing system where each stage continuously provides output to the next stage. When because of either data limitations or resource limitations a particular stage fails to produce a completely accurate output, the next stages are still provided some information from which to work. This results in performance degrading in a gradual rather than an all-or-nothing manner.

The inferences we will now draw are rooted in Norman and Bobrow's (1975) model of human information processing, that within the constraints of available resources and data, each stage in the processing stream continuously provides output for the higher stages. For the sake of this discussion we hypothesize that while the governor system of the schizophrenic is impaired, the allocation system, per se, is not. We make this assumption for the sake of analytic simplicity. At the end of this chapter we will consider how deviations in the allocation system might account for some of the behavioral deviation seen in schizophrenic patients. To examine the implication of an impaired governor system the following questions must be addressed. How does the allocation system function when the governor system does not provide it with sufficient capacity to meet task demands? How does this result in behavior that deviates from optimal performance?

Kahneman's (1973) general rules for the functioning of the allocation system generate predictions about how the schizophrenic's allocation system will deal with its resource limitations. Two principles are particularly relevant. First, processes that take attention involuntarily will supercede other functioning. For instance, motion in the periphery will attract visual attention. The second principle is that priority is given to finishing a single task when multiple tasks are competing for processing resources. One implication of this principle is that when some tasks in and of themselves require more capacity than can be generated, these tasks will be supplanted by tasks that can be successfully completed. So, for example, speeded processes that require large bursts of attention will be given low priority, and may very well fail completely, if other completeable processes are competing for attentional resources.

If, however, a high capacity-demanding task can be extended in time so that the capacity demanded in any moment in time is within the system's limit, then the process will be given a higher priority by the allocation system. There is a cost, though, to the overall functioning of the cognitive system when tasks are forced to be extended in time to avoid exceeding momentary capacity recruitment limitations. A process that is extended in time is more susceptible to interruptions by events that draw capacity involuntarily. This could, in part, explain the schizophrenic individual's sense of being flooded by uninterpreted percepts. He fails to complete time-extended processes such as object identification before environmental events cause processing capacity to be drawn to a new focus.

Extending processing in time to avoid capacity limitations produces another set of problems. Effort must be expended in place-keeping each time capacity is drawn away and then must be refocused on the original processing. These added place-keeping costs, in conjunction with overall reduced capacity, may explain in part the schizophrenic's problem in maintaining a line of thought.

A corollary of Kahneman's second allocation principle is that the system will give priority to automatized functions that are, by definition, less capacity demanding processes. An important consequence of this corollary is that when the demands on the cognitive system exceed its capacity, degradation of performance will first occur in the most capacity-demanding functions before occurring in automatized functions.

How might this orderly degradation of functioning appear in the language production of schizophrenic adults? Rochester (1978) has shown that in schizophrenics' speech the overlearned (automatic) syntactic rules of the language are not violated. Neither are local constraints on semantics, another automatized process in adults, violated. What is disrupted is the processing that requires the moving of information in and out of short term memory in a speeded manner. This type of processing involves more controlled, temporally extended processing that is not automatized. In schizophrenic adults this problem is manifest, not only in their poorly connected oral discourse, but also in their difficulties in laboratory tasks that require speeded lexical access.

The Chapmans (1973) argue that the essence of schizophrenic speech is the lack of sensitivity to listener needs and context effects. Assessments of the listener's needs or context effects require the processing in *real time* of another person's facial expressions, or queries at the same time that the speaker is producing language. If, as Rochester suggests, even the production of speech taxes the capacity of the schizophrenic's information processing system, certainly the schizophrenic individual's performance on a secondary task (monitoring the response of the listener) will fail. This conjecture is born out in studies of incidental learning in schizophrenics. The schizophrenic does poorly on central tasks and shows even greater limitations when his secondary or incidental learning is probed (Lawson, 1967).

THE COGNITIVE DISABILITIES OF THE SCHIZOPHRENIC CHILD

If we extend this analysis to the case of the schizophrenic child, the problems appear even greater than those of a schizophrenic adult. The child does not yet have a store of automatized skills, but rather is at a stage in life where learning and the acquisition of more sophisticated information-processing strategies is paramount. If, at this point in development, capacity limitations become excessive, not only will current functioning be impaired but cognitive development will be compromised. In middle childhood, children move from external stimuli controlling the allocation of attention (Kahneman's first rule) to internally- or goal-directed allocation of attention (Kahneman's second through fourth rules) (Pick, Christy, & Frankel, 1972; Hagen, Jongeward, & Kail, 1976).

If the child does not have sufficient cognitive capacity to perform and practice more complex cognitive functions, those functions will not become automatized. In other words, the basic units of information-processing to be worked with will remain more simple than those of normally developing children. Certain strategies and skills that will become automatized, and therefore demand only modest amounts of attention in the child's normal peers, will remain unpracticed and therefore highly capacity-demanding for the schizophrenic child. This is especially true since the child's ability to recruit capacity for cognitive work is already reduced (Strandburg et al., 1984).

Cognitive skills that cannot be extended in time to avoid overstepping capacity limits will not be well learned, while strategies or processes that require less cognitive effort or that can be extended in time will be learned. This will result in a pattern of strengths and weaknesses, abilities and inabilities that is the hallmark of the schizophrenic child. It distinguishes him from the retarded child or the younger, but normally developing, child. For example, in our studies the schizophrenic children performed at the level of the younger normal children on the partial-report version of the span of apprehension. However, the schizophrenic children, but not the younger normals, appeared to be using a search strategy similar to that used by the older children. The schizophrenic children, though, were less able to effectively employ this strategy than were the older normals.

On standardized intelligence tests, the schizophrenic child displays a characteristic pattern of strengths and weaknesses. Let us see if this pattern can be accounted for by this model, which assumes that schizophrenic children show impaired information processing abilities because of problems in the recruitment of attentional capacity. Schizophrenic individuals tend to perform consistently better on the verbal subtests of the WISC–R (Weschler, 1974), than on the performance subtests.

One of the major differences between subtests on which the schizophrenic child performs adequately, and on which he fails, have to do with whether the method of testing a particular set of abilities requires the child to perform in a speeded manner. Thus, among the verbal subtests, the schizophrenic children tend to perform poorly on such subtests as digit span while doing well on the vocabulary and information subtests. The digit span test is a time-limited task that requires the subject to maintain a set of items in working memory. This sort of active information processing requires large bursts of attentional capacity; if these "bursts" of attentional capacity are not recruited on the digit span, items will be lost from memory. In contrast, the vocabulary and information subtests assess the recall of overlearned facts. They do not measure problem solving abilities, and they are assessed in a nonspeeded manner. Success on these subtests does not require the recruitment of large amounts of attentional capacity at any moment in time.

How might this model of impairments in the recruitment of attentional capacity account for the major behavioral problems associated with schizophrenia in children: thought disorder, disordered social relations, and inappropriate and reduced affect? Schizophrenic speech may be characterized as digressive, vague, and circumstantial (Andreasen, 1979). We believe that a profitable way to understand these phenomena is to ask the question, how do children learn to avoid such failures in communication? To avoid these problems, the speaker must simultaneously solve multiple information-processing tasks. He or she must determine how the current topics pertain to what was said before and to his current intentions. He or she must monitor the listener's responses and help the listener see all of the relevant links. In order to accomplish this successfully, the speaker must rapidly move information in and out of short-term memory in order to see connections between current intentions and the just-prior conversation. He or she must rapidly update information on the listener's reactions to his or her statements. The speaker must use place-keeping and updating abilities to know exactly how much of his or her current stream of thought has been verbalized.

Our model predicts that the schizophrenic individual simply cannot succeed on these multiple updating and place-keeping tasks because of the burden they place on the ability to recruit additional capacity. The schizophrenic individual will lose his or her place in his or her stream of thought, and the listener will experience the speaker's thoughts as drifting. The impaired speaker will fail to make the necessary logical linkages for the listener, and fail to remind the listener of the referent of various pronouns. Speech will appear vague and digressive. The aspects of speech that will be spared from impairment are those that are less capacity-demanding. Highly overlearned aspects of speech such as syntax should be relatively intact. Also speech should appear logically consistent within small time units. Capacity demands only become great when information must be integrated over longer time intervals. Schizophrenic speech does indeed show these particular islands of ability.

How might the model account for another important disability seen in schizophrenic children, their social ineptness, particularly with peers? This model suggests that the schizophrenic child will be less able than other children to attend to a wide variety of cues at a given moment in time. The studies of children's friendship formation indicate the importance of empathy, the reading of interpersonal cues, and sensitivity to the affective reactions of others for developing successful friendships (Zahn-Waxler, Iannotti, & Chapman, 1982). Our model suggests that the schizophrenic child is uniquely unable to respond to this variety of cues presented in real time. Added to the schizophrenic child's lack of empathy is the fact that he or she may say many bizarre things that may frighten other children. The net result will be a child who becomes more and more socially isolated as his or her social skills progressively fall further and further behind those of his or her peers.

As developed in this chapter, the model of cognitive deficits associated with schizophrenia in children has focused on the issue of resource recruitment. We have followed this course in order to see how much of the research data, as well as the clinical symptomatology, could be accounted for by a parsimonious set of constructs. It is quite possible that schizophrenic individuals also have deviant rules for the *allocation* of cognitive resources. Schizophrenic children are preoccupied with internally generated ideas, and they engage in the performance of stereotyped behaviors. Both of these types of allocation deviancies will interfere even further with the child's cognitive functioning by draining his or her resources to nonproductive ends. These allocation problems will further impede the schizophrenic child's development of peer relations by interfering with the amount of cognitive capacity directed outward.

This model does not obviously account for the diminished or inappropriate affect of the schizophrenic child. In part this is a reflection of the current state of knowledge about the relation between affect and cognition. The two systems may be independent, one may be secondary to the other, or both may reflect the functioning of some underlying third system (Zajonc, 1980). In the case of the schizophrenic child, there may be some underlying problem that reveals itself both in reduced capacity for cognitive work and reduced affect.

This model can account for a broad range of the cognitive and social problems seen in schizophrenic children. It also seems to account for the varigated pattern of strengths and weaknesses that characterize the cognitive performance of schizophrenic children and that distinguish them from both normal and mentally retarded children.

By isolating what may be some of the core cognitive deficits associated with schizophrenia, the model also suggests directions for intervention. The schizophrenic child needs to be explicitly taught how to maintain a set, or task orientation. The importance of using self-instruction (self generated verbally mediated cues) to control attentional deployment has been described elsewhere (Asarnow & Asarnow, 1982; Asarnow & Watkins, 1982). In terms of the current model, these cues would not prevent the child's attention from being redirected involuntarily, or enhance the amount of capacity available for cognitive work. Instead, they would provide a means for the schizophrenic child to succeed better at place-keeping and thereby allow him or her a greater chance of returning to an appropriate place in interrupted tasks. In this way it provides the child a means of maintaining a task orientation.

Second, the schizophrenic child might benefit from explicit metacognitive training. Teaching the child how to monitor his or her own cognitive processes might increase control over his or her system for allocating cognitive resources. As with the case of self-instructional training, this would not alter the schizophrenic child's ability to recruit capacity for cognitive work. It might help the child reduce the amount of capacity squandered on stereotyped thoughts and behaviors at a given moment in time, thereby freeing more of his or her cognitive capacity for adaptive problem-solving and learning.

REFERENCES

Andreasen, NC. (1979). Thought, language, and communication disorders: I. Clinical assessment, definition of terms, evaluation of their reliability. *Archives of General Psychiatry, 36,* 1315–1321

Asarnow, R, & Asarnow, JR. (1982). Attention/information processing and vulnerability to schizophrenia: Implications for preventive intervention. In MJ Goldstein (Ed.), *Preventive intervention in schizophrenia: Are we ready?* Rockville, MD: Department of Health and Human Services

Asarnow, RF, & MacCrimmon, DJ. (1978). Residual performance deficit in clinically remitted schizophrenics: A marker of schizophrenia? *Journal of Abnormal Psychology, 87,* 597–608

Asarnow, RF, & MacCrimmon, D. (1981). Span of apprehension deficits during the postpsychotic stages of schizophrenia: A replication and extension. *Archives of General Psychiatry, 38,* 1006–1011

Asarnow, RF, & MacCrimmon, DJ. (1982). Attention/information processing, neuropsychological functioning and thought disorder during the acute and partial recovery phases of schizophrenia: A longitudinal study. *Psychiatry Research, 1* 309–319

Asarnow, RF, & Sherman, T. (1984). Studies of visual information processing in schizophrenic children. *Child Development, 55,* 247–262

Asarnow, RF, Steffy, RA, MacCrimmon, DJ, & Cleghorn, JM. (1977). An attentional assessment of foster children at risk for schizophrenia. *Journal of Abnormal Psychology, 86,* 267–275

Asarnow, RF, & Watkins, JM. (1982). Schizophrenic thought disorder: Linguistic incompetence or information processing impairment? *The Behavioral and Brain Sciences, 5,* 589–590

Cash, TF, Neale, JM, & Cromwell, RL. (1972). Span of apprehension in acute schizophrenics: Full-report procedure. *Journal of Abnormal Psychology, 3,* 322–326

Chapman, LJ, & Chapman, JP. (1973). *Disordered thought in schizophrenia.* New York: Appleton-Century-Crofts

Cromwell, RL. (1984). Preemptive thinking and schizophrenia research. In WD Spaulding (Ed.), *Nebraska Symposium on Motivation 1982–1983.* Lincoln, NE: University of Nebraska Press

Donchin, E, Ritter, W, & McCallum, W. (1978). Cognitive psychophysiology: The endogenous components of the ERP. In E Callaway, P Teuting, & S Koslow (Eds.), *Event related brain potentials in man* (pp. 349–442). New York: Academic Press

Friedman, D, Vaughan, HG, & Erlenmeyer-Kimling, L. (1982). Cognitive brain potentials in children at risk for schizophrenia: Preliminary findings. *Schizophrenia Bulletin, 8,* 514–531

Gjerde, P. (1983). Attentional capacity dysfunction and arousal in schizophrenia. *Psychological Bulletin, 93,* 57–72

Hagen, J, Jongeward, R, & Kail, R. (1976). Cognitive perspectives on the development of memory. In H. Reese (Ed.), *Advances in child development and behavior* (Vol. 10). New York: Academic Press

Kahneman, D. (1973). *Attention and effort.* Englewood Cliffs, NJ: Prentice-Hall

Koh, SD. (1978). Remembering of verbal materials by schizophrenic young adults. In S Schwartz (Ed.), *Language and cognition in schizophrenia.* Hillsdale, NJ: Erlbaum

Koh, SD, Kayton, L, & Berry, R. (1973). Mnemonic organization in young nonpsychotic schizophrenics. *Journal of Abnormal Psychology, 81,* 299–310

Koh, SD, Kayton, L, & Schwartz, C. (1974). The structure of word-storage in the permanent memory of nonpsychotic schizophrenics. *Journal of Consulting and Clinical Psychology, 42,* 879–887

Koh, SD, Kayton, L, & Streicker, S. (1976). Short-term memory for numerousness in schizophrenic young adults. *Journal of Nervous and Mental Disease, 163,* 88–101

Lane, EA, & Albee, GW. (1968). On childhood intellectual decline and adult schizophrenics: A reassessment of an earlier study. *Journal of Abnormal Psychology, 73,* 174–177

Larsen, SF, & Fromhalt, P. (1976). Mnemonic organization and free recall in schizophrenia. *Journal of Abnormal Psychology, 85,* 61–65

Lawson, JS. (1967). Distractibility in schizophrenia and organic cerebral disease. *British Journal of Psychiatry, 113,* 527–535

Naatanen, R, & Michie, P. (1979). Early selective attention effects on the evoked potential: A critical review and reinterpretation. *Biological Psychology, 8,* 81–136

Neale, JM. (1971). Perceptual span in schizophrenics. *Journal of Abnormal Psychology, 77,* 196–204

Neale, JM, & Cromwell, RL. (1970). Attention and schizophrenia. In BA Maher (Ed.), *Progress in experimental personality research* (Vol. 5). New York: Academic Press

Neale, JM, & Oltmans, TF. (1980). *Schizophrenia.* New York: Wiley

Norman, D, & Bobrow, D. (1975). On data-limited and resource-limited processes. *Cognitive Psychology, 7,* 44–64

Offord, DR, & Cross, LA. (1969). Behavioral antecedents of schizophrenia: A review. *Archives of General Psychiatry, 21,* 167–283

Pick, A, Christy, M, & Frankel, G. (1972). A developmental study of visual selective attention. *Journal of Experimental Child Psychology, 14,* 165–175

Posner, MI. (1978). *Chronometric explorations of mind.* Hillsdale, NJ: Erlbaum

Rochester, SR. (1978). Are language disorders in acute schizophrenia actually information processing problems? In L Wynne, R Cromwell & S Matthysse (Eds.), *The nature of schizophrenia: New approaches to research and treatment.* New York: Wiley

Roth, WT, Horvath, TB, Pfefferbaum, A, & Kopell, BS. (1980). Event-related potentials in schizophrenics. *Electroencephalography and Clinical Neurophysiology, 48,* 127–139

Ruchkin, DS, Munson, R, & Sutton, S. (1982). P300 and slow wave in a message consisting of two events. *Psychophysiology, 19,* 629–642

Schneider, W, & Shiffrin, RM. (1977). Controlled and automatic human information processing: Detection, search and attention. *Psychological Review, 84,* 1–66

Strandburg, RJ, Marsh, JT, Brown, WS, Asarnow, RF, & Guthrie, D. (1984). Event-related potential concomitants of information processing dysfunction in schizophrenic children. *Electroencephalography and Clinical Neurophysiology, 57,* 236–253

Syndulko, C, & Lindsley, DB. (1977). Motor and sensory determinants of cortical slow potential shifts in man. In J Desmedt (Ed.), *Attention, voluntary contraction and event related cerebral potentials, progress in clinical neurophysiology* (Vol. 1) (pp. 97–131). Basel: Karger

Szymanski, LS. (1980). Psychiatric diagnosis of retarded persons. In LS Szymanski & PE Tanguay (Eds.), *Emotional disorders of mentally retarded persons.* Baltimore, MD: University Park Press

Venables, PH. (1964). Input dysfunction and schizophrenia. In BN Matter (Ed.), *Progress in experimental personality research* (Vol. 1). New York: Academic Press

Wechsler, D. (1974). *Manual for the Wechsler intelligence scale for children—Revised.* New York: The Psychological Corporation

Zahn-Waxler, C, Iannotti, R, & Chapman, M. (1982). Peers and prosocial development. In K Rubin & H Ross (Eds.), *Peer relationships and social skills in childhood.* New York: Springer-Verlag

Zajonc, RB. (1980). Feeling and thinking: Preferences need no inferences. *American Psychologist, 35,* 151–175

Steven Reiss

9

The Mentally Retarded, Emotionally Disturbed Adult

The consequences of emotional and behavioral disorders in mentally retarded people include placement in restrictive environments, unemployment, and intense suffering (e.g., Eyman, Dingman, & Sabagh, 1966; Eyman, O'Connor, Tarjan, & Justice, 1972; Greenspan & Shoultz, 1981; Peckham, 1951). For example, depression is associated with suffering and, in some mentally retarded adults, has led to alcoholism, prostitution, and suicide. Aggression and conduct disorders are among the most frequently cited problems in providing adequate services for mentally retarded citizens. Schizophrenia and schizoid personality processes lead to withdrawal from the interpersonal environment and significantly impair the individual's quality of life. In this chapter, we will consider these and other topics related to the mental health of mentally retarded adults.

Much of what is known about emotional disturbances in mentally retarded people is based on professional experience supplemented by occasional scientific study. The professional experiences reported in this chapter were obtained by cofounding an outpatient developmental disabilities mental health program at the University of Illinois at Chicago. Throughout this chapter, I shall refer to this clinic as the *Illinois-Chicago clinic*. The clinic was started in 1980 with funds provided by the Illinois Department of Mental Health and Developmental Disabilities and the Illinois Institute for Developmental Disabilities.

The Illinois-Chicago clinic has demonstrated a significant consumer demand for mental health services for mentally retarded people (Reiss & Trenn, 1984). In the first 27 months that new clients were accepted for services, the clinic received 274 referrals from 63 agencies, hospitals, schools, and state offices (Reiss & Trenn, 1984). The demand for services increased in virtually every month of the clinic's operation until service capacities were exceeded and new clients no longer could be accepted. To a large extent, the clinic functioned

CHILDREN WITH EMOTIONAL DISORDERS AND DEVELOPMENTAL DISABILITIES ISBN 0–8089–1700–5

as a professional support service for mentally retarded adolescents and adults living in community-based facilities. Approximately two thirds of the clients were between the ages of 15 and 29, and approximately two thirds of the referrals came from community-based facilities.

The clients of the Illinois-Chicago clinic have ranged in age from 6 to 55 years and in level of mental retardation from mild to severe. Reiss (1982) reported a survey of the first 66 clients to the clinic, and Benson (1985) reported a follow-up survey of the first 130 clients. In the Benson survey, 77 of the clients were adults aged 21 years or older, whereas 53 were children or adolescents. Of the 77 adults, 59.7 percent were mildly retarded, 27.3 percent were moderately retarded, and only 13.0 percent were severely retarded. The adult sample included 52 males and 24 females; the sample consisted of 40 whites, 33 blacks, and 4 Hispanics.

CLINICAL FEATURES

A distinction is made between emotional disturbances in people with mild and moderate mental retardation versus those with severe and profound mental retardation (Reid, 1980). In mentally retarded people with IQs above 50, the symptoms of emotional disturbances are essentially the same as those seen in people who are not mentally retarded (Szymanski & Tanguay, 1980). For example, the symptoms of depression are very similar in mildly retarded and nonretarded adults. In contrast, emotional disturbances in severely and profoundly retarded people often appear discontinuous with that seen in both mildly retarded and nonretarded people. In people with severe or profound mental retardation, the symptoms of emotional disturbances tend to be highly individualistic and frequently are accompanied by demonstrable brain pathology and other organic conditions (Eaton & Menolascino, 1982). These problems often are called behavioral disturbances.

The full range of emotional disturbance is found in mentally retarded adults. The disorders commonly seen in clinical practice are depression, schizophrenia, antisocial behavior, and personality problems such as a lack of self-confidence, problems in managing anger, nonassertiveness, and discomfort in social situations. The professional literature includes reports of mentally retarded people with manic-depressive illness (Reid, 1972a), phobia (Matson, 1981), anxiety neurosis (Reiss, 1982), and anorexia nervosa (Hurley & Sovner, 1979), although these disorders are not seen very often in clinical practice.

Depression

Depression is among the more prevalent emotional disorders seen in mentally retarded adults. In a survey of all people in New York State who were receiving services for developmental disabilities, Jacobson (1982) found evidence of depression in 6.2, 3.6, and 2.4 percent of mildly, moderately, and severely retarded adults. The disorder was reported for 10.4 percent of the mentally retarded adults living independently. In the Benson (1985) survey of the Illinois-Chicago clinic, depression accounted for 20.7 percent (n = 16) of the first 77 adult clients. The disorder was evident in 28.3 percent of 46 mildly retarded adults, 9.5 percent of 21 moderately retarded adults, and 10.0 percent of 10 severely retarded adults. Of the 16 depressed clients, 11 were female and 5 were male. At least for the samples that have been reported thus far, depression seems to be more likely in mildly than severely mentally retarded people and in females than males.

Many of the symptoms of depression are the same for mentally retarded and nonretarded people (Hurd, 1888; Matson, 1983a). This includes certain emotions (sadness, loneliness, guilt, and anger), cognitions and beliefs (self-blame, self-criticism, indecisiveness, negativity), and physical complaints (sleep disturbance, loss of appetite, diminished sex drive, tiredness, weight loss, constipation). However, there may be some differences between depression in mentally retarded versus nonretarded people. For example, our experience at the Illinois-Chicago clinic suggests that literally not knowing how to enjoy oneself can be a factor in the mood of some mentally retarded people (O'Neil, 1982). Thus, instructions in the skills necessary to participate in leisure activities may be a more important component of therapy for depression in mentally retarded than nonretarded people.

The initial research on the mental health aspects of mental retardation has concerned the topic of depression. The available evidence suggests that mildly mentally retarded adults can self-report depressive symptoms in a reasonably reliable and valid manner (Kazdin, Matson, & Senatore, 1983; Reiss & Benson, 1984a). Conventionally-accepted self-report scales, including the Zung Self-Rating Depression Scale and the Beck Depression Inventory, have been used successfully with mentally retarded adults. However, some mildly retarded adults, and many moderately retarded adults, have difficulty understanding some of the items on the conventional scales for depression. For this reason, Matson and colleagues have been working on the development of a self-report inventory especially tailored to the mentally retarded adult population (Kazdin et al, 1983).

Case Example

Joan P was a mildly mentally retarded, 35-year-old woman when she was referred to the Illinois-Chicago clinic by her sister. The sister reported that Joan seemed depressed, became upset easily, and refused to discuss her problems with the family. Joan was single and living with her parents and her brother Stanley. Her father was retired, her mother apparently never worked outside the home, and Stanley was a bachelor employed at a local industrial plant. Joan also had two sisters and one older brother, all of whom were married. With the exception of one sister, all of Joan's siblings graduated from high school, and one brother also graduated from college. Although Polish was the primary language spoken in the parents' home, Joan spoke English with her brothers, sisters, and caseworker.

Joan attended school for two years in Poland before moving to Chicago at age nine years. She was enrolled in two parochial schools during her elementary years in Chicago and then attended a public high school for approximately a year and a half. According to her sister, Joan was evaluated in eighth grade and was found to be a "slow learner" who was working at a fourth grade level. [The results of psychological testing at the Illinois-Chicago clinic indicated a full-scale WAIS-R IQ of 60.] Joan reported that she had dropped out of high school because she was doing poorly and could not handle the work.

Joan had been employed as a factory worker for ten years prior to being seen at the Illinois-Chicago clinic. About two years prior to the referral, she began taking classes to pass an examination for a General Equivalency Diploma. She had taken the test a few weeks prior to being seen at the Illinois-Chicago clinic and had scored only 156 points, with 225 being the minimum needed to pass.

The findings of the personality testing, as well as interview and observational data, suggested that Joan suffered from depression. She reported feeling tired most of the day and having difficulty falling asleep at night. Other indications of depression included bouts of crying and a poor appetite. She viewed herself as stupid and as different from other people, was quick to identify her faults and areas of deficiency, and tended to deny the importance of her good qualities. She apparently felt sad and lonely most of the time. She felt left out of family decisions, had no friends in the community, and had few hobbies other than needlepoint. Her primary interest was passing the equivalency examination and obtaining a high school diploma. She stated that she wanted a high school diploma in order to "finish high school like other people."

Although Joan usually was lethargic and despondent, she became agitated at times, particularly when discussing her family. She had strong feelings of anger toward her parents whom she blamed for not allowing her to finish high school. Joan also reported anger toward family members because they treated her like a child. For example, they frequently ignored her presence in family conversations, did not allow her to visit her cousin by herself because they feared she would get lost, and discouraged her from pursuing her studies for a high school diploma.*

The case of Joan is typical of the depressed clients seen at the Illinois-Chicago clinic. Most of the major symptoms of depression found in nonretarded people were evident in Joan's behavior. This includes sadness, crying bouts, dependency conflict, anger toward those who gratify dependency needs, self-blame and negative self-concept, loneliness, and sleep difficulties. The depression was associated with anger and hopelessness regarding the stigmatization of being a "slow learner." The depression also was associated with low levels of social support, an unrealistic life-goal (obtaining a high school diploma), and a lack of interesting activities and hobbies in daily life.

Schizophrenia

The confidence with which we can diagnose schizophrenia in mentally retarded people varies with the individual's level of intellectual functioning. For mildly and moderately mentally retarded adults, the consensus is that schizo-

* Case based on a psychological report by Maggi Musico Reiss.

phrenia can be identified as a distinct type of psychosis (Eaton & Menolascino, 1982; Reid, 1972b). For severely and profoundly mentally retarded people, however, it can be very difficult to differentiate between schizophrenia and other types of psychoses. In this regard, Herskovitz and Plesset (1941) have noted the special importance of deterioration in diagnosing schizophrenia in severely/profoundly retarded adults. A severely mentally retarded adult who has episodes of rage and smears feces should be considered psychotic only when these symptoms represent a deterioration from the individual's usual or premorbid behavior.

The prevalence of active psychosis among mentally retarded people appears to be low and may not be higher than the figure for the general population. The results of Jacobson's (1982) survey of developmentally disabled people in New York State revealed a prevalence rate of 2.2 percent for delusions and hallucinations and 3.8 percent for disorientation to time/place. This finding of a low prevalence rate is consistent with the impressions formed by this author while working on the topic of dual diagnosis in the State of Illinois. Although I am aware of scores of mentally retarded, psychotic adults residing in state institutions in the Chicago metropolitan area, the total number of such cases is only a small fraction of the population of mentally retarded people residing in the area.

Among mentally retarded adults, schizoid behavior is much more prevalent than active psychosis. The prominent symptoms of schizoid behavior in mentally retarded adults are social withdrawal (extreme shyness; discomfort in social situations; spending a lot of time alone), extreme sensitivity to criticism, and bizarre behavior. Affect may be flat (the individual is emotionally nonresponsive and rarely smiles) or inappropriate (for example, the individual may act silly).

Two possible differences between schizophrenia in mentally retarded and nonretarded people may be noted. One difference is that schizophrenic defenses are much less sophisticated in mentally retarded than nonretarded people. Whereas an intellectually average person with schizophrenia might try to escape from interpersonal anxiety by "tuning out" the conversation of the other person, the mentally retarded individual with schizophrenia might actually run away. Another apparent difference is that psychotic episodes in mentally retarded people seem to be precipitated by more ordinary and seemingly minor events. For example, not being allowed to go to a party precipitated a psychotic episode in one of the outpatients at the Illinois-Chicago clinic. An older brother temporarily returning home from college precipitated a schizophrenic episode in another Illinois-Chicago client.

Case Example

Mary was born prematurely as the only child of two achievement-oriented, black parents. Her father was a medical technician, and her mother was a psychiatric social worker. Because neither parent had the time to deal with the special demands of raising a mentally handicapped child, residential placement was sought when Mary was six. The parents had been described by social workers as being guilt ridden over their decision to place Mary in an institution.

Mary experienced a large number of transfers from one residential facility to another. She was placed in a state institution in Chicago at age 6, transferred to a private institution at age 8, and returned to live with her parents at age 11. She was placed in a Wisconsin institution at age 19, transferred to a community-based residential facility at age 20, and returned home at age 21. She then was placed in a state mental hospital, transferred to a nursing home, and transferred again to a community agency. Mary had lived in seven different residential facilities in the first 23 years of her life. This high degree of social disruption and implicit rejection may have contributed to the development of her emotional problems.

Mary was 23 years old when first seen at the Illinois-Chicago clinic. She was diagnosed as both mildly mentally retarded and schizophrenic. The presenting symptoms were inappropriate laughter and giggling, flat affect (she rarely smiled and usually showed no emotion), social withdrawal (she spent a lot of time alone and was difficult to engage in conversation), and bizarre behavior (she was intensely interested in other people's attire). She was brought to the clinic by her father who expressed concern that Mary's behavior was regressing and becoming increasingly immature.

Shortly after referral to the Illinois-Chicago clinic, Mary did not menstruate for two months, and the staff at the nursing home where she resided began asking her many questions about sexual activities. Under intense questioning and false suspicion of being pregnant, Mary began having paranoid outbursts, first falsely accusing a staff member of raping her, and then falsely accusing her father of seeking to have sexual intercourse with her. These outbursts are continuing as of this writing.

Antisocial Behavior

Antisocial behavior is one of the most prevalent psychological problems seen in mentally retarded people. In his survey of developmentally disabled people in New York State, Jacobson (1982) found that 5.5 percent, 8.5 percent, 13.9 percent and 17.3 percent of the mildly, moderately, severely, and profoundly mentally retarded people, respectively, were rated as showing physical aggression. Moreover, Benson (1985) found that antisocial behavior accounted for 20.8 percent of the adult referrals to the Illinois-Chicago clinic. These antisocial problems included physical aggression, lying, stealing, and starting fires. Antisocial behavior was diagnosed at the Illinois-Chicago clinic more frequently in males than in females and more in children and adolescents than in adults.

Case Example

Andy was a 22-year-old, mildly mentally retarded man of Puerto Rican origin who was adopted when he was two weeks old. He was described as being close to his mother during childhood. She died when Andy was 12, and his father remarried when he was 13. Andy did not get along with his stepmother as she would holler at him and criticize him.

Andy's behavioral problems began at age 15 years when he was a student attending special classes at a vocational high school. He began arriving late for school, and he occasionally had temper tantrums when in class. A series of suspensions was followed by dismissal from school when his behavior failed to improve. Since both parents worked and his brother attended school, Andy often was at home alone with nothing constructive to do. He had some boyfriends with whom he would play ball, but he had no girlfriends and had never been out on a date. His father told him to get a job, earn a living, and move out of the house.

Andy was very sensitive about being mentally retarded. He felt that he was not as smart as other people (his full scale WAIS IQ was 68), and it bothered him that he could not get a driver's license. He wanted to go to work and earn a living like "normal" people; he felt that his inability to get a job was a sign that he was not normal. He was concerned that other people might make fun of him because he was mentally retarded, and he presented a good physical appearance as part of his effort to look as normal as possible.

Andy coped with anxiety by running away, avoiding situations, and pretending. He often was late for school because he was afraid the other students would make fun of him. He stopped going to a vocational workshop program because it reminded him of his status as a mentally retarded person. He attended therapy irregularly because he did not want to discuss his behavior and deal with his problems. By the time he was seen at the Illinois-Chicago clinic, he was running away from home for periods of several days per incident.

Andy went to jail for eleven days when he was 21 years old because he tried to steal a suitcase at a bus depot. When asked why he did this, he lied and claimed that he was only trying to help a passenger with her luggage. He was arrested for shoplifting several months after his release from jail. He began stealing money from his father and making up tall stories to account for his having money. For example, he told the therapist the following story as to how he obtained $160. He claimed that his watch was stolen when he was in jail; when he later saw the person who stole it, he hit the person over the head with a rock and took $160 from him to pay for the watch. Andy later admitted that the story was fabricated and that he stole the money from his father.

Personality Disorders

The personality problems most commonly seen in mentally retarded people are nonassertiveness, problems with dependency, difficulties managing anger, and a negative self-concept. At the Illinois-Chicago clinic, we diagnose a personality disorder only when the personality problems are the primary or most salient psychological problem shown by the individual. Of the 77 adult outpatients in the Benson (1985) survey of the Illinois-Chicago clinic, 12 (15.6 percent) were diagnosed as having a personality disorder other than a schizoid disorder (which was grouped with schizophrenia) or antisocial personality disorder (which was grouped with antisocial behavior problem). All but one of the 12 clients diagnosed as having a personality disorder were mildly mentally retarded. In Eaton and Menolascino's (1982) survey of a Nebraska clinic, 21 of 58 adults (36.2 percent) were diagnosed as having a personality disorder other than a schizoid or antisocial personality disorder. Thus, personality disorders are among the problems seen most frequently in clinical practice with mildly mentally retarded adults.

Estimates of the prevalence of personality disorders among mentally retarded people have been extremely high. Craft (1959) found that 33 percent of the mentally retarded people in an English institution had a personality disorder. Webster (1970) suggested that virtually all mentally retarded people have a personality disorder. Philips (1967) reported that some disordered and/or delayed personality functioning could be found in virtually all of the mentally retarded children he examined. In the experience of this writer, a very large number of mildly mentally retarded people show personality adjustments to the stigmatization of mental retardation. Although the percentage of mildly mentally retarded people in whom these adjustments are severe enough to be considered a personality disorder is nowhere near the 100 percent figure, it is nevertheless very high.

The following case history shows some of the problems diagnosing personality disorders in mentally retarded people.

Case Example

Judy was a mildly mentally retarded, 19-year-old woman whose inappropriate behavior included running away from home, noncompliance, tantrums, and refusing to take insulin. The state administrators for mental health services claimed that Judy's behavioral problems were consequences of her immaturity and mental retardation; their view was that the state administrators for developmental disabilities were responsible for services for Judy. The state administrators for developmental disabilities claimed that Judy's behavioral problems were an emotional disturbance; their view was that the state administrators for mental health were responsible for services for Judy. Judy was referred to the Illinois-Chicago clinic for an opinion on whether her behavioral problems justified a diagnosis of emotional disturbance in addition to mental retardation.

Judy was identified as mentally retarded at age 6 years and spent her entire school career in special education classes. As a child, Judy showed no behavioral problems at school, was unusually compliant, and rarely expressed anger. The behavioral problems started about two years prior to the referral when it was discovered that Judy was diabetic and needed to take insulin on a daily basis. Judy began quarreling with her mother and started running away from home. On one occasion, she ran away from home, neglected to take her insulin, and had to be hospitalized when found by the police.

Judy was placed in a state mental institution pending diagnostic evaluation. During her stay at the state institution, she ran away to visit her boyfriend, called her boyfriend many times each day, refused to take insulin, and had angry outbursts. A diagnostician at the state institution felt that Judy's behavioral problems were the result of her mental retardation. His view was that her running away to an older man indicated emotional immaturity and a failure to understand the consequences of being involved in a relationship. He attributed both the running away and the angry outbursts to a childish impulsivity he associated with mental retardation.

The psychologist at the Illinois-Chicago clinic disagreed with this opinion for four reasons. First, when Judy was younger and presumably even more immature, she did not present any serious problems controlling her impulses. Second, Judy's behavior was atypical of mentally retarded people her age; for example, very few mildly mentally retarded people would endanger their lives by refusing to take medication. Third, in calm moments Judy could accurately report the probable consequences of her inappropriate behavior. Fourth, Judy's behavioral problems constituted an entire syndrome of abnormal behaviors usually identified as a borderline personality disturbance.

Judy's behavior expressed conflict concerning dependency issues. She ran away from home and called her boyfriend many times each day because she could not tolerate being alone. She became angry and noncompliant primarily when her dependency needs were frustrated. Her refusals to take insulin constituted a history of self-damaging acts. These symptoms suggest a diagnosis of borderline personality disturbance. This disorder is evident in some people who are highly intelligent, some who are intellectually average, and some who are mentally retarded. The diagnostician at the state facility erred in suggesting that these behaviors could be viewed as a natural consequence of mental retardation.*

Other Emotional Disturbances

Mentally retarded adults are vulnerable to the full range of emotional disturbances. In addition to depression, schizophrenia, antisocial behavior, and personality disorder, this includes anxiety disorders, phobias, drug abuse (including alcoholism), sexual dysfunctions, and dissociative states.

There appears to be very little consumer demand for the treatment of fears and phobias in mentally retarded people. Only three clients were treated for phobia during a two-year period at the Illinois-Chicago clinic. Only one mentally retarded person was diagnosed as having a phobia during a three-year period at the Nebraska clinic (Eaton & Menolascino, 1982). This weak demand for therapy for phobia is surprising. Phobia is one of the few topics relating to the mental health aspects of mental retardation that has received some research attention (Sternlicht, 1979), and it is one of the disorders that can be treated successfully (Matson, 1981). The small number of referrals for phobia could mean that debilitating phobias are relatively unusual in mentally retarded people. The prevalence of debilitating phobia among women in the general population is slightly more than 1 case per 200 people (Costello, 1982). Although fears are quite common in both mentally retarded and nonretarded people, apparently it is unusual for a mentally retarded person to be debilitated by a fear.

Behavioral Abnormalities

Mentally retarded people show a wide range of behavioral abnormalities that often appear to be related to neurologic disease. These problems are much more prevalent among severely and profoundly mentally retarded people than mildly retarded people. Examples of the abnormalities are stereotypes, hyper-

* Case based on a psychological report by Rolf A. Peterson.

activity, echolalia, self-injurious behavior, and extreme irritability. Efforts to diagnose these behaviors in terms of a psychosis or some other severe emotional problem should be treated very cautiously since the diagnoses often are difficult to substantiate.

Reid, Ballinger, and Heather (1978) performed a cluster analysis on the behavioral abnormalities shown by 100 severely and profoundly mentally retarded adults. Of the eight clusters summarized in their report, two were relatively free of disturbed behavior, one was indicated by hyperactivity, one by stereotypic behavior, and another by severe behavior management problems. The remaining clusters were much more interesting from the perspective of possible emotional problems. Cluster 6 comprised a group of seven older people who were socially and emotionally withdrawn. Cluster 7 consisted of nine people who appeared to have depressed mood, and cluster 8 consisted of seven people who were anxious, socially withdrawn, and seemingly paranoid. The results of this interesting study still need to be replicated on other samples of mentally retarded people before they can be accepted as valid.

PSYCHOLOGICAL FACTORS

Very little research has been reported on the possible psychosocial factors in the development of emotional disturbances in mentally retarded people. The literature in this area consists mostly of theoretical discussion supplemented by occasional scientific study. Because of the need for much more research, much of what is proposed here needs to be substantiated by future scientific research before it can be accepted as valid.

Negative Social Conditions

Some instances of psychopathology in mentally retarded people may be reactions to negative social conditions such as rejection, social disruption, and stigmatization (Reiss & Benson, 1984b). These negative social conditions presumably result from attitudes and public policy toward mental retardation and deviance. Many mildly and moderately mentally retarded people become aware of these negative social conditions (Reiss & Benson, 1984b), and this awareness may motivate a variety of abnormal reactions. The possible abnormal reactions include rebellion against the negative social conditions (antisocial behavior), beliefs that the situation is hopeless (depression), withdrawal into a fantasy world (schizophrenia), and efforts to alleviate the emotional suffering directly (drug abuse). Which of these reactions occurs may depend on the individual's habitual style of coping with stress and the coping behaviors that happen to be reinforcing in the individual's environment.

At least seven negative social conditions are commonly experienced by mentally retarded people. These conditions are the stigma of being labeled *mentally retarded*, rejection and ridicule, segregation from nonretarded people, social disruption, infantilization, restricted opportunities, and victimization. These conditions include experiences such as being called "dummy" by peers (rejection and ridicule), having a workshop job paying a few dollars per week instead of a meaningful job paying minimum wage or more (segregation, restricted opportunities), and often being relocated from one residential facility to another (social disruption). The prolonged exposure to one or more of these negative social conditions may increase significantly the risk of emotional disturbance.

The possible importance of negative social conditions in the development of abnormal behavior is suggested by the high degree of awareness mentally retarded adults have of the stigmatization in their lives (Reiss & Benson, 1984b). This was exemplified in the case histories presented earlier in this chapter. For example, Joan expressed resentment toward her family because they treated her like a child, Mary recalled seven different residential placements by age 23, and Andy related in detail how he became angry at anything that reminded him of his status as a mentally retarded person.

We need only imagine life through the eyes of a mentally retarded person subjected to these negative social conditions to appreciate the potential for the development of emotional disturbances. Mentally retarded people are treated as objects to be avoided. They rarely are asked to express their opinions because other people erroneously assume that they are not smart enough to have opinions. Mentally retarded people have difficulty finding friends when they live at home and other mentally handicapped people do not live nearby. Although it often is assumed that low intelligence plays a significant role in the development of emotional disturbances in mentally retarded people, the emotional disturbances shown by mentally retarded people are very similar to what we should expect to see if a group of nonretarded people were subjected to negative social conditions for long periods of time.

Inadequate Social Support

Inadequate social support from significant others may be an important factor in the development of emotional problems in mentally retarded people. The mere presence of significant others can be anxiety-reducing and can increase tolerance for stress. Significant others also can help find solutions to difficult psychological problems and provide an objective appraisal of a situation. Unfortunately, mentally retarded people seem to have inadequate access to social support networks. Many mentally retarded children are separated from their parents and raised in community residences or state institutions. Some do not have an adequate opportunity to marry and/or to develop a close personal relationship with a member of the opposite sex. Mentally retarded adults living at home may have restricted opportunities for making friends if other mentally retarded people do not live nearby. Thus, some mentally retarded people may be forced to solve emotional problems without adequate emotional support from significant others.

The Reiss-Peterson Social Support Scale for Mentally Retarded Adults is a self-report instrument designed to measure the degree of social support available to mentally retarded adults. The scale is divided into two parts. In Part 1, the subject can identify up to seven significant others (spouse, mother, father, two family members with whom he/she gets along best, and two best friends). In Part 2, an interviewer asks the subject four questions about each of the individuals identified in Part 1. The questions are, How often do you see [name]? How often do you talk to [name] about your feelings? How much do you like [name]? and, How much does [name] help you with your problems? The Reiss-Peterson scale has a significant degree of test/retest reliability and is significantly correlated with informant ratings of social support.

Reiss and Benson (1985) and Schloss (1982) have obtained evidence relating inadequate levels of social support to depression in mentally retarded adults. The association between depression and low levels of social support is so strong that one is tempted to propose that depression is both a consequence and a cause of low levels of social support. Loneliness, the lack of intimate relationships, and the absence of other sources of social support, all may be important factors in depression in mentally retarded adults.

Deficient Social Skills

Deficiencies in social skills may be both causes and consequences of emotional disturbances in mentally retarded people. Deficiencies in social skills may cause emotional problems by increasing the person's exposure to negative social conditions such as social isolation, segregation, and unemployment (Greenspan & Shoultz, 1981). Deficiencies in social skills also may be consequences of emotional disturbances. For example, emotional problems may interfere directly with the performance of social behavior as in the case of an individual who is too nervous, self-centered, or depressed for socially adequate conversation.

Although the related topics of social intelligence, social competence, and social skills recently have received some attention from researchers in developmental psychology and in behavior modification (Greenspan, 1979; Gresham, 1981), very little attention has been paid to the possible role of deficiencies in social skills in the development of emotional problems in mentally retarded people. Virtually the only work in this area is clinical case reports of successful treatment outcomes of emotional problems by improving social skills. Much more research is needed.

At least three specific social skill deficiencies have been discussed as possibly relevant to the development of emotional problems in mentally retarded people. Perhaps the most important of these are deficiencies in social problem solving (Goldstein, 1977). Many mentally retarded people are deficient in generating appropriate solutions to everyday social problems. This suggests that interpersonal problems may remain unresolved and stressful for long periods of time, and this could increase the risk of an emotional disturbance. This consideration also suggests that mentally retarded people may be more likely to have chronic emotional disturbances than nonretarded people. Improving social problem solving skills and increasing social understanding may be an especially important component of therapy with mentally retarded adults.

Another social skill deficiency especially relevant to mental retardation is inappropriate assertiveness (Gentile & Jenkins, 1980; Ruderman, McNally, Levitan, & O'Neil, 1982). As noted previously, problems with dependency are common among mentally retarded people. Sometimes the problem is a lack of assertiveness and a tendency to be taken advantage of by others. Other times the problem is asserting oneself in ways that are hostile and offensive. In both cases, the lack of appropriate assertion skills is an important component of the individual's inadequate social adjustment.

Another noteworthy social deficiency is inadequate leisure skills or literally not knowing how to enjoy oneself (O'Neil, 1982). Training in appropriate leisure skills may be an important part of therapy with some depressed, mentally retarded adults (Adkins & Matson, 1980).

Interaction of Emotional and Intellectual Handicaps

Emotional and intellectual handicaps may interact so that mentally retarded people may be disabled by less severe and more ordinary problems than nonretarded people. For example, if the social/emotional adjustments of mentally retarded people tend to be more marginal than those of nonretarded people, mentally retarded people might be less able than nonretarded people to cope with stress and anxiety. Whereas very high levels of stress and anxiety must be present before emotional disturbances occur in nonretarded people, the presence of much lower levels of anxiety may be sufficient to cause an emotional disturbance in some mentally retarded people. In other words, the threshold for debilitation from an emotional problem may be much lower for mentally retarded than nonretarded people.

ISSUES RELEVANT TO SERVICE DELIVERY

Emotionally disturbed, mentally retarded people constitute an underserved population insofar as mental health services are concerned (Reiss, Levitan, & McNally, 1982). On the one hand, the presence of mental retardation seems to increase vulnerability to emotional disturbances. On the other hand, the presence of mental retardation decreases the opportunity for mental health services. Consequently, there is a need to increase significantly the supply of mental health services for mentally retarded people.

Prevalence

Our knowledge of the prevalence of emotional disturbances among mentally retarded people can be summarized as follows. First, the true prevalence of emotional disturbances among mentally retarded people is unknown. Although estimates vary considerably from one another, a conservative estimate is that between 15 and 20 percent of all mentally retarded adults also are emotionally disturbed. Second, under conditions of stress, mentally retarded people are much more likely than nonretarded people to develop emotional and behavioral problems. Third, emotional problems are probably more prevalent among mentally retarded than nonretarded people.

Prevalence Estimates

Although a few prevalence estimates for emotional disturbances among mentally retarded people have been very high or low (Grouse, Kessler, Pully, Avellar, Biskin, Payne, & Ahr, 1982; Webster, 1970), a conservative estimate would be that between 10 and 15 percent of all mentally retarded children and between 15 and 20 percent of all mentally retarded adults are also emotionally disturbed. For example, a recent survey of a community-based program for mentally retarded people in the Omaha, Nebraska area found that 14.3 percent of the mentally retarded people referred to the program also were emotionally disturbed (Eaton & Menolascino, 1982). In Jacobson's (1982) survey of 30,578 individuals receiving developmental disabilities services in New York State, 12.4 percent of the adults and 9.8 percent of the children were classified as both emotionally disturbed and mentally retarded. The rate for mildly mentally retarded adults was 17.7 percent. There are two reasons for regarding the Jacobson figures as underestimates of the true prevalence rates. First, the survey excluded certain types of emotional disturbances such as phobias and drug abuse. Second, portions of the results are implausible and suggest bias on the part of the raters of abnormal behavior. For example, the survey found that 3.1 percent of the mentally retarded people living at home were depressed compared to 10.4 percent of those living independently. This very large difference is difficult to accept on theoretical grounds and is inconsistent with our experience with depressed clients at the Illinois-Chicago clinic. Perhaps the difference reflects a discrepancy in the way in which information was obtained from the home and independent living environments so that the estimate for the home environment is too low.

Unpublished data obtained by the author from the Illinois State Board of Education are consistent with the Jacobson findings regarding children. Almost all mentally retarded children enrolled in special education classes in the State of Illinois during the school year 1980-81 were evaluated by school psychologists as part of the data included in the Individualized Education Programs. The evaluation results revealed that 188 of 1116 children identified as educable mentally handicapped (mildly mentally retarded) also had a behavioral disturbance, compared with 388 of 4521 children identified as trainable mentally handicapped. Thus, the prevalence estimates for behavioral disturbance were 16.8 percent for mildly mentally retarded school children and 8.6 percent for moderately mentally retarded school children. These are probably low estimates because school psychologists generally are suspected of tending not to make multiple diagnoses (Reiss, Levitan, & Szyszko, 1982).

Many more mentally retarded people need mental health services than those counted as "emotionally disturbed." The 15 to 20 percent range does not include people with problems such as a negative self-concept, deficient social skills, and many types of personality problems. Moreover, the percentage of mentally retarded who may develop an emotional disturbance sometime during their lives may be much higher than the percentage who are emotionally disturbed at any particular point in time.

Stress Conditions Effects

Because the incidence of emotional disturbances increase significantly under conditions of stress, the true vulnerability of the mentally retarded adult to emotional disorders would not necessarily be evident even if we could validly survey all mentally retarded people in the world. Such a survey might not provide information as to how mentally retarded people might function under less protected and/or different circumstances. For example, a mentally retarded person who cannot tolerate frustration may be likely over time to be placed in an environment relatively free of frustration in an effort to prevent behavioral outbursts. The person would not appear to be emotionally disturbed in the protected environment even though emotional problems would become evident in other environments.

The results of two studies support professional observations that mentally retarded people have much more difficulty than nonretarded people in coping with stress. Dewan (1948) reported a survey of 30,247 men tested for induction into the Canadian army. Emotional instability was found in 47.7 percent of the mentally retarded people and 19.7 percent of the nonretarded recruits. Weaver (1946) surveyed 8000 people with IQs below 75 who were inducted into the United States army during World War II and found that 44 percent of the men and 38 percent of the women developed psychiatric symptoms or committed repeated acts of misconduct. These data suggest that a large percentage of mentally retarded people have difficulty handling stressful situations such as an army induction or being in the army during time of war. Moreover, the results suggest that when large and relatively unbiased samples of mentally retarded and nonretarded people are compared under conditions of stress, emotional and behavioral problems are much more common among the mentally retarded than the nonretarded groups.

Diagnostic Overshadowing

Although many mentally retarded people suffer from an emotional problem requiring treatment, these people have limited access to mental health services. One possible reason for this is suggested by the experimental phenomenon called diagnostic overshadowing (Reiss, Levitan, & Szyszko, 1982). This term refers to instances in which the presence of mental retardation decreases the diagnostic significance of an accompanying emotional disorder. For example, psychologists tend to rate the same case description of schizophrenia lower on scales of psychopathology when the individual is mentally retarded versus nonretarded. As of this writing, four experimental demonstrations of the phenomenon have been reported in a series of three articles.

The first two experiments on diagnostic overshadowing established the basic finding and provided evidence of generality across measures and categories of psychopathology. The methodology of Experiment 1 presented a case description of a debilitating fear to three groups of psychologists. The groups differed only in terms of the information that was added to the case description of the debilitating fear. One group rated the fear for an individual who was suggested to be mentally retarded, another group rated the same fear for an individual who was suggested to be an alcoholic, and a third group rated the fear for an individual who was suggested to have average intelligence. The results indicated that the same debilitating fear was less likely to be considered an example of a neurosis or an emotional disturbance when the subject was suggested to be mentally retarded as compared to intellectually average. In other words, the presence of mental retardation overshadowed the diagnostic significance of an accompanying abnormal behavior usually considered indicative of an emotional disturbance.

The results of Experiment 2 extended findings of diagnostic overshadowing to cases involving schizophrenia and personality disorder. Clinical and school psychologists rated the same case descriptions of schizophrenia and avoidant personality disorder as less indicative of schizophrenia, a personality disorder, a psychotic disorder, a neurotic disorder, an emotional disturbance, a thought disorder, and a disorder needing long-term psychotherapy, when the individual was suggested to be mentally retarded as opposed to intellectually average.

Experiment 3 evaluated the role of professional experience with mentally retarded people in the occurrence of diagnostic overshadowing (Reiss & Szyszko, 1983). In a 3 × 2 factorial experiment, psychologists at state developmental disabilities facilities (High Experience Group), state mental health facilities (Moderate Experience Group), and clinical graduate students (Low Experience Group) rated a case description of schizophrenia on 11 scales of psychopathology. Half of the subjects within each group were presented with information suggesting mental retardation in addition to schizophrenia; the client was described as intellectually average for the remaining subjects. The results indicated that diagnostic overshadowing occurred for groups with a high, moderate, and low degree of professional contact with mentally retarded people. In other words, the total amount of professional experience with mentally retarded people was not related to diagnostic overshadowing.

Experiment 4 demonstrated the generality of diagnostic overshadowing across professional disciplines (Levitan & Reiss, 1983). The subjects in this experiment were advanced graduate students in psychology and social work. The results indicated that the same disabling fear was rated as less neurotic, less irrational, and less likely to require desensitization therapy for a client who was mentally retarded versus a client with average intelligence. There were no significant differences in the ratings of the students in clinical psychology versus social work.

An evaluation of the practical implications of diagnostic overshadowing should take into consideration the nature of the decision-making process relevant to the delivery of a publicly-supported mental health service. As we noted in Reiss and Szyszko (1983),

> Service delivery typically requires an interdisciplinary staffing leading to a diagnosis of an emotional problem and a recommendation for treatment, a case manager who acts on the recommendation, state administrators who recognize the emotional aspects of mental retardation to be sufficiently important to fund appropriate services, and community clinics capable of providing the relevant services. If overshadowing is interpreted as a tendency to view emotional problems in mentally retarded people as less important than they really are, the phenomenon can influence the delivery of services at any of a variety of points in the case management process. For example, even in instances in which a diagnosis and treatment recommendation are made, the service might not be delivered if the case manager assumes that the recommendation for psychotherapy is less important than the recommendation for other services (p. 401, with permission*).

Disputed Ownership

Another reason for the inadequate level of mental health services for mentally retarded people is the absence of administrative ownership of the issue. Historically, state and federal services for mentally retarded people were administered by mental health professionals who were primarily interested in helping mentally ill people. Mentally retarded people did not get their fair share of the service dollar, and advocates demanded that the administration of services for mental retardation be separated from the administration of services for mental health. Although this separation generally has benefited mentally retarded people, one disadvantage has been the inadequate level of mental health services for mentally retarded people. The mentally retarded, emotionally

---

* From Reiss S & Szyszko J. (1983). Diagnostic overshadowing and professional experience with retarded persons. *American Journal of Mental Deficiency, 87,* 396–402, with permission.

disturbed individual now falls through a gap in the service system between mental health centers serving mentally ill people and developmental centers serving mentally retarded people.

The problem of disputed ownership has been particularly severe in states in which administrators actively plan ways of avoiding responsibility for the issue. The mental health administrators do not perceive themselves as owning the problem because the clients being served are mentally retarded. These administrators believe that the administrators for developmental disabilities should fund mental health services for mentally retarded people. The administrators for developmental disabilities have argued that mentally retarded people should have access to the same community services as anyone else. Accordingly, these administrators believe that the community mental health centers should provide mental health services for mentally retarded people. The result of the dispute has been a stalemate in which neither group of administrators is funding a minimally adequate level of services. Consequently, the dually diagnosed population constitutes one of the most underserved in the United States from the perspective of mental health services (Reiss, Levitan, & McNally, 1982).

Appropriateness of Therapy

Another obstacle to increasing the supply of mental health services for mentally retarded people has been the assumption that psychotherapy is ineffective with this population (Fine, 1965). This assumption was based on clinical impressions of unsuccessful outcomes with insight-oriented therapy during the 1940s and 1950s (Colby, 1951; Fenichel, 1945; Healy & Bronner, 1939). Not surprisingly, both psychoanalysis and client-centered therapy as traditionally practiced did not seem to work with mentally retarded people who appeared to lack the intelligence necessary to discuss their problems in psychodynamic concepts. Although many other therapies have been tried successfully with mentally retarded people, the general impression that these people are unsuited for psychotherapy has remained influential even though it is invalid.

Almost all therapies except the insight-oriented approaches are appropriate for mildly mentally retarded adults. This includes supportive psychotherapy (Fine, 1965), group psychotherapy (Szymanski & Rosefsky, 1980), assertion and social skill training (Matson & Adkins, 1980), reinforcement therapy (Matson, 1983b), and drug therapy (Breuning, Davis, & Poling, 1982). The primary treatment alternatives for severely mentally retarded adults are reinforcement therapy, drug therapy, activity therapy, and Prouty's (1976) pretherapy. Which therapy should be offered depends on the skills of the therapist, the client's level of functioning, and the type of emotional disturbance being treated.

An important program for training anger management skills has been reported (Benson, Johnson, & Miranti, 1984). The treatment package includes training mentally retarded people to identify problem situations, training appropriate self-talk to cope with anger, and relaxation training. This work is demonstrating that some techniques of cognitive–behavior therapy can be adapted for use with mentally retarded adults.

The professional literature includes numerous case reports of successful outcomes in therapy with mentally retarded people and several controlled studies suggesting positive outcomes (Matson, 1981; Menolascino, 1970; Silvestri, 1977; Szymanski & Tanguay, 1980). The assumption that the emotional problems of mentally retarded people cannot be treated successfully is inconsistent with the experience of a large number of therapists. This experience supports the need to increase mental health services for mentally retarded people.

Service Programs

Recent interest in the mental health aspects of mental retardation has stimulated the development of a number of service models (Holmes, 1984). These models include mental health as a component of early diagnostic and treatment programs (Menolascino, 1965; Philips & Williams, 1975), community-based day programming (Smull, Fabian, & Shanteau, in press), residential units in state institutions (Charlton & Ziegelman, 1982), and outpatient community mental health clinics (Benson, 1985; Reiss, 1982). Each of these models serves a different clientele and potentially is an important component of a total system for providing mental health services for mentally retarded adults.

One type of service model is the special unit for dually diagnosed persons in state institutions. The goal of these units varies somewhat across the U.S. Some units are intended primarily for the purposes of providing a residential environment for the stabilization and observation of individuals whose behavior has become psychotic and/or out of control. Other units, such as Fran Cella's pioneering program at Elgin State Mental Health Hospital in Illinois, are treatment-oriented and provide extensive rehabilitative services. The special inpatient unit for the dually diagnosed is needed to help the individual who is both mentally retarded and severely emotionally disturbed.

Another type of service model is the outpatient developmental disabilities mental health clinic demonstrated at the University of Illinois at Chicago (Reiss & Trenn, 1984). This model provides professional support services for community-based facilities serving mentally retarded people; hence, the model is especially relevant in places where the goal is to help mentally retarded people adjust to the community. As has been noted previously, the Illinois-Chicago clinic has demonstrated a significant degree of previously unmet consumer demand for outpatient mental health services for mentally retarded people.

Although it will take years before a minimally adequate level of services can be put into place, some progress has been made in recent years. The mental health needs of mentally retarded people are receiving much more attention than was the case in the past. Let us hope that this progress will continue.

REFERENCES

Adkins, J, & Matson, JL. (1980). Teaching institutional mentally retarded adults socially appropriate leisure skills. *Mental Retardation, 18,* 249–252

Benson, BA. (1985). Behavior disorder and mental retardation: Association with age, sex, and levels of functioning in an outpatient clinic sample. *Applied Research in Mental Retardation*

Benson, BA, Johnson, C, Miranti, SV. (1984). *Effects of anger management training with mentally retarded adults.* Paper presented at the 17th Annual Gatlinburg Conference on Research in Mental Retardation and Developmental Disabilities

Breuning, SE, Davis VJ, & Poling, AD. (1982). Pharmacotherapy with the mentally retarded: Implications for clinical psychologists. *Clinical Psychology Review, 2,* 79–114

Charlton, M, & Ziegelman, M. (August, 1982). *A treatment program for dual diagnosed adolescent residents.* Paper presented at the annual convention of the American Psychological Association, Washington, DC

Colby, KM. (1951). *A primer for psychotherapists.* New York: Ronald Press

Costello, CG. (1982). Fears and phobias in women: A community study. *Journal of Abnormal Psychology, 91,* 280–286

Craft, M. (1959). Mental disorder in the defective: A psychiatric survey of in-patients. *American Journal of Mental Deficiency, 63,* 829–834

Dewan, JG. (1948). Intelligence and emotional stability. *American Journal of Psychiatry, 104,* 548–554.

Eaton, LF, & Menolascino, FJ. (1982). Psychiatric disorders in the mentally retarded: Types, problems, and challenges. *American Journal of Psychiatry, 139,* 1297–1303

Eyman, RK, Dingman, HF, & Sabagh, G. (1966). Association of characteristics of retarded patients and their families with speed of institutionalization. *American Journal of Mental Deficiency, 71,* 93–99

Eyman, RK, O'Connor, G, Tarjan, G, & Justice, RS. (1972). Factors determining residential placement of mentally retarded children. *American Journal of Mental Deficiency, 76,* 692–698

Fenichel, O. (1945). *The psychoanalytic theory of neurosis.* New York: Norton

Fine, RH. (1965). Psychotherapy with the mentally retarded adolescent. *Current Psychiatric Therapies, 5,* 58–66

Gentile, C, & Jenkins, JO. (1980). Assertive training with mildly mentally retarded persons. *Mental Retardation, 18,* 315–317

Goldstein, H. (1977). Reasoning abilities of mildly retarded children. In P Mittler (Ed.), *Research to practice in mental retardation: Education and training* (vol. 2). Baltimore: University Park Press

Greenspan, S. (1979). Social intelligence in the retarded. In NR Ellis (Ed.), *Handbook of mental deficiency: Psychological theory and research.* (2nd ed). New York: Erlbaum, pp. 483–531

Greenspan, S, & Shoultz, B. (1981). Why mentally retarded adults lose their jobs: Social competence as a factor in work adjustment. *Applied Research in Mental Retardation, 2,* 23–38

Gresham, FM. (1981). Social skills training with handicapped children: A review. *Review of Educational Research, 51,* 139–176

Grouse, AS, Kessler, BL, Pully, EN, Avellar, JW, Biskin, DS, Payne, D, & Ahr, PR. (May, 1982). *Dual diagnosis: Fact or fiction.* Paper presented at the annual convention of the American Association of Mental Deficiency

Healy, W, & Bronner, AF. (1939). *Treatment and what happened afterward.* Boston: Judge Baker Guidance Center

Herskovitz, H, & Plesset, MR. (1941). Psychoses in adult mental defectives. *Psychiatric Quarterly, 15,* 574–588

Holmes, PA. (1984, December). *Final report dual diagnosis program study: Mr/mi state-of-the-art service delivery.* Report to the Developmental Disabilities Planning Council, Project No. 2050, State of Michigan

Hurd, HM. (1888). Imbecility with insanity. *American Journal of Insanity, 45,* 261–269

Hurley, AD, & Sovner, R. (1979). Anorexia nervosa and mental retardation: A case report. *Journal of Clinical Psychiatry, 40,* 480–482.

Jacobson, JW. (1982). Problem behavior and psychiatric impairment within a developmentally disabled population. I. Behavior frequency. *Applied Research in Mental Retardation, 3,* 121–140

Kazdin, AE, Matson, JL, & Senatore, MSW. (1983). Assessment of depression in mentally retarded adults. *American Journal of Psychiatry, 140,* 1040–1043

Levitan, GW, & Reiss, S. (1983). Generality of diagnostic overshadowing across disciplines. *Applied Research in Mental Retardation, 4,* 59–64

Matson, JL. (1981). A controlled outcome study of phobias in mentally retarded adults. *Behaviour Research & Therapy, 19,* 101–108

Matson, JL. (1983a). Depression in the mentally retarded: Toward a conceptual analysis of diagnosis. In M Hersen, R Eisler, & PN Miller (Eds.), *Progress in behavior modification.* New York: Academic Press

Matson, JL. (1983b). The treatment of behavioral characteristics of depression in the mentally retarded. *Behavior Therapy, 13,* 209–218

Matson, JL, & Adkins, J. (1980). A self-instructional social skills training program for mentally retarded persons. *Mental Retardation, 18,* 245–248

Matson, JL, DiLorenzo, TM, & Adraskik FA. (1983). A review of behavior modification procedures for treating social skill deficits and psychiatric disorders of the mentally retarded. In JL Matson & F Andrasik (Eds.), *Treatment issues and innovations in mental retardation.* New York: Palladium

Menolascino, FJ. (1965). Emotional disturbance and mental retardation. *American Journal of Mental Deficiency, 70,* 248–256

Menolascino, FJ. (1970). *Psychiatric approaches to mental retardation.* New York: Basic Books

O'Neil, M. (August, 1982). *Depression and mental retardation.* Paper presented at the annual convention of the American Psychological Association, Washington, DC

Peckham, RA. (1951). Problems in job adjustment of the mentally retarded. *American Journal of Mental Deficiency, 56,* 448–453

Philips, I. (1967). Psychopathology and mental retardation. *American Journal of Psychiatry, 124,* 29–35

Philips, I, & Williams, N. (1975). Psychopathology and mental retardation. I. Psychopathology. *American Journal of Psychiatry, 132,* 1265–1271

Prouty, G. (1976). Pre-therapy—A method of treating preexpressive psychotic and retarded patients. *Psychotherapy: Theory, Research and Practice, 13,* 290–294

Reid, AH. (1972a). Psychoses in adult mental defectives. I. Manic depressive psychoses. *British Journal of Psychiatry, 120,* 205–212

Reid, AH. (1972b). Psychoses in adult mental defectives. II. Schizophrenic and paranoid psychoses. *British Journal of Psychiatry, 120,* 213–218

Reid, AH. (1980). Diagnosis of psychiatric disorder in the severely and profoundly retarded patient. *Journal of the Royal Society of Medicine, 73,* 607–609

Reid, AH, Ballinger, BR, & Heather, BB. (1978). Behavioural syndromes identified by cluster analysis in a sample of 100 severely and profoundly retarded adults. *Psychological Medicine, 8,* 399–412

Reiss, S. (1982). Psychopathology and mental retardation: Survey of a developmental disabilities mental health program. *Mental Retardation, 20,* 128–132

Reiss, S, & Benson, BA. (March, 1984a). *Stability and measurement of depression in mentally retarded adults.* Paper presented at the 17th Annual Gatlinburg Conference on Research in Mental Retardation and Developmental Disabilities

Reiss, S, & Benson, BA. (1984b). Awareness of negative social conditions among mentally retarded, emotionally disturbed outpatients. *American Journal of Psychiatry, 141,* 88–90

Reiss, S, & Benson, BA. (1985). Psychosocial correlates of depression in mentally retarded people. I. Minimal social support and stigmatization. *American Journal of Mental Deficiency, 89,* 331–337

Reiss, S, Levitan, G, & McNally, R. (1982). Emotionally disturbed, mentally retarded people: An underserved population. *American Psychologist, 37,* 361–367

Reiss, S, Levitan, G, & Szyszko, J. (1982). Emotional disturbance and mental retardation: Diagnostic overshadowing. *American Journal of Mental Deficiency, 86,* 567–574

Reiss, S, & Szyszko, J. (1983). Diagnostic overshadowing and professional experience with retarded persons. *American Journal of Mental Deficiency, 87,* 396–402

Reiss, S, & Trenn, E. (1984). Consumer demand for outpatient mental health services for mentally retarded people. *Mental Retardation, 22,* 112–115

Ruderman, AJ, McNally, RJ, Levitan, GW, & O'Neil, M. (May, 1982). *Effects of social skills training on vocational adjustment of mentally retarded people.* Paper presented at the convention of the American Association on Mental Deficiency, Boston

Schloss, PJ. (1982). Verbal interaction patterns of depressed and nondepressed institutionalized mentally retarded adults. *Applied Research in Mental Retardation, 3,* 1–12

Silvestri, R. (1977). Implosive therapy treatment of emotionally disturbed retardates. *Journal of Consulting and Clinical Psychology, 45,* 14–22

Smull, MW, Fabian, EF, & Shanteau, FB. (in press). A special program for mentally retarded/mentally ill citizens: The Rock Creek Foundation. In FJ Menolascino & J Stark (Eds.), *The handbook of mental illness in the mentally retarded.* New York: Plenum

Sternlicht, M. (1979). Fears of institutionalized mentally retarded adults. *The Journal of Psychology, 101,* 67–71

Szymanski, LS, & Rosefsky, QB. (1980). Group psychotherapy with retarded persons. In LS Szymanski & PE Tanguay (Eds.), *Emotional disorders of mentally retarded persons.* Baltimore: University Park Press

Szymanski, LS, & Tanguay, PE. (1980). *Emotional disorders of mentally retarded persons.* Baltimore: University Park Press

Weaver, TR. (1946). The incident of maladjustment among mental defectives in military environment. *American Journal of Mental Deficiency, 51,* 238–246

Webster, TG. (1970). Unique aspects of emotional development in mentally retarded children. In FJ Menolascino (Ed.), *Psychiatric approaches to mental retardation.* New York: Basic Books

SECTION III

Assessment and Treatment of the Child with Dual Disabilities

The last section of this volume reviews assessment and treatment procedures used with emotionally disturbed, mentally retarded children and adolescents. Methods of assessing level of cognitive functioning and the nature and severity of emotional disorders are presented. The issue of diagnosis of mentally retarded individuals is introduced as a prelude to the discussion of treatment approaches. Chapter 15 focuses on family issues related to mental retardation and the use of family therapy for the prevention and amelioration of emotional disorders in mentally retarded individuals.

Mary J. O'Connor

10

Cognitive Assessment of the Dual Diagnosis Young Child

The seriousness of the job of psychological assessment of the child cannot be overemphasized. Often practitioners are asked to see a child for the child's first assessment and find themselves in the sensitive position of being the first to convey information to the parents about the child's development. Once the assessment and parent feedback process is over, psychologists may also be asked to provide recommendations for future treatment or intervention. The psychologist's job becomes even more difficult when a child is not only retarded but also has severe behavioral or emotional problems.

For these reasons, the psychological assessment of a child should provide an accurate and optimal picture of the child's functioning. In addition, care should be taken to see the child more than once in order to examine the reliability of the child's performance and the test instruments used in assessment. The psychologist should be thoroughly familiar with the strengths and limitations of the test measures employed in assessing children. All too often, tests with poor or inadequate psychometric properties are used to assess children who are difficult to test, simply because the tests are short and easy to administer. Unfortunately, it has been our experience that the diagnosis of mental retardation or normality has been made by practitioners using a single measure such as the Leiter Test of International Performance or the Peabody Picture Vocabulary Test. Although the test authors warn against such overgeneralization from their tests, many practitioners ignore these warnings when testing difficult-to-test mentally retarded youngsters. In reviewing records of previous psychological evaluations received by our inpatients at NPI, it is our

CHILDREN WITH EMOTIONAL DISORDERS AND DEVELOPMENTAL DISABILITIES ISBN 0–8089–1700–5

impression that the use of inadequate assessment tools is more prevalent when a behaviorally disordered mentally retarded child is evaluated. It is also apparent that the more difficult the child is to test, the more inclined the examiner is to ignore the test scores obtained and to speculate that the child is of average intelligence if it could only be measured. The rationale behind this kind of conclusion is faulty and all too often does a disservice to a child desperately in need of special services.

Sometimes an examiner will administer tests with less than adequate psychometric properties simply because, for certain children at certain levels of developmental functioning, there is nothing better available. A skillful practitioner, with an adequate understanding of his or her test tools, can provide useful information about the child providing the results are interpreted conservatively and serve as a description of the child's actual behavior so that interventions can be planned.

The purpose of this chapter is to familiarize the reader with tests and techniques for testing mentally retarded youngsters who also manifest severe emotional or behavioral problems. The chapter begins with a survey of tests including test descriptions and comments on limitations and strengths of each test. Methods for testing dual diagnosis children are presented along with common misconceptions regarding diagnosis and assessment of these very special youngsters.

The discussion will focus on tests that we use at the UCLA Neuropsychiatric Institute to assess the psychological functioning of children in our care. The reader will note that some tests with which they may be familiar are omitted. Our rationale for discussion of tests we currently use is that clinical practice has shown these tests to be the most useful, valid, and reliable in assessing our population. Years of experience has gone into choosing these particular tests, although the shortcomings of each are also recognized. Tests will be described along with a discussion of reliability and validity. Suggestions as to the appropriate tests for various clinical populations will be made. In general, screening tools and measures used for specific language evaluation are not included in this discussion although they are often used when assessing our patients.

MEASURES USED TO ASSESS DUAL DIAGNOSIS CHILDREN

Intelligence Tests

Probably the most valuable and the most psychometrically sound tests available today are those that measure intelligence. It is also these tests that are of unique importance to the psychologist whose job it is to assess the cognitive functioning of the retarded child.

Currently, there is much debate concerning the advisability of using intelligence tests to classify children, particularly minority children (Sattler, 1982). While many arguments presented are valid, critics of intelligence tests fail to consider that these tests have many practical uses. The most important use is that they allow us to assess a child's areas of strength and weakness in order to plan educational interventions. They give us a fairly good sample of the child's behavior in an educational/achievement related situation and allow us to advocate for children who truly need special programs. Tests should be used carefully and interpretations made cautiously by individuals with a sound background in psychometric testing. It is only when one has such a background that one can appreciate the shortcomings of the measures we have at our disposal and, therefore, be less inclined to overinterpret the test results to the detriment of the child.

In practice, the three intelligence tests most frequently used with children are the Stanford-Binet—Revised (1972), the Wechsler Preschool and Primary Test of Intelligence (WPPSI), and the Wechsler Intelligence Scale for Children Revised (WISC–R). A fourth test, the McCarthy Scales of Children's Abilities is also proving to be a useful tool but is less popular than the Stanford-Binet, WPPSI, and WISC–R.

The Stanford-Binet has a long history beginning in 1905 with the construction of the Binet-Simon Test (Binet & Simon, 1905). The test was published in the United States by Terman in 1916 following revision and standardization. This revision was called the *Stanford Revision and Extension of the Binet-Simon Intelligence Scale* (Terman, 1916). In 1960, a new revision was introduced by Merrill (Terman & Merrill, 1960) that replaced conventional ratio IQ scores with deviation IQs. During 1971–1972 the norms for the Stanford-Binet were revised on a standardization group of 2100 children between the ages of 2 and 18 years. Approximately 100 children were tested at each Stanford-Binet year level. White and nonwhite English-speaking children were included in the standardization sample.

When compared to the 1960 norms, the 1972 norms yield lower IQs for comparable mental ages particularly in the younger age groups (2 to 5 years). Thus, a 4-year-old child who obtains a mental age of 4 receives a 98 deviation IQ using the 1960 tables and an 88 IQ using the 1972 revision tables. The differences in deviation IQs between the two revisions become progressively smaller after age 5 years until age 10 years and then rise again in the older age groups. Therefore, the examiner should be aware that the 1972 norms result in IQs that are usually lower than those of the 1960 norms for the same mental age levels for a specific chronological age group. For this reason, it is important to use the 1960 tables when evaluating tests given prior to the 1972 revision and when examining children who have been tested longitudinally prior to 1972. The 1972 revised norms are the most recent and should be used for all current testing and testing after 1972. If the examiner is not aware of these changes, there is a danger that he or she could incorrectly report a decline in IQ score solely as a function of using improper norms.

Another result of the 1972 revision of the Stanford-Binet is that the mental age score obtained by the child lost its significance as a reflection of what children do at particular chronological ages. This is because the average mental age score no longer corresponds to the child's chronological age. Thus, the mental age score is now simply a raw score that represents the sum of the total number of items passed by the child after a basal is established. However, a corrected or true mental age score can be found using the following procedure. Using the child's obtained mental age score, the examiner goes down the chronological age rows in the norm tables until he or she finds an IQ of 100; the chronological age at that point then becomes the corrected mental age (Shorr, McClelland, & Robinson, 1977). Using the previous example, for a child receiving a mental age score of 4 years 0 months, the corrected mental age would be 3 years 6 months. This true (or corrected) mental age score reveals more accurately the age level performance of the child and should be reported along with the obtained mental age score.

A major problem with the Stanford-Binet is that it yields a single mental age or IQ score, which is the sum of a number of items representing diverse and unrelated cognitive functions. Factor analysis of the Stanford-Binet suggests that it measures more diverse areas of functioning at the lower age levels containing increasingly more verbal items in the upper age levels. At younger ages it measures such functions as verbal reception and expression, visual–motor coordination and memory. At the upper age levels, the test measures verbal fluency and reasoning (Sattler, 1982).

The Binetgram, introduced by Sattler (1982), provides a profile of the child's performance in one of seven categories: language, memory, conceptual thinking, reasoning, numerical reasoning, visual–motor, and social intelligence. Sattler's system is based upon groupings of tests according to test content or face validity. This classification scheme is suggested by Sattler as an aid in making interpretations but is not intended to be used to report special abilities or deficits since it is not based upon empirical or statistical standardization procedures.

Major criticisms of the Stanford-Binet include its heavy reliance on verbal and rote memory skills, too few items measuring general intelligence, skills not sampled at every age level, and the already mentioned provision of only one IQ score to reflect complex mental functions (Sattler, 1982). In spite of these criticisms, the scale provides a valid and reliable measure of intelligence for retarded populations (Silverstein, 1982) and can be useful as one measure in a battery of tests. Indeed, it is usually the Stanford-Binet that is most often used as a criterion measure against which the concurrent validity of other tests is measured.

The Wechsler Intelligence Scale for Children was first published in 1949 as a downward extension of the adult intelligence scale, the Wechsler-Bellevue

Intelligence Scale. In 1974 the scale was revised and standardized on 2200 white and nonwhite children stratified according to the 1970 United States Census (Wechsler, 1974). The Wechsler Intelligence Scale for Children–Revised (WISC–R) covers ages 6-0 to 16-11 years and is composed of six verbal subtests and six performance subtests. Following is a list of the subscales and what they are intended to measure.

Verbal Subtests

Information:	Range of general factual knowledge
Similarities:	Logical abstract or conceptual thought
Arithmetic:	Concentration and simple arithmetic skill
Vocabulary:	Expressive word knowledge and semantic language skill
Comprehension:	Understanding of social convention, knowledge of coping skills
Digit Span:	Short-term auditory memory and attention

Performance Subtests

Picture Completion:	Visual alertness and attention to detail, long-term visual memory
Picture Arrangement:	Temporal sequencing ability; anticipation and planning of social actions and consequences
Block Design:	Nonverbal concept formation; visual–spatial perception; perceptual–motor coordination
Object Assembly:	Visual–spatial perception and visual–motor coordination
Coding:	Psychomotor accuracy and speed; short-term visual memory; ability to associate sign and symbol
Mazes:	Visual–spatial planning

A scaled score with a mean of 10 and standard deviation of 3 is obtained for each subtest. Subtest scores are added in order to obtain Verbal, Performance and Full Scale IQ scores. These deviation IQ scores (with a mean of 100, and SD of 15) are based upon 10 of the 12 subtests with Digit Span and Mazes considered as supplementary tests.

Although verbal subtests tend to correlate with one another as do performance subtests, the results of an extensive factor analytic study by Kaufman suggests that three rather than two factors may better explain what the test is measuring (Kaufman, 1975). These factors are Verbal Comprehension, Perceptual Organization, and Freedom from Distractibility. The Verbal Comprehension factor is composed of the subtests Vocabulary, Information, Similarities, and Comprehension. The subtests loading heavily on the Perceptual Organization factor are Block Design, Object Assembly, Picture Completion, Picture Arrangement, and Mazes. The third factor, Freedom from Distractibility, consists of the Arithmetic, Digit Span, and Coding B subtests. For some children, particularly those suspected of having attentional problems, the Freedom from Distractibility factor may be useful to interpret in addition to the verbal and performance scores. Nevertheless, it has been noted that the third factor is less stable in clinical populations and highly dependent upon the chronological age of the child and should be interpreted with caution (Groff & Hubble, 1982; Petersen & Hart, 1979).

The classification scheme used by Bannatyne (1971) for organizing WISC subtests is also applicable to the WISC–R. These categories are Verbal–Conceptualization Ability (Similarities, Vocabulary, Comprehension), Spatial Ability (Picture Completion, Block Design, Object Assembly), Sequencing Ability (Arithmetic, Digit Span, Coding), and Acquired Knowledge (Information, Arithmetic, Vocabulary). When retarded children are administered the WISC–R, some studies show that they demonstrate relative strength in Spatial Ability and weakness in Acquired Knowledge (Kaufman, 1979; Van Hagen & Kaufman, 1980). The rank order of WISC–R subtests from least to most difficult for retarded children has been reported as follows: (1) Object Assembly, (2) Picture Completion, (3) Block Design, (4) Coding, (5) Similarities, (6) Comprehension, (7) Picture Arrangement, (8) Information, (9) Arithmetic, and (10) Vocabulary (Kaufman, 1979; Kaufman & Van Hagen, 1977).

Recently, investigators have shown that retarded and nonretarded children do not differ substantially in the patterning of intellectual abilities (Groff & Hubble, 1982; Groff & Linden, 1982). The results of the studies of Groff and associates suggest that the factor structure of the WISC–R for young mentally retarded children (9–11 years) is the same as that for normal children (Groff & Hubble, 1982). Furthermore, when children are matched on mental and/or chronological age, no differences in the intellectual strengths and weaknesses of retarded and nonretarded groups are evident (Groff & Linden, 1982). Differences found in previous studies are explained by the fact that children were heterogenous with regard to chronological age. Groff and Linden (1982) found that young children (8–11 years) showed no elevation in their Perceptual Organization scores whereas older children (13 to 16 years) demonstrated comparative strength in this area. Therefore, studies demonstrating relative strength in perceptual organization by retarded children may have been describing a pattern attributable only to older children. Differences in sample selection may also explain differences in study results in that Groff and associates used only children who had no known organic or emotional impairment.

Test-retest reliability for the WISC–R has been shown to be adequate for both normal and retarded populations (Wechsler, 1974; Vance, Blixt, Ellis, & Debell, 1981). A study by Vance et al. (1981) that included retarded and learning-disabled children yielded comparable but somewhat lower reliability coefficients than those reported by Wechsler in normal children. Retarded children also showed less average increase in IQ scores over time than normal children.

The WISC–R also appears to be a valid measure of intelligence when compared to other intelligence scales such as the Stanford-Binet and the Wechsler Preschool and Primary Scale of Intelligence. It also has been shown to be highly related to school achievement (Sattler, 1982).

The WISC–R is useful in evaluating relative strengths and weaknesses in retarded children but it does have some limitations. The most problematic is the limited range of the test. Full Scale IQs of less than 40 are not computable, making it difficult to assess the overall intelligence of moderate to severely retarded youngsters. Even for children who are functioning in the mild to borderline range, only a small sample of the child's abilities can be measured because of the paucity of items available for administration at lower levels. Wechsler recommended that intelligence quotients not be computed unless a child obtains a raw score of greater than 0 on at least three of the subtests of the Verbal and Performance Scales. While this may give a rough estimate of intellectual functioning, it is our suggestion to choose another test. The test chosen should be one that adequately samples the child's abilities so that appropriate interventions can be selected.

With retarded children, it is sometimes useful to use mental-age equivalents in order to develop programs and to understand the child's behavior better. Although Wechsler rejected the notion of "mental age," he did provide test–age equivalents as guides to facilitate test performance interpretation.

The Wechsler Preschool and Primary Scale of Intelligence (WPPSI), published in 1967, is designed for children between the ages of 4 and 6.5 years (Wechsler, 1967). The WPPSI was standardized on 1200 children stratified according to the 1960 US Census. Children were tested cross-sectionally at six month intervals with 200 children (equated on sex) at each age period. The WPPSI shares most features of the WISC–R and eight of the subtests are the same as those on the WISC–R. These subtests are Information, Vocabulary, Arithmetic, Similarities, Comprehension, Picture Completion, Mazes, and Block Design. Three subtests, Sentences, Geometric Design, and Animal House, are unique to the WPPSI.

While the WPPSI has been shown to have excellent psychometric properties (Sattler, 1982), its use may be limited for retarded populations. The reasons for this are numerous, including its limited floor (similar to WISC–R), restricted age range, possible sociocultural bias, and relatively long administration time. Furthermore, a search of the literature revealed no studies on the use of the WPPSI with retarded children, suggesting that we do not know how valid or reliable a measure it is for this population. Until more information is available, it is recommended that an alternative test, like the Stanford-Binet be used instead for 4 to 6.5 year old retarded children.

The McCarthy Scales of Children's Abilities, developed in 1972, seems to be a promising new tool for measuring the cognitive ability of children between the ages of 2.5 to 8.5 years (McCarthy, 1972). Although the test yields a General Cognitive Index (GCI) rather than an Intelligence Quotient, many abilities tapped by the test are the same as those measured by intelligence tests. The GCI is derived from three scales, the Verbal, Perceptual–Performance, and Quantitative scales. The GCI is a standard score with a mean of 100 and a SD of 16. Other unique developmental abilities such as hand dominance and gross motor skill are assessed but not included in the GCI. The McCarthy Scale has good test-retest reliability and concurrent validity for normal children (Harrison & Wiebe, 1977; Kaufman, 1975). However, in spite of its strengths and some innovative improvements over traditional intelligence tests, the McCarthy Scales have a number of limitations when applied to retarded populations. Levenson and Zino (1979) and Naglieri and Harrison (1979) found that the mean McCarthy indexes were about 20 points below mean Stanford-Binet (1972) IQs for mentally retarded children but not for matched normal controls. Similarly, Naglieri (1980a) found that while the WISC–R Full Scale IQ and the McCarthy Index were highly correlated for retarded children ($r = .82$), the McCarthy Index was 7 points lower than the WISC–R IQ in this sample. In contrast, there was less than 1 point difference between the two tests for the normal controls. These results suggest that GCI's are not interchangeable with WISC–R or Stanford-Binet IQ's in retarded populations and that school placement decisions should not be based upon results of the McCarthy Scales. The Scales have other limitations but should still be considered useful for assessing cognitive and motor abilities of young children following more extensive research and standardization.

Adaptive Behavior Measures

Adaptive functioning is as important to assess in retarded populations as is intelligence. Children with delayed or below average intelligence also have difficulty adapting to the demands of the environment. Unlike intelligence tests, adaptive behavior measures are not entirely based on direct observation of the child's behavior. Information is generally obtained through parent interview or by interviewing people most familiar with the child. We have found that parents are generally accurate in their assessment of the child's adaptive functioning and information from the adaptive behavior scales we employ is valid when compared with direct observation of the child's behavior (Petty & Hansen, personal communication).

All children entering our program are assessed using either the AAMD Adaptive Behavior Scale for Children and Adults (for children 7 or older) or the AAMD Adaptive Behavior Scale for Infants and Early Childhood (for children less than 7 years of age).

The 1974 revision of the Adaptive Behavior Scale (ABS) is divided into two parts (Nihira, Foster, Shellhaas, & Leland, 1974). Part I measures ten behavioral domains necessary for independence in everyday life. These include independent functioning, physical development, economic activity, language development, numbers and time, domestic activity, vocational activity, self-direction, responsibility, and socialization. Part II measures fourteen domains focusing on maladaptive behavior. The test was standardized on 4000 institutionalized children and adults. Test-retest reliabilities are not provided for the scale and while interrater reliability for Part I is high, it is low for Part II. Other problems with Part II have been described (McDevitt, McDevitt, & Rosen, 1977) and Part II has proven to be of little use with autistic children (Sloan & Marcus, 1981). We too have found Part II to be unreliable with our population, but Part I provides a clinically useful measure of competence in various areas of independent and social functioning. Part I of the ABS has been shown to correlate highly with the Vineland Social Maturity Scale in a group of retarded children and adults (Roszkowski, 1980).

We also use the AAMD Adaptive Behavior Scale—Public School Version (ABS–PSV), standardized by Lambert, Windmiller, Cole, and Figueroa (1975) on 2600 public school children, to aid us in suggestions for school placement. The test was standardized on children aged 7 to 13 years who were representative of the California school population. School placements include regular, educable mentally retarded, and trainable mentally retarded classes. Part I and Part II are comparable on the Public School Version to the ABS with the exception of domestic activity, which is omitted from the School Scale. Using the Public School Version of the ABS, the child's percentile scores on various domains are compared with the scores of children of the same chronological age in regular and special education classrooms.

The recent development of the AAMD Adaptive Behavior Scale for Infants and Early Childhood has allowed for the measurement of adaptive functioning in children between the ages of 2 weeks and 6 years. This scale is also divided into two parts. Part I measures behavior in seven domains including independent functioning, physical development, communication skills, conceptual skills, play, self-direction, and personal responsibility/socialization. Part II deals with maladaptive behavior and suffers from the same problems as Part II of the ABS.

A final measure that we use is the Alpern-Boll Developmental Profile (Alpern & Boll, 1972). This scale is designed to assess the developmental competence of children in 5 areas: physical, self-help, social, academic, and communication. Unlike the ABS Scales that provide percentile scores, the Alpern-Boll provides developmental age scores, and items on the test are ordered according to developmental functioning at progressive age levels. The Scale was standardized on 3008 normal children between birth and 12.5 years of age. The sample was representative of the United States population according to the 1970 Census. Items that discriminated on the basis of sex, race, and socioeconomic status were eliminated. There is good interrater reliability and reported behavior compares favorably with observed behavior. The scale is useful as a screening measure, as a measure for use in program planning and evaluation, and as a tool for parent feedback regarding the child's development. The Scale provides an IQ equivalent based upon the results of the Academic Scale but this score does not appear to be accurate in our experience and it does not meet the criteria necessary to make it a valid estimate of intelligence. For these reasons, we do not recommend that the IQ conversion score be used. The Scale also provides tables for determining the degree of developmental delay associated with different chronological and developmental age levels. These tables were not based upon empirical data but rather on clinical judgment and should not, in our opinion, be used in the interpretation of the child's functioning. The Alpern-Boll is an improvement over the Vineland Social Maturity Scale both in terms of its psychometric properties and its ability to provide descriptive behavioral information on young children. Unlike the Vineland, the Scale does not yield a single Social Age score. Nevertheless, we have found the Alpern-Boll extremely useful in working with young children and their parents.

Infant Assessments

During the late 1930s and early 1940s many tests designed to measure infant development were introduced. Most notable were the Gesell Developmental Schedules: the California First Year Mental Scale, later to become the Bayley Scales of Infant Development; and the Cattell Infant Intelligence Scale.

The Gesell Scale, developed by Arnold Gesell at the Yale Clinic of Child Development, is the oldest infant scale and has served as the prototype of all newer scales. Gesell did not regard his measure as an intelligence test but rather as an observational tool to assess individual maturation and development. The original schedules have been criticized for poor standardization and lack of research on reliability and validity. Nevertheless, most infant tests in use today include items originated by Gesell. In 1977, the Gesell was standardized by Knobloch in collaboration with Stevens and Malone. The new schedules, the *Revised Gesell and Amatruda Developmental and Neurologic Examination*, were standardized on over 900 infants and children between the ages of 1 to 36 months. Children were tested at 20 age levels. Like the old schedules, the new test assesses development in five areas: language, personal-social, adaptive, fine motor, and gross motor. Language items measure both expressive vocalization and verbal comprehension. The Personal/Social scale reflects the child's response to social interaction and acquisition of self-help skills. For example, the scale assesses the child's reactions to people, imitative ability, as well as signs of independence as reflected in feeding and toileting behavior. Adaptive behavior involves the way in which the child problem-solves in his or her use of objects, and is considered the scale most closely associated with intellectual outcome (Knobloch & Pasamanick, 1974). Fine motor behavior consists of the facility of the small muscles particularly the use of the fingers and hands. Gross motor skills include sitting, walking, jumping, and other activities involving large muscle groups. The schedules yield Developmental Quotients or DQs obtained by dividing the developmental or mental age by the chronological age of the child.

The authors report the interrater reliability of the Gesell as quite high but do not give test-retest reliabilities. No mention is made of the exam's concurrent validity although it is compared with the previous version of the Gesell. In general, exam items are passed earlier by today's infants when compared with age values from the original Gesell. Thus, the old version of the Gesell will yield DQs that are higher when compared with the revised version. Our experience in testing normal clinic children is that the average DQ can vary as much as 10 points when the two exams are compared. In spite of some of the as yet unknown psychometric properties of the Revised Gesell, the test is an invaluable tool for the clinician interested in the observation and description of infant behavior as the infant evolves over the first three years of life.

In 1933, Nancy Bayley published the California First Year Mental Scale to be used to determine whether or not there was a relationship between early infant development and later intelligence. The 1969 revision, which is the latest revision of the Bayley scales and now called the Bayley Mental and Motor Scales of Infant Development was standardized on a stratified US sample of 1962 children between the ages of 2 months and 2.5 years (Bayley, 1969). The test is divided into a Mental Scale and Psychomotor Scale, each yielding a Developmental Index with a mean of 100 and SD of 16. There is also an Infant Behavior Record that can be used for rating behavioral observations of the child.

The Mental Scale contains 163 test items designed to measure "sensory–perceptual acuities, discriminations . . . the early acquisition of object constancy and memory, learning and problem-solving ability; vocalizations and the beginning of verbal communication; . . . the ability to form generalizations and classifications; which is the basis of abstract thinking" (Bayley, 1969, p. 3). The Psychomotor Scale contains only 81 items and covers such gross and fine motor tasks as finger grasp, sitting, walking, and jumping.

Currently, the Bayley Scales of Infant Development is the best researched and standardized infant test available. Nevertheless it does have some limitations. Unlike the Gesell, which includes many items within five areas of behavioral development, the Bayley samples relatively fewer behaviors at each age period. Furthermore, behaviors are broken down into two rather gross categories labeled Mental and Psychomotor.* Within the Psychomotor scale, fine motor development is assessed infrequently with no fine motor skills sampled beyond 9 months of age.

---

*These scales have been factor analyzed and broken down further by Kohen-Raz to include an Eye–Hand Scale, Manipulation Scale, Object Relation Scale, Imitation and Comprehension Scale, and Vocalization–Social Contact Scale, but there are too few items included in these factors to amply sample the domains.

Because of these shortcomings, the Scales are not as useful to the clinician who is interested in assessing an individual's strengths and weaknesses in order to program-plan. If program planning is the goal of assessment, then the Gesell is a better instrument to use. If the primary goal is to assess global cognitive functioning, the Bayley is a good research tool.

The Bayley appears to have fair concurrent validity with the Stanford-Binet (r = .57). Test-retest reliability coefficients are somewhat low but explainable by the fact that one is using the test on a quickly developing and fairly unreliable subject. Unlike the Gesell, which allows mother's report to be scored in addition to actual observed behavior, the Bayley uses only observable behavior produced by the child either spontaneously or on command. Because young children often choose not to respond, particularly to requests for language or motor performance, the test does not yield completely comparable results from one test session to another.

An infant scale that closely parallels the Bayley Scales is the one developed in 1940 by Psyche Cattell, the Cattell Infant Intelligence Scale. Cattell (1940; 1960) drew heavily from the Gesell test items, using only those that showed a regular increase in percent passed from one age to another. Cattell eliminated gross motor items and those personal/social items related to self-help skills such as feeding and toileting. The standardization was based on a total of 1346 examinations administered longitudinally to 274 lower-middleclass children tested at 3 month intervals up to a year and then 6 month intervals thereafter to 30 months. The Scale yields a mental age score that can be converted to an IQ equivalent by dividing the obtained mental age by the child's chronological age. The test has several limitations including outdated standardization, the use of IQ ratio scores rather than deviation IQs, and behaviors interpolated rather than observed across 3 to 6 month age intervals (Honzik, 1976).

The advantages of the Cattell is that it is short and interesting, the directions for administration and scoring are very clear and the test was designed to be a downward extension of the Stanford-Binet. Thus, after 22 months, items from the 1937 Stanford-Binet Form-L are used. Because the 1937 edition of the Stanford-Binet is now out-of-date, those items that appear in the latest revision that are the same or that parallel the 1937 items must be employed. Caution must be used, however, in estimating IQ scores in this way, and if an examiner sees that a child can pass enough Stanford-Binet items to get a basal, the Stanford-Binet rather than the Cattell should be used instead. The Cattell has its most use in those cases where the child is performing somewhere between 24 and 36 months. The reason is that, for some children who function in this developmental range, it is not possible to get a ceiling on the Bayley or a basal on the Stanford-Binet. In this instance, the Cattell can be used to accurately reflect the full range of the child's developmental functioning. Furthermore, the Cattell has been shown to be so similar to and to correlate so highly with the Bayley Mental Scales as to be considered interchangeable when used to evaluate retarded young children (Erikson, Johnson, & Campbell, 1970).

The overriding concern of most clinicians is how valid are infant tests for later prediction of mental functioning. In answer to this question there are several generalizations that can be made based upon the research literature. In neurologically intact normal infants, global scores obtained on infant tests in the first year of life are not very predictive of later intelligence (Bayley, 1955, 1969; McCall, 1979; Stott & Ball, 1965). However, prediction becomes better in the second year. Prediction can be made much earlier than two years for low scoring infants no matter what the cause of their developmental disability. For example, Knobloch and Pasamanick (1960, 1967) found that the correlation between 9 month Gesell DQs and the three year Stanford-Binet was .74 for neurologically- or intellectually-impaired children. Werner, Bierman, and French (1971) found that the accuracy of clinical prediction of poor school performance in 5- to 9-years-olds from 20 month ratings by pediatricians could be improved from 46 to 75 percent if Cattell IQs were taken into account. Furthermore at 10 year follow-up, the best single predictor of school achievement and IQ was the Cattell administration at 20 months.

Goodman and Cameron (1978), using the Bayley Scales on children with mental ages of 30 months or less, demonstrated remarkable stability over two year periods with correlations ranging from .72 to .92. An additional finding was that the lower the child's IQ, the higher the predictive validity. Similar results of high predictive validity over a 1 to 3 year period for retarded children are reported by Vander Veer and Schweid (1974).

Measures of Visual–Motor Functioning

The most popular visual–motor test used today is the Bender Visual Motor Gestalt Test (Bender, 1938). The Bender Gestalt Test was developed by Loretta Bender in 1938 and consists of nine figures, which are presented one at a time to the subject who is asked to copy them on a blank sheet of paper. Bender used a developmental approach in analyzing children's protocols but did not provide an adequate objective scoring system for the test. In the 1960s, Koppitz (1963) developed a scoring system using composite scores for all nine figures. Normative data were collected from the Bender records of over 1100 children aged 5 to 10 years. This scoring system was then applied to protocols of groups of children with emotional problems, brain injury, learning difficulties, and/or mental retardation. In addition, records were analyzed for indicators of emotional problems. The scoring system was restandardized in 1975 (Koppitz, 1975). The new norms are based on 975 children between 5 and 12 years of age. Test-retest reliabilities are adequate, but according to Sattler (1982) the reliability of the test is "not high enough to permit diagnostic decisions based on the test alone, or on only one administration of the test" (p. 292). The test has concurrent validity when compared with other tests of visual–motor coordination like the Beery Developmental Test of Visual Motor Integration ($r = .82$). The test is not highly correlated with measures of intelligence.

While the Bender is sometimes used as a measure for diagnosis of organicity, its validity to be used in this way is questionable (Sattler, 1982). Furthermore, the Bender cannot be used to diagnose mental retardation, although retarded individuals do tend to obtain lower scores on the Bender than normal children (Koppitz, 1963).

The Beery-Buktenica Developmental Test of Visual Motor Integration is a perceptual–motor coordination test developed for children between the ages of 2 to 15 years. The test consists of 24 geometric figures arranged in increasing difficulty, which the child must copy. The total score, based upon the number of figures drawn successfully, is converted into a developmental age equivalent. The test was standardized on 1039 normal children from 3 to 14 years of age in 1964. For each figure, a developmental age estimate is given according the sex of the child. The test-retest reliability and concurrent validity of the test is satisfactory. Specifically, the test scores correlate .89 with chronological age and .80 with perceptual skill (Beery & Buktenica, 1967).

In a study comparing Bender and Beery Developmental Test protocols in a group of school-aged retarded children, Krauft and Krauft (1972) found the two tests to be highly similar. The Beery, however, represents an improvement over the Bender in that it covers a wider age range and can be used with individuals functioning as young as two years developmentally.

The Frostig Developmental Test of Visual Perception reportedly allows for the assessment of eye–hand coordination, figure–ground perception, form constancy, and perception of position in space and spatial relationships (Frostig, Maslow, Lefever, & Whittlesey, 1964). The test was standardized on 2116 middle class white children between the ages of 3 and 9 years. It is recommended, however, that the test be used with children between the ages of 4 and 7 years since the reliability of the test for other ages is unknown. Because the test requires a minimum of language, it can be used with deaf and non-English speaking children, although there are no studies on the use of this measure with these populations. Furthermore, physically handicapped children may be able to complete some of the subtests simply by pointing to the answers.

Although the authors claim that the test measures five discrete areas of visual processing for which a training program can be specified, factor analytic studies have shown that the subtests load heavily on only one factor, which is best described as visual perception (Silverstein, 1972). Furthermore, the low test-retest reliabilities of individual subtests suggest that they are unreliable and the overall perceptual quotient is the most stable score and the one recommended for use. Because of the psychometric and validity problems of the Frostig, Sattler (1982) has recommended the test be used as a screening device and not be used to prescribe specific remediations.

In our own hospital, we have found the Frostig useful in monitoring the behavioral consequences of neuroleptic medication on psychotic children. For example, the subtest measuring eye–hand coordination can give us some idea of extrapyramidal effects of certain phenothiazines whereas other subtests can help us assess attention and perceptual accuracy. Used systematically, the test can be useful in determining both harmful and helpful effects of medication. The test, however, should never be used as the sole measure of medication effects.

Other tests measuring perceptual–motor functioning that also measure visual memory for designs are the Graham-Kendall Memory for Designs Test (1973) and the Revised Visual Retention Test (Benton, 1963; Rice, 1972).

Tests Used With Nonverbal Children

The Peabody Picture Vocabulary Test (PPVT) was developed by Dunn in 1959 for use with the mentally handicapped (Dunn, 1965). The PPVT—Revised was completed in 1981 and appears to be a useful measure of receptive vocabulary (Dunn & Dunn, 1981). The PPVT–R was standardized on 4200 children between the ages of 2.5 to 18 years and 828 adults between 19 and 40 years. The sample was stratified according to the 1970 United States Census and all racially, culturally, or sexually biased words from the previous PPVT were eliminated. The test has two versions (Forms L and M) with 175 plates for each. Each plate consists of 4 pictures. The examiner reads the child a word and the child must choose the picture that represents that word. The test is highly useful for physically handicapped nonverbal children.

The test yields a standard score mean of 100 with a standard deviation of 15. Like other tests, however, the range of the test from 40 to 150 is somewhat restricted and may not be useful for extremely retarded children.

Alternate form reliabilities for the 1959 version of the PPVT are not high and there are no reliability data for the 1981 revised version in normal populations. Nevertheless, alternate form reliabilities are high for mentally retarded children (Dunn & Dunn, 1981).

Studies comparing the 1959 PPVT scores to Stanford-Binet and Wechsler IQs consistently show that the tests do not yield comparable results in samples of special children (Covin, 1976, 1977a, 1977b; Hodapp & Hodapp, 1980; Vance, Prichard, & Wallbrown, 1978). Similarly, Prasse and Bracken (1981) reported that the PPVT–R yielded a significantly lower mean score than the WISC–R for a sample of mentally retarded children. A more careful study by Naglieri (1982), however, found a high level of concordance between WISC–R IQs and PPVT–R Standard Score Equivalents in retarded children. The corrected validity coefficients were also high. Niglieri, however, cautions that the

> two tests should not be considered interchangeable because of the wider range of information assessed by the WISC–R. The PPVT–R appears to be most appropriate as a measure of verbal comprehension, which does not require verbal expression, that may be used in conjunction with other tests in a psychoeducational battery. (p. 637)

The advantages of the PPVT–R are that it can be administered quickly by an examiner with no special testing experience. It is a useful screening tool for children with limited or no expressive language. The revised version appears to be more difficult than the old PPVT; therefore, scores from the 1959 version should not be compared with scores from the 1981 version in discussions of test-retest performance.

The Leiter International Performance Scale (Leiter, 1948) is a nonverbal test designed to be used with children who have language problems and/or sensory/motor deficits. The Scale consists of 54 items arranged in an age scale format from 2 to 18 years. The Scale yields a mental age score and an adjusted ratio IQ. The test is not timed and is administered using gestures only. The child's task is to select blocks and insert them into a test frame in order to match certain designs or pictures. The test contains items that most consistently reflect perceptual organizational and discrimination skill. Many items can be completed successfully simply by visual matching.

No standardization data are provided by Arthur (1962) on the latest revision of the Leiter; however, test-retest reliabilities for handicapped children appear to be high (Spellacy & Black, 1972). Large differences between Leiter and WISC–R IQs have been found (Sattler, 1982). In particular, deaf children score significantly lower on the Leiter than on the WISC–R Performance Scale (Bonham, 1974). Furthermore, our experience has been that the Leiter overestimates the intelligence of autistic and retarded children. This is particularly true for retarded autistic children who are relatively skilled in visual matching. With these special children, the Leiter can be considered an aid in clinical diagnosis but never as a measure of general intelligence.

Other limitations of the test include its outdated norms; inadequate standardization; uneven item difficulty at different age levels; limited sampling of behavior at each age level; and use of ratio rather than deviation IQs. In addition, the test requires fine motor coordination sometimes absent in younger, physically disabled, or more retarded children.

The Merrill-Palmer Scale of Mental Tests (Stutsman, 1948) covers an age range from 18 to 71 months. Since the test can be administered with little language, it can be used with deaf, asphasic, or autistic children, although there are no norms for these groups. The test measures fine motor coordination, visual spatial skill, visual matching, shape discrimination, self-representation, physical imitation, and memory and response to simple words or word groups. The test is made up of several older tests including the Sequin-Goddard Formboard, Pinter Maniken Test, and Wallin Pegboards.

The test items are arranged in six-month intervals and ranked supposedly according to difficulty. Although the test is designed as a Guttman scale, there are no data presented in the manual that would support this assumption, nor has it been our experience that all items are appropriately placed developmentally. Furthermore, unlike the Gesell, which examines the unfolding of certain skills in a developmental fashion, the Merrill-Palmer is scored on a timed or pass/fail basis with little regard to developmental successive approximations.

The Merrill-Palmer was last standardized in 1931 on 631 children equated on sex. No information is provided on the ethnic or socioeconomic backgrounds of the sample children. Scores are reported in Mental Age or percentile rank and although not recommended by the author, IQ equivalents can be computed using a ratio IQ computation.

Reading the manual, one is struck by how outdated and lacking in standardized methodology the test is. Some items were not administered to subjects if they appeared fatigued, some notions about what the test measures are no longer valid considering what we know now about child development, and the language of the test is derogatory. For example, children are referred to as "bright" or "stupid."

Further problems include the allowance of refusals and omissions left to the examiner's discretion and time-limited items, which may penalize slower, less motivated children. Test-retest reliability is variable but concurrent validity appears high, particularly for retarded children. Like the Leiter, however, the Merrill-Palmer overestimates intelligence in autistic children and should not be used without other tests.

The test's strengths include a wide age range, measurement of nonverbal performance particularly in children with limited language, and it is a test in which children easily engage. The nonverbal items of the Merrill-Palmer Scale are useful in assessing children who have severe impairment of language, who are retarded (Gould, 1977; Rutter & Bartak, 1973).

The usefulness of tests like the Merrill-Palmer that involve visuospatial skill in the absence of symbolic language for determining intelligence, however, is questionable. For example, Gould (1977) found that, depending upon which test was used in a battery including the Reynell Developmental Language Scales, the Vineland Social Maturity Scale, and the Merrill-Palmer, the same child would be classified as mildly/moderately retarded on one and profoundly retarded on another. These results suggest that in populations of exceptional children, marked discrepancies can occur among different areas of cognitive, language, and social functioning. The profiles obtained from children using different tests must be assessed according to the quality of the tests used and the areas of functioning measured. Educational planning should be based upon a thorough understanding of the limitations of assessments used and the skills needed for the child to function in society. Thus, an autistic child who obtains a score of 80 on a nonverbal visuospatial test like the Merrill-Palmer or the Leiter, but who obtains a Verbal IQ of 50, Performance IQ of 66, and Full Scale IQ of 58 on the WISC–R should not be placed in a classroom of nonretarded aphasic children but, rather in a classroom with other retarded children with language deficits. The rationale for this decision would be based upon the fact that the WISC–R is a better measure of intellectual functioning than either the Leiter or the Merrill-Palmer, both of which measure an area of performance in which autistic children excel but which has little practical significance for further learning or independent functioning.

Tests Based On Piagetian Principles

As an alternative to standardized intelligence tests, Piaget-based scales of early cognitive–intellectual development have been suggested for use with retarded children (Robinson & Robinson, 1976; Wachs, 1970). The Robinsons (1976) have suggested that Piaget's work represents a truly developmental approach to the assessment of cognition that is not reflected in many intelligence tests in use today. According to the Robinsons many items from current intelligence tests "have largely been chosen on a trial-and-error basis and not because they are representative of central intellectual processes characteristic of different age levels" (p. 260). In contrast, Piaget's system "is by far the most comprehensive and detailed stage-analytic theory of cognitive development in existence . . . This is particularly true of the three periods which are most relevant to the field of mental retardation, those of sensorimotor, preoperational, and concrete-operational intelligence" (p. 254*).

The Infant Psychological Development Scale (Uzgiris & Hunt, 1975), is designed to measure intellectual growth during the sensorimotor period. There are eight subscales consisting of separate ordinal steps, with each step delineating a stage in the development of the ability measured by the subscale. The subscales measure the development of means–ends relations, foresight, schemas in relationship to objects, causality, objects in space, vocal imitation, gestural imitation, and object permanence. The Scale was designed to be administered to infants 2 weeks to 24 months of age; however, it has been demonstrated that the scale is useful for testing older retarded children (Kahn, 1976; Wachs, 1970).

Another scale, developed in France and standardized in the United States, is the Casati-Lezine Scale of Sensorimotor Development (Kopp, Sigman, & Parmelee, 1974). The scale, like the Uzgiris-Hunt Scale, consists of separate ordinal subscales covering the period from 6 to 24 months. The subscales include exploration of objects, search for hidden objects (object permanence), use of intermediaries, use of an instrument, use of the relationship between an object and its support, and combination of objects. All subscales are designed to measure the child's problem-solving abilities at different stages during the sensorimotor period. The American version of the Casati-Lezine consisted of 336 tests administered longitudinally to 24 infants from 7 to 18 months. The scale meets criteria for being an ordinal invariant Guttman scale (Kopp, Sigman, & Parmelee, 1973). There are no data reported on the use of this scale with older retarded children.

While no formal scales are available to measure development beyond the

---

* Robinsons quotes on this page and on pages 222, 223 from: Robinson NM, & Robinson HB. (1976). *The mentally retarded child: A psychological approach* (2nd ed.). New York: McGraw-Hill Book Company, © 1976; by permission.

sensorimotor period, the use of other Piagetian tasks examining preoperational and concrete–operational thought have been shown to be highly correlated with mental age as opposed to chronological age in mentally retarded individuals (Gruen & Vore, 1972; Patterson & Milakofsky, 1980).

Although the use of Piagetian-based measures is attractive, current tests and Piagetian tasks have not been subjected to adequate standardization procedures and lack psychometric properties essential for adequate assessment tools. Nevertheless, tests based upon Piagetian principles would represent a major advance in the testing field. Furthermore, performance on such tests could be used in order to suggest educational interventions.

Other Tests Used to Assess Cognitive Functioning

The Goodenough-Harris Draw-a-Man test (Harris, 1963) is based upon the assumption that children's drawings are an indication of intellectual maturity. The test requires that the child simply draw a human figure. The standardization sample for the Harris scoring procedure consisted of 2975 children stratified according to the 1960 United States Census. Children were sampled at each age level from 5 to 15 years of age, although it is preferable to use the test with children between the ages of 5 and 10 years. Although test-retest reliabilities are fairly good, validity studies suggest that the Draw-a-Man test should not be used as a measure of intelligence (Sattler, 1982). Inherent in the use of the test is the possibility that factors reflecting motivation and emotional processes can influence the quality and complexity of a child's human figure drawing. The test can be viewed as a measure of complex processes involving perceptual, fine motor, cognitive, and social/emotional factors. As such, it can be used as part of a battery of tests designed to assess overall functioning.

Few studies examine the relationship between intelligence and figure drawings in retarded children but it has been shown that, when compared with WISC–R IQs, the IQs derived from the Draw-a-Man Test overestimate intelligence in children who have below average IQs (Lehman & Levy, 1971). Furthermore, the test is not valid as a predictor of IQ in children with emotional and/or significant organic problems (Ables, 1971). The test does seem to provide some insight into the retarded child's self-concept and body image, particularly when size is a factor. Children with smaller self-drawings tend to have poorer self-attitudes (Ottenbacher, 1981). Our own experience has been that, in general, the human figure drawings of retarded children reflect developmental level. In other words, a child who functions like a 3.5-year-old would produce a drawing characteristic of that developmental age. This relationship between figure drawings and developmental level decreases with age and milder intellectual impairment.

In an attempt to provide a more balanced assessment of minority children from lower socioeconomic backgrounds, the SOMPA or System of Multicultural Pluralistic Assessment developed by Mercer (Mercer, 1979; Mercer & Lewis, 1978), is a battery of measures designed to correct for psychosocial differences and health factors. The standardization sample for the SOMPA was composed of 2085 children ranging from 5-0 to 11-11 years. The sample consisted of an approximately equal number of black, hispanic and white California children. The SOMPA battery is divided into two parts consisting of a parent interview and direct testing of the child. A thorough description of the test is given by Mercer (1979) and Sattler (1982), but the main goal of the battery was to reduce the overrepresentation of minority students in educational programs for the mentally retarded. The SOMPA reportedly allows for a comprehensive view of the child by eliminating cultural bias. In order to do this, WISC–R IQs are adjusted using the scores from four Sociocultural Scales to arrive at an Estimated Learning Potential (ELP). Thus, a child from a large lowerclass family who is culturally isolated from the majority population can obtain an ELP Full Scale IQ that is substantially higher than his original WISC–R IQ. In addition, the SOMPA provides measures of vision, audition, physical growth, perceptual–motor, and adaptive functioning.

In examining the current literature on the SOMPA, Sattler (1982) concludes that while "the ELP I.Q. may be of some interest, its use in placement and clinical situations is not supported by current studies," (p. 281). Furthermore, Reschly (1981) reports that the use of the ELP and adaptive behavior measures of the SOMPA greatly reduces the number and percentage of children falling in the mildly retarded range, regardless of racial group, below currently accepted prevalence rates. Reschly found that when scores were corrected using the ELP for white, black, hispanic, and American Indian children, fewer children from all social groups could be classified as mildly retarded. This finding suggests that far fewer children than suggested by traditional prevalence rates would be eligible for services if sociocultural variables are considered in placement decisions. The author concludes that the SOMPA must be used with care when placement decisions are being made so as not to deny needed services to eligible children. This would be true for all children regardless of race or cultural background.

APPROACHES TO TESTING CHILDREN

The goal in any testing situation is to obtain an accurate sample of the child's behavior upon which to base conclusions and recommendations about the child's overall development and psychological functioning. In testing children with behavioral problems, our task becomes more difficult in that we must engage the child in the testing situation to the point that the child's maladaptive or difficult to manage behaviors do not interfere with an adequate assessment of the child's abilities. Thus, as clinicians we must be able to manage the unique behavioral problems that many of our children manifest in order to maximize their performance in the testing situation. We do this in two ways. First, we provide a testing situation for the child that is free of potential distractors and that allows us to contain the child in a highly structured environment. Second, we introduce behavioral management techniques that reduce behaviors that interfere with the child's test performance. We also teach the child test-taking skills. These behaviors include general skills such as attending behavior and more specific skills such as pointing or nodding.

Test Setting

The test setting should be one in which the child and the examiner can have optimal interaction. Ideally it should be well-lighted with a minimum of furniture and distracting stimuli. The child should be seated at a table in a chair that is appropriate for his size. It may be necessary to have another adult in the room seated beside the child in order to help manage him. For highly distractible youngsters who are also very active, we have found it useful to have the examiner sit across from the child with the testing table placed against a wall. Another adult sits beside the child blocking his exit from the table.

Behavioral Management

The behavioral technique that we most frequently employ is the use of positive reinforcement in the form of primary reinforcers (food) and social reinforcers (verbal praise). There is controversy in the literature regarding the use of reinforcement in the standardized testing situation. Critics of this practice argue that because tests were not standardized using reinforcers of this kind, the results obtained are not valid.

The decision to use behavioral techniques in the evaluation of a child depends upon what the examiner wishes to accomplish from such an assessment. In the case of behaviorally-disturbed mentally retarded children, you are usually not asking how the child compares with normal children. You already know that the child is not functioning like children upon whom the tests were standardized. The more appropriate question to answer in the evaluation procedure is, what is the child capable of achieving in an environment designed to optimize performance? Ideally, you would want the child's performance to reflect the child's potential as closely as possible. Test results perceived in this way serve as behavioral descriptors and could suggest educational programs based upon the child's capacity under ideal conditions.

A second consideration when introducing behavioral reinforcers is what are the consequences of such reinforcers on performance. The literature is fairly clear that mentally retarded children often have motivational problems and difficulty in mastery-oriented situations (Harter & Zigler, 1974). Harter and Zigler (1974) have argued that because the retarded child has a life history of failure experiences, he may have a high need for social reinforcement in order to motivate performance. Harter (1977) has demonstrated that given a choice, retarded children are more likely to choose easier tasks than more difficult ones even though they may be capable of more difficult task performance. Normal children, in contrast, show more pleasure over successful completion of more difficult tasks. Harter attributes these differences to the fact that task mastery motivation in retarded children has been attenuated in the course of their development and that other motives such as fear of failure and low expectancy for success have become more salient. Thus, the goal of reinforcement should not be aimed at increasing the child's intelligence score by teaching him the test, rather to increase motivation for task mastery.

Saigh and Payne (1978) have demonstrated that positive reinforcement serves to keep the retarded child on task, resulting in an increased number of test items attempted and answered successfully. They concluded that reinforcers result in a more reliable estimate of test performance.

In addition to providing a testing situation to optimize motivation for task completion, it is often necessary to try to decrease maladaptive behaviors that interfere with successful performance. We have found that the best way to extinguish maladaptive behavior is through active or passive ignore procedures. In active ignore, the examiner actually turns away from the child and does not attend to him until he ceases the inappropriate behavior and complies with task demands. In passive ignore, the examiner remains engaged with the child, ignores his inappropriate behavior, and repeats requests for task completion.

Other techniques that have been particularly useful in optimizing test performance include short and frequent testing sessions and returning to items previously failed or refused. It is important to remember that no child is "untestable" and that a good examiner is one who can maximize the child's performance by increasing the child's motivation while decreasing behaviors that interfere with an adequate assessment of the child's functioning.

Assessment Procedure

The complete assessment of the child should include the following components: parent interview; medical screening (hearing, vision, physical condition); behavioral observations/mental status of the child; and formal testing including measures of cognitive, perceptual–motor, adaptive, and personality functioning. All formal evaluations are then analyzed and interpreted based upon all information gathered about the child.

The parent interview is an extremely important component in the assessment of the child. Parents are the people most intimately involved with the child and can provide a wealth of information about the total child. Parents as informants, however, will provide the most valuable information only if asked the right questions. Thus, it takes a skillful clinician to elicit information that will provide insight into the child's problems.

The parent interview usually begins with a discussion of the child's presenting problems as the parent sees them. When discussing the child's problems it is important that the parent be asked to describe specific behaviors and situations under which these behaviors occur (antecedents) along with events that serve to maintain the behaviors (consequences). No useful information is provided by the general statement, "He's a bad boy." In the course of the parents' delineation of specific behaviors, the clinician can begin to formulate plans for intervention.

Another important aspect of the parent interview is the developmental history of the child beginning with pregnancy, labor, and delivery. Possible biologic or psychological trauma are explored along with major environmental stressors such as separation, death, or multiple moves.

An important aspect of the developmental history includes an assessment of the rate of attainment of developmental milestones. While this part of history-taking is highly valuable when assessing a retarded child, it is often an area neglected or inadequately covered by clinicians. The reasons for this failure are numerous but the most common are an inadequate knowledge of normal child development on the part of the clinician and skepticism about the parents' reliability as historians. The first issue can only be solved when child development is required as part of the learning experience of every clinician. The second issue, in our experience, has not been a great problem. Parents, in general, are adequate historians and generally describe their child's development accurately. It is often helpful, however, to have them bring in a baby book and pictures of the child to facilitate their memory of the child's development. It is also useful to ask them to estimate their child's developmental age based upon the behavior of siblings or other children they know. Questionnaires such as the AAMD Adaptive Behavior Scale or the Alpern-Boll Developmental Profile are also useful in gathering developmental information.

Social and school behaviors is another area to cover in the parent interview. School reports and discussion of the child's behavior with his or her teacher are also fruitful.

The medical evaluation of the child should include medical history, physical/neurologic examination, laboratory workup, and vision/hearing screening. Medical history should include any medical insults the child has experienced along with a description of similar behavioral/developmental conditions in other family members. The physical examination should focus on neurologic functioning and an examination of the child's overall physical condition that might suggest certain clinical syndromes. The laboratory studies should be requested in order to answer specific questions about the child's developmental problem. Although we frequently receive requests from referrants for a "thorough neurologic workup" including CAT scans and EEGs, it has been our experience that if there are no clinical manifestations of an organic problem when the child is examined, that further diagnostic measures such as CAT scans are not very useful. Furthermore, an abnormal EEG, in and of itself, is often not helpful either in diagnosis or treatment of a developmental problem.

Vision and hearing screening, on the other hand, has had tremendous payoff in aiding our understanding and treatment of mentally retarded or developmentally disabled youngsters. It is frighteningly common that we will see a child diagnosed as autistic only to find out that he or she has a sensory deficit. For this reason and because there are fairly reliable techniques for assessing sensory functioning, we recommend that all children receive vision and hearing screening.

Once the parents have been interviewed and the child examined by a physician, the clinician should interview the child and observe the child's behavior in several common environmental situations. Behavioral observation is particularly important when dealing with children who do not or cannot talk. The child interview should include observations about the child's appearance, behavior, thought process and thought content, cognition, mood and affect, language, reality orientation, interpersonal interactions, and play behavior. Observations of the child's play and interaction with the parents gives considerable insight into developmental level and parent–child relationship.

Most commonly, the clinician observes the child's behavior in the office or in the institution to which the child is referred. The reason for this limited perspective on behavioral observation is the assumption that the child will act similarly across many environmental conditions. This assumption has proven inaccurate, thus leading many practitioners to suggest that assessment should take place in the child's natural environment. For this reason, we often make home and school visits in order to more adequately access the child's problems and to offer suggestions for treatment. On the other hand, behavior problems are sometimes pervasive in all situations and can be handled or treated as they occur in the office or on the ward. For certain behaviors, rating scales or checklists are useful. Commonly used scales are the Behavior Problem Checklist (Quay & Peterson, 1967), the Conner's Scales (Goyette, Conners, & Ulrich, 1978), and the Child Behavior Checklist (Achenbach, 1979).

Choice of Test Instruments

Once the clinician has interviewed the parents, examined and observed the child, he or she is then ready to test the child using test instruments. The first task the clinician is faced with is what instruments are appropriate for evaluating the child. With children of normal intelligence and few behavioral problems, the decision is simple and based upon the child's chronological age. With the developmentally disabled child, the task becomes more difficult. The choice of inappropriate test measures not only wastes time but also can result in an extremely frustrating experience for the child. Since we cannot use chronological age alone as a guide to test selection for the retarded child, a first step in test selection is to establish the child's developmental or mental age level. Based upon interviews with the parents and interaction with the child, the examiner should have some rough idea of the child's general level of developmental functioning. Although different children with the same mental age may vary a great deal in the quality of their intellectual development, a rough assessment of overall developmental functioning is necessary in order to guide the examiner in test selection so that he or she will not select a test that is too easy or difficult for the child. One must be able to select a test instrument that provides an adequate sample of behavior, including both basal and ceiling performance levels. For example, suppose an examiner saw a 2.5-year-old mildly retarded youngster with a developmental age of 18 months. Suppose the examiner decided to use the Stanford-Binet based solely upon the child's chronological age. Because the Stanford-Binet is designed to measure the development of children whose skills are like those of normal children with a chronological age of two years or older, the examiner of this particular child would be unable to obtain a basal age and the test results would be useless. However, if the examiner made his test selection based upon his estimate of the child's developmental age of 18 months, he would choose an infant intelligence test such as the Cattell or Bayley and would have no trouble obtaining basal and ceiling levels.

Measures of adaptive functioning, in contrast to intelligence tests, are chosen based upon the child's chronological age and the child is compared with other children of his chronological and developmental age.

A second important consideration in instrument selection is the psychometric features of the tests to be used. As discussed earlier in this chapter, certain tests are much better than others in terms of their standardization, reliability and validity. Whenever possible it is advisable to choose the most psychometrically sound test instrument when assessing any child. However, there may be times when the clinician must choose tests that are poorly standardized because there are no better tests available. When this occurs, the examiner must decide how best to use the results. It is our preference that when such tests are used, a description of their limitations be included in the psychological report. In addition, test results should be interpreted more conservatively, and behavioral descriptions rather than intelligence test scores should be included in the test report.

A guide to test selection for children of varying developmental ages is provided in Table 10-1. Tests recommended, in our experience, have provided the best information for each developmental age represented. Of course there are times when tests will be added to these basic batteries in order to answer more specific questions about the child's development. The reader will also note that although we have not focused on projective or personality measures in this chapter, we use such measures on children who are verbal enough to respond to them. We have found the use of projectives enormously helpful in diagnosing more extreme forms of psychopathology and in understanding interpersonal problems or intrapsychic conflicts in retarded youngsters. A comprehensive discussion of the use of projectives with dual diagnosis children is presented in Chapter 11.

Table 10-1
Suggested Test Batteries Based On Developmental Level

Developmental Level	Chronological Age	Test Name	Designed to Measure
2 months to 2.5 years	2 months to 12 years	Bayley Scales of Infant Development* or:	Measures mental and motor development; yields a Mental Development Index (MDI) and Psychomotor Development Index (PDI)
		Cattell Infant Intelligence Scale (if no ceiling can be obtained on the Bayley)	Mental age score and intelligence quotient equivalent or ratio IQ
		Alpern-Boll Developmental Profile	Measures physical, self-help, academic, social, and communication skills; yields developmental ages
2.5 to 6 years	2 to 12 years	Stanford-Binet Intelligence Scale (Revised)	Mental age and deviation IQ
		Merrill-Palmer Scale of Mental Tests	Nonverbal performance measure, yields mental age score and percentile score
		AAMD Adaptive Behavior Scale for Infants and Early Childhood (Chronological Ages to 6 years only)	Measures independent functioning, physical development, communication skills, conceptual skills, play, self-direction, personal responsibility, and socialization; yields percentile scores
		Beery Buktenica Visual Motor Integration Test	Measures visual motor integration; yields a Visual Motor Index (VMI) in years and months

≥7 years	6.5 to 12 years	Weschsler Intelligence Scale for Children—Revised	12 subtests measuring specific areas of verbal and nonverbal functioning; yields subtest scaled scores and Verbal, Performance, and Full Scale deviation IQs
		AAMD Adaptive Behavior Scale, 1974 Public School Version (Use with school-aged children)	Assesses 9 behavioral domains including independent functioning, physical development, economic activity, language development, numbers and time concepts, vocational activity, self-direction, responsibility, and socialization. Yields percentile scores based on norms for children in regular, EMR or TMR classrooms
		Bender Visual Motor Gestalt Test for Children (Chronological age to 10 years) or: Beery Buktenica Visual Motor Integration Test	Measures visual motor integration; yields a raw score and mental age equivalent using the Koppitz scoring method

* For children with a chronological age greater than 2.5 years, an approximate developmental age can be estimated using a conversion procedure explained in the manual.

PROBLEMS IN DIAGNOSIS OF THE DUAL DIAGNOSIS CHILD

This chapter concludes with a discussion of common problems in diagnosis of the dual diagnosis child, in order to emphasize the importance of proper understanding and assessment of these unique individuals. Experience has been that these children represent a diagnostic enigma to practitioners involved in their identification and treatment. The major drawback to diagnosis of many of these children has to do with the desire to classify them as either mentally retarded or behaviorally/emotionally disordered, as though the two diagnoses were mutually exclusive.

According to Robinson and Robinson (1976),

> Severe emotional disturbances in retarded children range from short-lived, episodic reactions which emerge only under unusual stress to long-term, continuous, bizarre and intractable psychotic behaviors. Although intellectual handicap and emotional maladjustment are clearly not related . . . in any simple fashion, the incidence of some degree of emotional disturbance is apparently a great deal higher in retarded children than in others of average or superior intellect. (p. 196)

Estimates of the frequency of psychiatric disturbance in retarded children range from 25 to 100 percent (Menolascino, 1965; Webster, 1970). The frequency of finding emotional disturbance in a retarded population varies with the nature of the sample and the mental health facility in which they are diagnosed. Thus, in our hospital, a nationally known, inpatient, brief treatment and diagnostic center, it is uncommon for us to see a retarded child with no emotional maladjustment since it is probably the child's unusual behavior rather than his or her level of retardation that resulted in the need for inpatient hospitalization in the first place. In very young preschool children, Webster (1970) was unable to find a child who was simply retarded without emotional disturbance. However, investigators studying older children find a much lower incidence of disturbance (Menolascino, 1965).

It should be noted that there is considerable controversy concerning the diagnosis of childhood psychopathology and the wisdom of differentiating the primary and secondary roles of mental retardation and emotional disturbance when both are present. It has been this author's experience that in severe forms of psychopathology, retardation and behavioral disorders develop concomitantly from very early in life. Indeed, when parents are asked about their child's development they will often describe developmental delays and associated atypical emotional/social behaviors. There are also cases reported of schizophrenic individuals with clearly documented clinical histories of both mental retardation (primary disorder) and schizophrenia. Recently, Eaton and Menolascino (1982) described 21 percent of their retarded population as having schizophrenia. In this sample, retardation was not secondary to personality regression but rather preceded the onset of the psychiatric disturbance.

It appears that mental retardation and emotional disorder are often so closely associated that many clinicians feel that an accurate differential diagnosis is not possible (Cantor, 1961; Milgram, 1972). Others argue that it is both possible and necessary (Halpern, 1970). A level-headed approach to the debate comes from the recommendation of the Robinsons (Robinson & Robinson, 1976).

> Given the current state of our knowledge and the evidence of the intimate relationship between mental retardation and emotional disorder, the diagnostic goal in most cases should be not to discover whether emotional disturbance or mental retardation is "primary" but rather to determine the depth and nature both of the child's emotional troubles and of his intellectual deficit. (p. 206)

They go on to say that,

> mental retardation is a symptom and not a syndrome. If a child is functioning at a retarded level, then he is retarded, for the time being at least, whether the symptom is associated with permanent organic damage or malfunction, with a chronic illness, with a familial disorder, with cultural deprivation, or with psychosis.... *To refuse to describe these children as mentally retarded because the retardation can be related to emotional factors would be to draw a misleading and incomplete picture of the nature of their behavior.* (p. 206)

We have come to accept the fact that mental retardation and emotional disturbance coexist in many children and to believe that treatment should focus on all aspects of the child's functioning. Unfortunately, what we see in practice is that either the retardation or the emotional disturbance rather than both are addressed. As pointed out in Chapter 6, the emotional needs of many retarded youngsters are ignored because of misconceptions and prejudices concerning psychotherapy with these children. Conversely, some emotionally disturbed retarded children are denied vital services because it is assumed that their retardation is due to a psychiatric disorder. Implicit in this assumption is the idea that if the emotional disorder were not there, the child would function normally. This has not been our experience. A psychiatrically disturbed child may have periods of higher adaptive functioning, but his overall cognitive functioning rarely improves to the point that he no longer needs special services. The reasons for this are numerous but relate to the fact that the earlier the onset of psychopathology, the more severe it is likely to be. In severe forms of psychopathology, retardation and behavioral disorders develop concomitantly from very early in life. Although psychiatric disorders in adults such as schizophrenia involve a period of deterioration or regression from previous levels of functioning, evidence on schizophrenia in children suggests no such dramatic decline in cognition but rather consistent subaverage performance throughout life (Baker, 1979).

Another problem in the early detection of dual-diagnosis children is that often their disturbed behavior interferes with attempts to assess their cognitive functioning. Thus, many examiners will attempt testing, report that the child is untestable but probably of normal intelligence. This conclusion is strikingly frequent in diagnosing children who do not have the physical stigmata or "dull appearance" that many practitioners erroneously ascribe to retarded children. Thus, many mildly retarded children (the majority of the retarded population) who do not have syndromes and who are not dysmorphic but who have behavioral problems are often misdiagnosed as having normal intelligence.

Another fallacy that impedes early and accurate diagnosis is the belief that children are too young to test, or that infant tests are unreliable and not predictive of future intellectual potential. This misconception arises from a failure to appreciate the different predictive power of developmental testing in retarded, as opposed to normal children. As described in this chapter, infant tests used prior to two years of age are not successful in predicting intelligence in normal children; however, infant tests are predictive of later retardation if the child's functioning is quite delayed in infancy (Holden, 1972; Knobloch & Pasamanick, 1960, 1967; Werner, Honzik, & Smith, 1968). Thus, children suspected of showing developmental delay should be followed closely and tested at periodic intervals in order to establish an early diagnosis so that intervention can begin.

In this chapter, I have attempted to describe the tests that we have found useful in the evaluation of the dual-diagnosis child. I have also recommended approaches to testing and highlighted common problems in evaluating this population. I would like to conclude by saying that I hope this chapter has been helpful in pointing the way to sensitive and accurate assessment and I encourage practitioners working in this area to continue in their dedication to this difficult but rewarding group of young people.

REFERENCES

Ables, BS. (1971). The use of the Draw-A-Man Test with borderline retarded children without pronounced pathology. *Journal of Clinical Psychology, 27,* 262–263

Achenbach, TM. (1979). The Child Behavior Profile: I. Boys aged 6-11. *Journal of Consulting and Clinical Psychology, 47,* 223–233

Alpern, GD, & Boll, TJ. (1972). *Developmental profile.* Indianapolis, IN: Psychological Development Publications

Arthur, G. (1962). *The Arthur Adaptation of the Leiter International Performance Scale.* Washington, DC: Psychological Services Center Press

Baker, AM. (1979). Cognitive functioning of psychotic children: A reappraisal. *Exceptional Child, 45*(5), 344–348

Bannatyne, A. (1971). *Language, reading and learning disabilities.* Springfield, IL: Charles Thomas

Bayley, N. (1955). On the growth of intelligence. *American Psychologist, 10,* 805–818

Bayley, N. (1969). *The Bayley Scales of Infant Development.* New York: Psychological Corporation

Beery, KE, & Buktenica, NA. (1967). *Developmental Test of Visual-Motor Integration manual.* Chicago: Follett Publishing Company

Bender, L. (1938). A visual motor gestalt test and its clinical use. In *Research monographs No. 3. American Orthopsychiatric Association.* New York: AOA

Benton, AL. (1963). *Benton Visual Retention Test* (Rev. ed.) New York: Psychological Corporation

Binet, A, & Simon, T. (1905). Méthodes nouvelles pour le diagnostic du niveau intéllectuel des anormaux. *L'Année Psychologique, 11,* 191–244

Bonham, SJ. (1974). Predicting achievement for deaf children. *Psychological Service Center Journal, 14,* 35–44

Cantor, GN. (1961). Some issues involved in Category VIII of the AAMD Terminology and Classification Manual. *American Journal of Mental Deficiency, 65,* 561–566

Cattell, P. (1940, rev. 1960). *The measurement of intelligence of infants and young children.* New York: Psychological Corporation

Covin, TM. (1976). Correlation between the Pinter, Otis-Lennon, Peabody and Wechsler Intelligence Scale for Children—Revised. *Psychological Reports, 39,* 1058

Covin, TM. (1977a). Relationship of Peabody and WISC-R IQs of candidates for special education. *Psychological Reports, 40,* 189–190

Covin, TM. (1977b). Relationship of the SIT and PPVT to the WISC-R. *Journal of School Psychology, 15,* 259–269

Dunn, LM. (1965). *Expanded manual for the Peabody Picture Vocabulary Test.* Circle Pines, MN: American Guidance Service

Dunn, LM, & Dunn, LM. (1981). *Peabody Picture Vocabulary Test—Revised.* Circle Pines, MN: American Guidance Service

Eaton, LF, & Menolascino, FJ. (1982). Psychiatric disorders in the mentally retarded: Types, problems, and challenges. *American Journal of Psychiatry, 139*(10), 1297–1303

Erickson, MT, Johnson, NM, & Campbell, FA. (1970). Relationship among scores on infant tests for children with developmental problems. *American Journal of Mental Deficiency, 75*(i), 102–104

Frostig, M, Maslow, P, Lefever, DW, & Whittlesay, JRB. (1964). The Marianne Frostig Developmental Test of Visual Perception, 1963 standardization. *Perceptual and Motor Skills, 19,* 463–499

Goodman, JF, & Cameron, J. (1978). The meaning of IQ constancy in young retarded children. *Journal of Genetic Psychology, 132*(1), 109–119

Gould, J. (1977). The use of the Vineland Social Maturity Scale, the Merrill-Palmer Scale of Mental Tests (non-verbal items) and the Reynell Developmental Language Scales with children in contact with the services for severe mental retardation. *Journal of Mental Deficiency Research, 21*(3), 213–220

Goyette, CH, Conners, CK, & Ulrich, RF. (1978). Normative data on revised Conners Parent and Teacher Rating Scales. *Journal of Abnormal Child Psychology, 6,* 221–236

Graham, FK, & Kendall, BS. (1973). *The Perceptual and Motor Skills Memory for Designs Test: Revised general manual.* St. Louis, MO: Washington University School of Medicine

Groff, M, & Hubble, L. (1982). WISC-R factor structures of younger and older youth with low IQs. *Journal of Consulting and Clinical Psychology, 50*(1), 148–149

Groff, MG, & Linden, KH. (1982). The WISC-R factor score profiles of cultural–familial mentally retarded and nonretarded youth. *American Journal of Mental Deficiency, 87*(2), 147–152

Gruen, E, & Vore, DA. (1972). Development of conservation in normal and retarded children. *Developmental Psychology, 6*(1), 146–157

Halpern, AS. (1970). Some issues concerning the differential diagnosis of mental retardation and emotional disturbance. *American Journal of Mental Deficiency, 74,* 796–800

Harris, DB. (1963). *Children's drawings as measures of intellectual maturity: A revision and extension of the Goodenough Draw-A-Man Test.* New York: Harcourt, Brace & World

Harrison, KA, & Wiebe, MJ. (1977). Correlational study of McCarthy, WISC-R, and Stanford-Binet scales. *Perceptual and Motor Skills, 44,* 63–68

Harter, S. (1977). The effects of social reinforcement and task difficulty level on the pleasure derived by normal and retarded children from cognitive challenge and mastery. *Journal of Exceptional Child Psychology, 24*(3), 476–494

Harter, S, & Zigler, E. (1974). The assessment of effectance motivation in normal and retarded children. *Developmental Psychology, 10,* 169–180

Hodapp, AF, & Hodapp, JB. (1980). Correlation of the PPVT and WISC-R: A function of diagnostic category. *Psychology in the Schools, 17,* 33–36

Holden, RH. (1972). Prediction of mental retardation in infancy. *Mental Retardation, 10*(1), 28–30

Honzik, M. (1976). Value and limitations of infant tests: An overview. In M Lewis (Ed.), *The origin of intelligence: Infancy and early childhood.* New York: Plenum

Kahn, J. (1976). Utility of the Uzgiris-Hunt scales of sensorimotor development with severely and profoundly retarded children. *American Journal of Mental Deficiency, 80,* 663–665

Kaufman, AS. (1975). Factor analysis of the WISC-R at 11 age levels between 6-1/2 and 16-1/2 years. *Journal of Consulting and Clinical Psychology, 43,* 135–147

Kaufman, AS. (1979). *Intelligent testing with the WISC-R.* New York: Wiley-Interscience

Kaufman, AS, & Van Hagen, J. (1977). Investigation of the WISC-R for use with retarded children: Correlation with the 1972 Stanford-Binet and comparison of WISC and WISC-R profiles. *Psychology in the Schools, 14*(1), 10–14

Knobloch, H, & Pasamanick, B. (1960). An evaluation of the consistency and predictive value of the 40-week Gesell Developmental Schedule. *Psychiatric Research Reports, 13,* 10–31

Knobloch, H, & Pasamanick, B. (1967). Prediction from the assessment of neuromotor and intellectual status in infancy. In J Zubin & GA Jervis (Eds.), *Psychopathology of mental development.* New York: Grune & Stratton

Knobloch, H, & Pasamanick, B. (1974). *Gesell and Amatruda's developmental diagnosis* (3rd ed.). Hagerstown, MD: Harper & Row

Kopp, CB, Sigman, M, & Parmelee, AH. (1973). Ordinality and sensorimotor series. *Child Development, 44,* 821–823

Kopp, CB, Sigman, M, & Parmelee, AH. (1974). Longitudinal study of sensorimotor development. *Developmental Psychology, 10,* 687–695

Koppitz, EM. (1963). *The Bender Gestalt Test for Young Children.* New York: Grune & Stratton

Koppitz, EM. (1975). *The Bender Gestalt Test for Young Children: Research and application, 1963–1973* (Vol. 2). New York: Grune & Stratton

Krauft, VR, & Krauft, CC. (1972). Structured vs unstructured visual-motor tests for educable retarded children. *Perceptual & Motor Skills, 34*(3), 691–694

Lambert, NM, Windmiller, M, Cole, L, & Figueroa, RA. (1975). Standardization of a public school version of the AAMD Adaptive Behavior Scale. *Mental Retardation, 12*(2), 3–7

Lehman, EB, & Levy, BI. (1971). Discrepancies in estimates of children's intelligence. WISC and human figure drawings. *Journal of Clinical Psychology, 27,* 74–76

Leiter, RG. (1948). *Leiter International Performance Scale.* Chicago: Stoelting

Levenson, RL, & Zino, TC. (1979). Assessment of cognitive deficiency with the McCarthy Scales and Stanford-Binet: A correlational analysis. *Perceptual and Motor Skills, 48,* 291–295

McCall, RB. (1979). The development of intellectual functioning in infancy and prediction of later I.Q. In JD Osofsky (Ed.), *Handbook of infant development.* New York: Wiley

McCarthy, D. (1972). *Manual for the McCarthy Scales of Children's Abilities.* New York: Psychological Corporation

McDevitt, SC, McDevitt, SC, & Rosen, M. (1977). Adaptive Behavior Scale, Part II: A cautionary note and suggestions for revisions. *American Journal of Mental Deficiency, 82,* 210–212

Menolascino, FJ. (1965). Emotional disturbance and mental retardation. *American Journal of Mental Deficiency, 70,* 248–256

Menolascino, FJ. (1969). Emotional disturbances in mentally retarded children. *American Journal of Psychiatry, 126,* 168–176

Mercer, JR. (1979). *System of Multicultural Pluralistic Assessment technical manual.* New York: Psychological Corporation

Mercer, JR, & Lewis, JF. (1978). *System of Multicultural Pluralistic Assessment.* New York: Psychological Corporation

Milgram, NA. (1972). MR and mental illness: A proposal for conceptual unity. *Mental Retardation, 10*(6), 29–31

Naglieri, JA. (1980a). Comparison of McCarthy General Cognitive Index and WISC-R IQ for educable mentally retarded, learning disabled, and normal children. *Psychological Reports, 47*(2), 591–596

Naglieri, JA. (1980b). WISC-R subtest patterns for learning disabled and mentally retarded children. *Perceptual and Motor Skills, 51*(2), 605–606

Naglieri, JA. (1982). Use of the WISC-R and PPVT-R with mentally retarded children. *Journal of Clinical Psychology, 38*(3), 635–637

Naglieri, JA, & Harrison, PL. (1979). Comparison of McCarthy General Cognitive Indexes and Stanford-Binet IQs for educable mentally retarded children. *Perceptual and Motor Skills, 48,* 1251–1254

Nihira, K, Foster, R, Shellhaas, M, & Leland, H. (1974). *AAMD Adaptive Behavior Scale* (rev. ed.). Washington, DC: American Association on Mental Deficiency

Ottenbacher, K. (1981). An investigation of self-concept and body image in the mentally retarded. *Journal of Clinical Psychology, 37*(2), 415–418

Patterson, HO, & Milakofsky, L. (1980). A paper-and-pencil inventory for the assessment of Piaget's tasks. *Applied Psychological Measurement, 4*(3), 341–353

Peterson, CR, & Hart, DH. (1979). Factor structure of the WISC-R for a clinic-referred population and specific subgroups. *Journal of Consulting and Clinical Psychology, 47*(3), 643–645

Prasse, DP, & Bracken, BA. (1981). Comparison of the PPVT-R and WISC-R with urban educable mentally retarded students. Psychology in the Schools, *18*(2), 174–177

Quay, HC, & Peterson, DR. (1967). *Manual for the Behavior Problem Checklist.* Champaign, IL: University of Illinois, Children's Research Center

Reschly, DJ. (1981). Evaluation of the effects of SOMPA measures on classification of students as mildly mentally retarded. *American Journal of Mental Deficiency, 86*(1), 16–20

Rice, JA. (1972, September). *Benton's Visual Retention Test: New age, scale scores, and percentile norms for children.* Paper presented at the meeting of the American Psychological Association, Honolulu, HI

Robinson, NM, & Robinson, HB. (1976). *The mentally retarded child: A psychological approach* (2nd ed.). New York: McGraw-Hill

Roszkowski, MJ. (1980). Concurrent validity of the Adaptive Behavior Scale as assessed by the Vineland Social Maturity Scale. *American Journal of Mental Deficiency, 85,* 86–89

Rutter, M, & Bartak, L. (1973). Special educational treatment of autistic children. *Journal of Child Psychology and Psychiatry, 14,* 165–179

Saigh, PA, & Payne, DA. (1978). Effect of reinforcement of response on internal consistency of selected WISC-R subtests. *Psychological Reports, 43,* 756–758

Sattler, JM. (1982). *Assessment of children's intelligence and special abilities* (2nd ed.). Boston, MA: Allyn & Bacon

Shorr, DN, McClelland, SE, & Robinson, HB. (1977). Corrected mental age scores for the Stanford-Binet Intelligence Scale. *Measurement and Evaluation in Guidance, 10,* 144–147

Silverstein, AB. (1972). Another look at sources of variance in the Developmental Test of Visual Perception. *Psychological Reports, 31,* 557–558

Silverstein, AB. (1982). Note on the constancy of the IQ. *American Journal of Mental Deficiency, 87*(2), 227–228

Sloan, JL, & Marcus, L. (1981). Some findings on the use of the adaptive behavior scale with autistic children. *Journal of Autism and Developmental Disorders, 11*(2), 191–199

Spellacy, F, & Black, FW. (1972). Intelligence assessment of language-impaired children by means of two nonverbal tests. *Journal of Clinical Psychology, 28,* 357–358

Stott, L, & Ball, R. (1965). Infant and preschool mental tests. *Monographs of the Society for Research in Child Development, 30*(3, No. 101)

Stutsman, R. (1948). *Mental measurement of preschool children.* New York: Harcourt, Brace & World

Terman, LM. (1916). *The measurement of intelligence.* Boston: Houghton Mifflin

Terman L, & Merrill, M. (1960). *Stanford-Binet Intelligence Scale: Manual for the third edition, form L-M.* Boston: Houghton-Mifflin

Uzgiris, IC, & Hunt, MMcV. (1975). *Assessment in infancy: Original scales of psychological development.* Urbana, IL: University of Illinois

Vance, HB, Blixt, S, Ellis, R, & Debell, S. (1981). Stability of the WISC-R for a sample of exceptional children. *Journal of Clinical Psychology, 37*(2), 397–399

Vance, HB, Pritchard, KK, & Wallbrown, FH. (1978). Comparison of the WISC-R and PPVT for a group of mentally retarded students. *Psychology in the Schools, 15,* 349–351

Vander Veer B, & Schweid, E. (1974). Infant assessment: Stability of mental functioning in young retarded children. *American Journal of Mental Deficiency, 79*(1), 1–4

Van Hagen, J., & Kaufman, A.S. Factor analysis of the WISC-R for a group of mentally retarded children and adolescents, *Journal of Consulting and Clinical Psychology,* 1980, *43*(5), 661–667

Wachs, TD. (1970). Report on the utility of a Piaget based infant scale with older retarded children. *Developmental Psychology, 2,* 449–458

Webster, TG. (1970). Unique aspects of emotional development in mentally retarded individuals. In FJ Menolascino (Ed.), *Psychiatric approaches to mental retardation.* New York: Basic Books

Wechsler, D. (1967). *Manual for the Wechsler Preschool and Primary Scale of Intelligence.* New York: Psychological Corporation

Wechsler, D. (1974). *Wechsler Intelligence Scale for Children—Revised.* New York: Psychological Corporation

Werner, EE, Bierman, JM, & French, P. (1971). *The children of Kauai: A longitudinal study from the prenatal period to age 10.* Honolulu: University of Hawaii Press

Werner, EE, Honzik, MP, & Smith, RS. (1968). Prediction of intelligence and achievement at 10 years from 20-month pediatric and psychologic examination. *Child Development, 39,* 1063–1078

Martha Jura
Marian Sigman

11

Evaluation of Emotional Disorders Using Projective Techniques With Mentally Retarded Children

Clinical work with emotionally disturbed children and adolescents often involves an initial assessment of psychological processes. In most treatment facilities, such an assessment would include not only evaluation of cognitive and perceptual abilities but also an analysis of emotional and psychological functioning. In general, this analysis would be based on the responses of the child to a battery of projective techniques.

The emotional problems of the mentally retarded child are rarely evaluated in this manner. In the literature on projective testing (Anastasi, 1954; Beck, 1945, 1952; Beck, Beck, Levitt, & Molish, 1961; Klopfer, 1956; Klopfer, Ainsworth, Klopfer, & Holt, 1954; Rapaport, Gill, & Schafer, 1968; Schafer, 1948) there is no discussion of how these techniques might be adapted for use with the mentally retarded individual. The major concern has been one of differential diagnosis, with a focus on distinguishing psychosis from mental retardation. This might be seen as an extension of the original impetus for the development of psychological tests, which Anastasi (1954) has described as the identification of the feebleminded. Once the diagnosis of mental retardation is made, aberrant response patterns are often attributed to cognitive deficits. There has been little realization that projective tests are as powerful tools for the assessment of the emotional problems in mentally retarded individuals as in individuals of normal intelligence.

As a result, there is little literature on the use of projective tests with mentally defective individuals. There is however, an extensive literature on the

CHILDREN WITH EMOTIONAL DISORDERS AND DEVELOPMENTAL DISABILITIES ISBN 0–8089–1700–5

relationship between intelligence and integration of percepts on the Rorschach. Exner (1974) reviews this literature and notes that form and organizational level are related to intelligence. On this basis, good performance on the Rorschach is seen as contradicting a diagnosis of retardation. Recently, Exner and Weiner have described the limited determinants and poor organization seen in the percepts of retarded individuals. Consistent with this observation is the use of the Rorschach to identify retardation. Exner and Weiner (1982) have suggested, "if the Rorschach of a subject with severe intellectual limitation is not impoverished it may be appropriate to explore areas of cognitive functioning more thoroughly" (pp. 286–287). They go on to conclude that the Rorschach may be useful in the case of those with severe intellectual deficit, but that it can "probably contribute more to the planning for those cases in which the subject is not truly retarded, but rather is limited in talent," (p. 287).

In our child psychiatric service, we have made extensive use of projectives as part of a full battery of tests among truly retarded patients. In reviewing admissions to our inpatient ward over a two-year period, we found that projectives, including the Rorschach and Thematic Apperception Test, were not used in only 2 of approximately 100 cases. Thus, projectives are routinely administered to our mentally retarded inpatients at NPI. This is done not only in order to distinguish between mental retardation and other disabilities, but in order to identify psychological disturbances that might be present in addition to mental retardation, and to describe the dynamic functioning of dual diagnosis patients that might have implications for treatment.

THE USE OF DEVELOPMENTAL LEVEL IN INTERPRETATION

The concept that makes it possible to interpret the projectives of retarded adolescents is the concept of developmental level. It is our working assumption that has been supported by our experience that the developmentally delayed individual will provide an immature performance that reflects his developmental rather than his chronological level. This concept is important in understanding all projectives of this population, but it is particularly important in the case of the Rorschach. The question we ask ourselves is, "To what extent does this patient's cognitive or mental age account for this performance?" It should be noted that this process is full of approximations. Our estimate of developmental level is just that, an estimate, based primarily on intellectual testing. The responses to the Rorschach and other protocols are compared to the responses of other individuals of similar developmental level.

The justification for analyzing responses in this manner is suggested by research indicating a relationship between intelligence and sophistication of integration on the Rorschach (Exner, 1974; Exner & Weiner, 1982). In addition, some data on fantasy suggest that the content described, such as fears expressed, are related to cognitive maturity rather than chronological age (Derevensky, 1979).

Of course, the nature of responses to the projective tests is only partly a function of developmental level, and many other factors are influential. Chronological age is in fact one of these factors. Social and emotional development vary to some extent with an individual's chronological age regardless of his intelligence. Although the individual may have the cognitive capacities of a person of his mental age, he has still had experiences and impulses like a person of his chronological age. The heterogeneity in level of experiences and motivating impulses produces inconsistencies in the performance of mentally retarded individuals on projective tests. These inconsistencies appear in the type of vocabulary used as well as in expressed interests and concerns.

For example, a 17-year-old boy with a long history of moderate retardation was referred for inpatient evaluation for behavior problems. His most recent IQ Score was 43, making his mental age about 6-5. Other recent cognitive testing placed him at the 5- to 6-year-old level. His story to one of the TAT cards reflects the range of his concerns. "The girl is talking to the man. She says, 'Do not go . . . do not talk to strangers, and no hitch hiking, OK?' " On the one hand, this story gives the impression of a young child trying to internalize the prohibitions of the adults around him, and, on the other hand it ends with a concern of boys his own age.

Because of the variability in expected responses, interpretation of projective material has to be more flexible than is usual with projective material from individuals of normal intelligence. Although we are able to score responses on the Rorschach with any of the well-known systems (Beck, 1945, 1952; Beck et al., 1961; Exner, 1974, 1978; Klopfer et al., 1954; Klopfer, 1956), until recently the scoring could not be easily used to make interpretations in the manner described by the formulators of these systems because of the lack of valid and current norms for children. Even with better norms, interpretation of quantitative scores is still difficult. Without norms generated on mentally retarded individuals of varying chronological and mental ages, interpretation of responses to projective tests for retarded persons must necessarily be more individualized. However, by using developmental level to modify our understanding of the patient's "age" in assessing projective material, we can make a start in teasing apart cognitive disability and emotional disturbance. Without correcting for intellectual level, one either could not use projectives or one would run the risk of overestimating the degree of psychological disruption.

In order to estimate developmental level, any of the standard intelligence tests reviewed in the previous chapter can be used. Mental age can be estimated for the WISC-R using Table 21 of the manual. The method of calculating mental age on the Stanford-Binet has been described in the previous chapter. Because our estimate of developmental level is an approximation, we often try to base it not only on mental age but also modify it based on achievement levels reported by school or measured on achievement tests.

PROJECTIVE TESTS ADMINISTERED

We use the full range of projective assessments with retarded individuals that are commonly used with nonretarded individuals. We routinely administer the Thematic Apperception Test and the Rorschach as well as the Sentence Completion, Draw-a-Person, and Draw-a-Family. The MMPI is essentially never given because of its verbal demands. Besides overall cognitive levels, the richness of the material depends on the patient's specific verbal level and communication style. As with the projective material of young children, the projective material of retarded individuals is immature and restricted in various ways. As a result, the examiner often has to be more active than usual in eliciting important thematic material and supporting the productive efforts of the patient. We make the accommodations one often does in explaining and administering the tests to young children. For example, we often give the inquiry right after the free association on the Rorschach.

The usefulness of this effort is often unknown before it has been attempted and sometimes the results are unexpected. One retarded patient was asked to respond to the Sentence Completion. He said it made him mad that he couldn't read, and stated, "My greatest fault . . . is fall down, fall down, hit yourself in the head. Brain damage," suggesting his theory of what had happened to him. Once the testing is completed, the results are presented for the retarded patient, much as they would be for other patients.

GENERAL APPROACH

One of the major aims of the test interpretation is to specify whether the individual suffers from emotional disorders and, if so, to describe the extent and nature of these disorders. Another aim is to understand the kinds of feelings or difficulties experienced by the individual. The projective material is useful for both aims. In order to illustrate our general approach, we will present a case example.

PF was a 13-year-old boy referred for behavior and learning problems. His mother was having difficulty managing him at home as was his teacher at school. On the Stanford-Binet, he had an IQ of 44 and a mental age of 5-4. His range of function was between the ages of 4-6 and 6 years. His graphic material was consistent with this estimate of cognitive age. The Bender-Gestalt included numerous problems with distortions and integration and was like the performance of a child of 5-6 and 5-8 years. The Draw-a-Person depicted a head with major features, with legs and feet protruding from the head, and was like the rendering of a 4-5–year-old child. Thus, all measures of cognitive and visual-motor skills were consistent in placing this boy's developmental level at about 5 years of age. The Rorschach responses were as follows: Card I. Butterfly. II. Don't know. III. It looks like men. IV. Skunk. V. Bird. VI. Dragonfly. VII. Spider. VIII. On a Bike. IX. Picking up weights. X. Burn.

To the TAT, he told a number of stories involving people who were angry. To the picture of the boy with the violin, he said "He is thinking; try to do his own work. I don't know what else." When asked how the boy feels, PF replied, "He is mad." To the picture of a man and woman, he said "The man is mad. He wants to leave his mother. She don't want him to leave." The other stories also described people who have a desire to be able to do things and go places but are prevented by their own disabilities or other people's wishes so that they end up angry. His responses to the Sentence Completion also emphasized problems with acceptance and affection. The phrase, "I like people who," was ended, "nice." "Everything I do," was completed with "hug my mom." "If only my father" was ended with "would be nice to me." "The worst thing I ever did" was completed with "hug my mom." Despite his obvious difficulties with formulating responses, on all the projective material, he was able to provide informative thematic material.

In order to determine the extent of his emotional pathology, the kinds of responses he gave were compared to what might be expected for a child of a developmental age about 5 years. In this light, his responses to the Rorschach and other projective tests were a bit immature, but not bizarre. While his responses to some of the Rorschach blots were less appropriate and well-integrated than his response to others, this seemed to be specific to particular areas of conflict. Thus, based on his overall level of responses, we saw his difficulties as reflecting problems in adjustment rather than serious psychiatric illness. In order to understand the kinds of difficulties he was experiencing, the content of the material was used. He expressed very ambivalent feelings about dependency and closeness, particularly to maternal figures. In the Sentence Completion and TAT, he clearly showed that a central problem for him was his overdependency on his mother. Based on these results and some observations of the boy over time, counseling was recommended for the boy and the mother to help them to work out a facilitating relationship in general and a program of limits and responsibilities in particular.

THE USE OF THE RORSCHACH WITH DUAL DIAGNOSIS POPULATIONS

We would like to focus on the Rorschach because it has been used more than other projective tests with the mentally retarded, albeit in the identification of mental retardation rather than emotional disorders. As noted earlier, because of the relationship between the organization of the percepts and developmental or intellectual level, professionals have felt able to contradict the diagnosis of mental retardation when they observed an unexpectedly high performance on the Rorschach. A number of investigators have noted an association between low form level and mental retardation (Beck, 1932; Klopfer & Kelly, 1942). Jolles (1947) identified a relationship between "feeblemindedness" and measures of organization. Hemmendinger (1953, 1960) has found a relationship between developmental level and differentiation of Rorschach percepts. More recently Exner and Weiner (1982) have described the protocols of retarded individuals as "impoverished" in some general way. We would agree with this and the protocol quoted above might be characterized in this way.

Exner and Weiner (1982, p. 286) have provided the most detailed information about the Rorschach responses of individuals with IQs below 75. They describe these protocols as restricted in that the protocols are brief, contain mostly pure form responses, and show few figures in movement. If chromatic color is used, it is poorly integrated and color naming occurs relatively frequently. The quality of the form responses is weak and, as a result, the percentage of adequate responses tends to be low. Few responses that synthesize various portions of the percept are produced. The contents tend to be restricted and emphasize botany, animals, and landscape. On the whole, the number of popular answers is lower than average. These characterizations seem valid for the Rorschach protocols we have seen from mentally retarded individuals.

On the other hand, Exner and Weiner (1982) suggest that the variations between protocols will be slight for the retarded population (IQs below the mid 70s), and this does not agree with our observations. Even with the limitations noted above, there is wide variability in response patterns, as will be clear from the case examples provided throughout this chapter. It is this variability that allows us not only to confirm or contradict the diagnosis of retardation, but that allows us to approach a variety of other diagnostic issues as well.

METHODS FOR ASSESSING RORSCHACH PROTOCOLS

Three general methods are used in analyzing Rorschach responses. First, as mentioned previously, the responses are scored and the scores compared to those of children at a similar developmental level. For this purpose, the norms provided by Exner and Weiner (1982) for children from age 5 to 16 years are particularly useful. In addition, they have described the important developmental shifts that take place over this time span. Another set of descriptions of the Rorschach protocols of children and adolescents has been generated by Ames and her colleagues (Ames, Learned, Metreax, & Walker, 1952; Ames, Metreax, & Walker, 1971). These note the responses most frequently given by children and adolescents. The "popular" responses listed by adolescents (Ames, et al., 1952) are similar to those noted by Exner (1974).

Another method of analyzing Rorschach responses is to contrast one response with another. With this method, the use of each blot is compared with the others so that levels of integration can be specified. In this way, the patient's higher functioning can be contrasted with lower functioning. This allows a judgment of variability and also provides information about the situations that are difficult for the patient.

This method is particularly useful for assessing the degree of regression that a patient manifests from previous levels of functioning. If responses are very variable in terms of level of integration, the assumption is that the patient has been better able to organize his thoughts in the past. Using this method, psychopathology was identified in one retarded patient who saw a "butterfly" or named the colors on virtually all the blots but one (III), where she said, "they're pulling." The reference to two people was vague, but after further elaboration, was sufficient to indicate an entirely different, and higher, developmental level. This type of analysis of regression in the Rorschach is very useful in the assessment of degree and type of disturbances in retarded patients. In general, in the case of neurotic types of problems, the modal level is appropriate to the cognitive level and other levels represent regressions triggered by specific conflicts or concerns. An example is the protocol given previously (PF, page 232). His responses were particularly poor to Card VII and to the colored cards, suggesting greater difficulty with emotionally arousing situations. The psychotic patient (unless perhaps severely regressed) is expected to show even greater variability in level of functioning. A contrast between responses of an appropriate developmental level with more immature responses makes the presence of regression and disrupting factors clear. This is in contrast to the patient whose sole problem is an intellectual deficit. In the case of mental retardation, much less variability will be seen from one blot to another and modal level of responding will approximate estimates of cognitive abilities. As will be seen with later examples, the patient with characterologic problems may tend to show little variability across blots, but the overall level will commonly be more primitive than might be anticipated based on intellectual abilities.

A third approach to the Rorschach analysis, which is a direct outgrowth of the first two, is to be sensitive to responses or response patterns that do not reflect any developmental level at all. That is, some responses would not be regarded as normal or appropriate at any age. Such responses are often experienced as bizarre, and those sensitive to even the most immature performances will find these percepts and comments unusual. For example, one adolescent with an IQ of 65 saw on Rorschach III "Two insects craving a hoe (or whore)." It is hard to imagine a developmental level at which this would be an appropriate response.

All of these approaches involve looking at a number of determinants, but for our purposes as presented here, it is particularly fruitful to focus on the formal structural characteristics of individual percepts (the form level) and unusual features of language or logic (what Exner codes as "special scores").

ASSESSING SEVERE PSYCHOPATHOLOGY

The approaches described above are particularly useful in assessing the Rorschachs of the most disturbed patients, those with very disordered functioning, including odd thinking and verbalizations. Their cognitive confusion often raises the issue of schizophrenia. Despite the simplicity of the Rorschachs of retarded individuals, it is frequently possible to assess their protocols for the response pattern often associated with the symptoms of schizophrenia. Interestingly, we are not often asked to help clarify the diagnosis of affective disorder in retarded patients. In assessing schizophrenia, we basically use the Exner criteria as guidelines after we have corrected for developmental level. Little correction is necessary in terms of form level because of the tendency of children to see the world like their elders, starting as young as five years of age. That is, we expect approximately 80 percent of the responses to show acceptable form across a wide range of developmental ages starting at 5 years. In assessing thought disorder, we count the number of critical logical errors in excess of the number allowed for based on the individual's developmental, not chronological, age. In the end, if the form level is less than 70 percent and if more responses are minus than weak, and if the patient shows the critical special scores much in excess of expectation, we consider the possibility that the patient may be schizophrenic. (The reader is referred to Exner and Weiner [1982] for a discussion of the exact criteria.) The reason for using these criteria as guidelines is to determine whether the patient's thinking is deviant as well as immature. Bizarre and illogical thinking have not been reported as the result of retardation alone.

One young man was referred for strange and aggressive behavior as well as hallucinations about hearing the Devil and delusions which focused on his genitalia and anus. He had been functioning in the retarded range for many years. In 1977 his IQ Scores on the Wechsler had been Verbal 58, Performance 52, and Full Scale 52. In 1981 after a seizure his IQ was estimated to be below 32 and our estimate of his IQ on the Binet was also under 32. Although a young adult, his mental age was about 5-0. However, he did not see the world as one of his chronological age, like one of his original mental age (between 8 and 10), or like one of his later mental age (about 5 years). His percepts were very deviant and dysphoric, including a perseverative reference to bones that included a reference to "bones in the eye" of one skeleton. He did, however, give some appropriate responses, including a large animal on IV, and spiders and lobsters on X. The basic simplicity of his percepts suggested his retardation. The perseveration might be due to disturbance or organicity. The dysphoric and illogical content clearly related to his extreme psychopathology. This was manifested both in terms of problems with reality testing (F + % = .50, X + % = .36) and thought disorder (10 special scores).

The Rorschach is most successfully used in conjunction with the patient's history and presentation. When the diagnosis is not clear based on hallucinations and delusions as seen in behavior and poor reality testing plus thought disorder as seen on the Rorschach, the diagnosis is more difficult. In these cases, the Rorschach can sometimes help to establish a preponderance of evidence. However, in each case, the presentation, history and projectives must all be assessed together in making a determination of any diagnosis, particularly of schizophrenia.

Some retarded patients have been diagnosed schizophrenic without clear evidence of hallucinations or delusions, based on disordered thinking and behavior in the context of history. It should be noted that when thinking is immature to begin with as it is with retarded patients, it is often difficult to identify thought disorder proper, and this criteria is used cautiously with retarded individuals. While a determination or diagnosis is never made based on testing, the test data has often contributed to our understanding of these as well as other patients. The Rorschach has in these cases reflected very deviant and not just immature thinking.

For example, an 18-year-old girl was seen for bizarre behaviors, including constant talking to herself and eating dogfood out of the dog's dish. She had been in TMR class, and at the time of hospitalization, her IQ on the Binet was 38. Her mental age was about 6 years 5 months. Even the more structured material included incongruous elements. To a TAT picture showing a boy sitting in front of a violin, she saw a boy "reading his book." The Rorschach responses were poorly conceived and showed problems with reality testing. When given more time she could respond more appropriately on some of the more simple and structured blots. She became completely disorganized on the more complex and arousing cards. She saw spiders on VIII and a monkey on X. The rainbow seen on IX might have been forgiven as a function of her overall developmental age. However, other responses were not just immature, but unusual, illogical, bizarre, and dysphoric. For example, she saw a "body of a horse" and "horsemeat" on III. It was concluded that her problems on the projective material were not accounted for by her cognitive deficits, and that specific features of the Rorschach suggested serious emotional disturbance in addition to mental retardation. Even allowing for her mental age, her responses were acceptable on only four blots of ten, and the degree of disruption in reality testing alone was sufficient to describe her functioning as psychotic. Her bizarre and dysphoric responses (as well as presentation and history) suggested she might well be schizophrenic as well as retarded.

On the other hand, some patients might be diagnosed retarded and schizophrenic based on clear evidence of hallucinations or delusions (in the absence of indications of affective disorder), but their protocols are so simple or regressed for a variety of reasons, that it would be difficult to get a clear diagnostic impression based on the testing.

Sometimes, however, the presentation, history and protocol are all so nonspecific that it would be difficult to specify the diagnosis from even all three. We often see patients early in their adolescence, and it is apparent that they are overwhelmed by the need to integrate new impulses and increasing stimulation and demands. It is not clear whether they are struggling with truly "schizophrenic" thought processes, or are impaired individuals who are regressing in almost a reactive way because of psychological stresses in the context of cognitive and possibly neurologic impairment. In particular, our ability to make diagnostic distinctions decreases when the intellectual capacities of the individuals are very limited. It is our impression that a certain intellectual level is necessary for discrete thought disorder to clearly manifest itself as "schizophrenia," and be identified as such. For this reason, many of these retarded adolescents who present with diffuse problems in behavior and thinking are diagnosed as atypical psychosis.

One such patient was a 17-year-old boy who presented with aggressive and unusual behavior. He had threatened his mother with a knife at home. In the hospital, he spoke of his friendship with a movie actor who had been dead for years. At times he was seen moving his lips and it appeared that he might be speaking to someone, perhaps this actor. Despite this, it was not clear whether he was in fact delusional and hallucinating or disorganized in some other way. He had a long history of developmental delay. There was some question of organic dysfunction, but he had been exposed to environmental trauma as well, and had grown up under fire in a war zone. His family psychiatric history was unclear. The intellectual results placed his functioning below 45 on the WISC–R. The picture of a primitive and impoverished individual cognitively and emotionally was supported by the Rorschach. He saw birds, bears, dogs, and horses more like a young child than a maturing adolescent. There was nothing dysphoric about the content, or bizarre about his verbalizations. The most malignant aspect of his performance was his perception of two bears on II who seemed to be involved in some fight (based on the red area). Most striking, however, was the fragmentation of his percepts on the Rorschach. The form level on the Rorschach was uniformly poor, suggesting that this boy had significant difficulty interpreting what he saw. The occasional presence of good fit of percept and blot (the woman on I and the animals on VIII) suggests that he had glimpses of what was going on around him. The nature of the confusion he revealed suggested that he had difficulty differentiating between aspects of himself, other objects, and other individuals in almost every conceivable way. On the Rorschach, number VII was seen as "A person, three people, four people." The patient could not clarify the locations of these, ultimately, four individuals, and eyes stared out from the grey areas, and feet and ears poked out at the perimeters. In addition, he added a bird, noting two wings. It was clear that this patient was profoundly confused and disorganized, but it was not clear he was typically schizophrenic, so he was diagnosed as atypical psychosis, based on all the data.

From our experience using projective tests, we have come to realize that the percepts of autistic children and adolescents differ from those of schizophrenic individuals and that the Rorschach is helpful in assessing these individuals. While the typical patient with symptoms of schizophrenia shows illogical thought and poor reality testing, the patient with the syndrome of autism often shows unusual thinking in the context of appropriate reality testing. The protocols of autistic patients usually show immature form but it is appropriate to either their own developmental level, or to some even more immature but recognizable stage. That is, even if the percepts are immature based on their cognitive level, the responses are recognized as those of young children ("pumpkin," I; "face," II; "frog," III; "tree," IV; etc.) If this is not true of the most disordered protocols (and diagnostically problematic cases), even these usually show the patient's commitment to external reality.

It is our impression that the schizophrenic is so confused and responsive to his own concerns that his responses have a curious relationship to the blot and his thinking is illogical. On the other hand, the individual with autism makes every attempt to be true to this blot in some way although he thinks about his experience in peculiar ways. The differences between these groups is often seen in the nature of their poor form level. While the schizophrenic often scores with distorted responses (more minus than weak) the patient with autism shows vague or concrete responses. For example, an autistic 11-year-old boy (who was obsessed with helicopters, and engaged in much spinning and whirring behavior) had cognitive abilities like those of a 6–7-year-old, but described every blot as a butterfly.

A 13-year-old boy referred for bizarre behavior and verbalizations, with an IQ of 83, gave a protocol with good fit of percept to blot but described one blot as "two ladies hanging onto the birdbath" and another as "two birds talking to each other." Another teenage boy with overall cognitive abilities at about 6–7 years, showed particular skill in reproducing visual images on the Object Assembly and Block Design although his drawings on the Bender Gestalt were less sophisticated. His responses to the Rorschach were immature but more or less appropriate to the structure of the blots. However, some of his verbalizations were odd. To the third Rorschach card, he described a pumpkin and then went on to add "It makes witches." His Draw-a-Person and TAT stories revealed a kind of cognitive and emotional vacancy. To the TAT picture of the boy with the violin, he said "He feels happy. This is a violin. This is a paper and that's it." When asked what the boy was happy about, he said "Nothing."

Thus, autistic children and adolescents produce odd verbalizations in the presence of "acceptable" form level. Unlike schizophrenic children, they seem to perceive their environment correctly but their interpretations are faulty. These patterns of strengths and weakness have been described in research studies as well (see Chapter 7).

Of course, it is not always this simple. One patient was diagnosed autistic after much debate whether she was hallucinating or not, and whether she should be diagnosed schizophrenic. Her Rorschach reflected some of the same diagnostic confusion. On Rorschach III she saw a monster with a "ribbon blood nose." She elaborated saying "and blood's coming out of the head and it doesn't have a head." Other responses included dysphoric intrusions, including some about poison. Thus, autistic individuals who develop symptoms of schizophrenia later in life, such as hallucinations and loose associations, may tend to show features in their Rorschach protocols more like those of schizophrenics.

UNDERSTANDING PROBLEMS IN BEHAVIOR

Frequently, the aim of the assessment is to clarify the basis for behavioral disturbances in mentally retarded individuals. Behavior problems may appear in the form of overdependency, with the individual clinging to his parents and fearing separation. Alternatively, or in addition, the individual may have temper tantrums and show aggressive behavior with or without provocation. Certain response patterns on the Rorschach are characteristic of impulsive people, who have limited capacities to respond in a controlled fashion to emotionally arousing stimuli. These individuals tend to report percepts that use the color of the blot unintegrated with the form, and to see little human movement. They may also respond to blots as diffuse wholes rather than in a differentiated fashion. Their poor judgment is sometimes reflected in a paucity of responses that are frequently reported by others (the "populars"). Behavioral problems can be traced to particular ego deficits in the capacity for impulse control, but they are also attributable to other factors. In some cases, the individual may be acting inappropriately because of limited knowledge of situations or more appropriate actions. As mentioned above, behavior problems can also be associated with psychosis. Finally, inappropriate behaviors or loss of control may result from more emotional or characterologic deficits. Projective tests are very useful in differentiating between these alternative bases for inappropriate behavior patterns. The following case illustrates how immature thinking can be associated with inappropriate behavior.

An 11-year-old boy was referred for inappropriate and aggressive social behavior. He had a long history of retardation, probably associated with a neurologic disorder. He also puzzled his parents with claims of the superpowers of heroes, and had frightened them (understandably) when he climbed to a window ledge and announced he would fly away. There was a need to understand whether this boy's behavior was due to thought disorder or gross immaturity. At the time of evaluation, he was functioning well within the retarded range overall with a Full Scale IQ Score of 48 (Verbal 59 and Performance 45) on the WISC–R. There was some inter- and intratest scatter but it was not marked. Despite this, other cognitive evaluations indicated that he was functioning across a range of age levels, from about 5 to 8 years. His social behavior seemed lower than that. The Rorschach was helpful because it made clear how concrete he was, and that his symbolic thinking was very immature. When asked what the blots looked like to him, he responded as if they were in fact what they appeared to be. On the first, he noted it was like gum, and then while tracing it, touched it with his finger and noted "It won't come off." He responded in a similar manner to other blots. He seemed delayed differentially across a number of cognitive areas, but this symbolic immaturity was crucial. It was felt that the boy was not thought-disordered because there was nothing primitive or bizarre about the protocol, but that his thought patterns were extremely immature. It was recommended that he be carefully supervised, and that his exposure to fantasy be carefully monitored. He was not a child who could be left in front of a TV set to watch whatever came on without trouble later.

In other cases, acting-out or aggressive, impulsive behavior does not seem to be attributable to cognitive deficits but more to personality disorders. Unlike the boy discussed above, who was cognitively immature, these children act impulsively not because they do not understand situations but because they have learned inappropriate behavior patterns. An example of such a case, a socially infantalized boy, is given below.

A 12-year-old boy was referred for behavior problems in his residential placement. His behavior had become increasingly aggressive and self-abusive. He showed inappropriate approach behavior, kissing, and hugging the adults and peers he encountered. This annoyed and frightened other children and was responsible for provoking a number of fights. Previous testing on the WISC–R had placed his IQ in the moderate range of mental retardation with a Full Scale IQ Score of 41 (Verbal 49 and Performance 45). His Vineland showed a social quotient of 57. His difficulties with gross and fine motor coordination were suggestive of neurologic dysfunction. The inpatient evaluation suggested discrepancies between his cognitive and behavioral level. On the ward he seemed like a child of two or three. However, his mental age seemed to be above that with perceptual–motor functioning between four and five years, and auditory–verbal functioning about six years. Similar contrasts between behavioral and cognitive level were seen during testing. As we went to the testing room, this patient held the tester's hand and asked what "toys" she had in her office. However, the general developmental level of the Rorschach was consistent with a mental age between 5 and 6 years. He saw the differentiated percepts on II and III, along with human content and movement. However, even here his manner of presentation was infantile, and he identified the two figures on III as "Mommys." At this, he made the *Mmm* sound, in the manner of a cow going *Moo.* Based on this data the patient seemed to have been infantalized in some way, or had remained immature for some defensive reason. Although most of his percepts were benign enough on the Rorschach, he did see a shark on IX "because it has teeth." The percept was not well-justified. He also had more difficulty structuring the percepts thought to have female stimulus value suggesting that his relationship with female figures might have been disrupted. The failure of this defensively immature and infantalized boy to integrate negative affect seemed associated with some of his losses of control.

A third basis for behavioral disorders is a characterologic problem that interferes with the patient's capacity to function and control emotional responses. Such patients have not learned specific behaviors; their behaviors spring from a general psychological primitiveness.

A 17-year-old was referred for inappropriate behavior and socialization responses. He had a history of retardation and hyperactivity. At the time of hospitalization he was lying and stealing. He spoke in a loud, whining voice and interacted with peers by touching and grabbing them. At times he had tantrums that involved hitting, kicking, and biting staff. On the Stanford-Binet this patient achieved a mental age of 8-6 with a chronological age of 17-11, yielding an IQ of 52. On the Rorschach he showed little ability to perceive reality as others did except on the most structured cards. His worst responses were to the colored cards and to the colored portions of the cards where his responses showed evidence of impulsivity ("Blood, blood, blood") and anxiety. Many of his responses described the insides of bodies and "fires going up." In general, the material suggests that he felt like a vulnerable and defenseless (a shelless, headless "turtle") individual surrounded by chaos and hostility. He showed little distance from the percepts, roaring like a crocodile on I. To the first TAT card, his story was told in the first person "I am sitting there. He feels mad. Good bye." To the tester's inquiry as to what this boy was thinking, he replied, "He is mad like me, and I am madder." The material suggested that he was overwhelmed by his own anxieties and concerns, with little ability to modulate affect. Despite the primitive intrusions into his percepts, there was very little developmental contrast between the blots, and there was no evidence that he had ever functioned at higher developmental levels than he did at the time of evaluation. In behavior he showed no evidence of hallucinations or delusions. The absence of psychotic symptomatology, the limited variability of percepts, and the primitive protocol suggested long-standing characterologic problems.

Other patients seem psychologically intact, but show the eruption of impulses associated with specific emotional concerns and conflicts.

A 16-year-old patient was referred for "inappropriate behavior" including obvious sexual advances, stealing from her parents, yelling at her teachers, and making up stories for her friends. The evaluation suggested an intellectually immature girl dealing with adolescent issues. The intellectual testing indicated that her IQ scores were in the mildly retarded range (WISC–R Verbal 54, Performance 57, and Full Scale 51). The Bender with 3 errors and problems of distortion and integration was consistent with her estimated mental age of about 8. The projectives revealed no serious psychiatric illness, and she appeared to be responding to the blots in a way that was consistent with her information processing ability. Like many latency age protocols it included many populars (people III and VII, animals IV and VIII) and human form and movement (talking, giggling, sitting). She also showed her distress as other school-age children might. She used no color, although the presence of color did not disorganize her percepts. She was able to use and structure texture ("bear fur" on VI). Other responses revealed the unique nature of her own predicament. The data suggested that she was a girl in conflict over interpersonal relationships. On the one hand she seemed attracted to others (she saw III as two people warming their hands). On the other hand, something about this disturbed her; she saw black smoke coming from the wood "underneath the fire." Other data suggested that sexual relationships and issues in particular were difficult for her. Her percepts included the identification of VI as a bear "stomping, coming," his legs "going in and out." At this point the patient regressed and saw a "tree," much as a younger child would. She gave the impression she would like to get close to the interpersonal "fire," but she is not prepared to deal with the sexual implications of doing this. Her TAT stories also included themes of heterosexual relationships, which were maintained in some magical way despite a stormy course.

DIFFERENTIATION OF PERCEPTUAL, LANGUAGE, AND MOTOR PROBLEMS FROM PSYCHOPATHOLOGY

As discussed in a previous chapter, mental retardation is often associated with specific disorders in perception, language, ability, and motor functions. Frequently, such adolescents will show inappropriate behaviors. In these instances, it is important to determine whether the individual's problems are compounded by a psychotic process. Projective test material can be useful in distinguishing between perceptual or language disorder and loss of appropriate reality contact. In those instances in which psychosis is ruled out by the projective material, disorders of behavior may be attributed to the individual's difficulties in perceiving the world or expressing thoughts and feelings. The treatment implications can become apparent when projective tests are used in this manner. An example of a boy suffering from perceptual problem is presented below. The perceptual difficulties were obvious from all the testing, but the projective material was particularly useful in ruling out psychosis.

A 15-year-old boy was referred for evaluation of psychosis. Although his Full Scale IQ was in the retarded range (60), there was a significant difference between his Verbal (78) and Performance (46) scores. The Bender showed serious problems with perceptual-motor integration. The overall performance was very immature. The most complex figure seemed crushed and bent out of shape. He rendered a diamond (a task suitable for 7-year-olds) inconsistently. His problems included telling the most outlandish stories, which struck observers as possibly delusional. He claimed to be the leader of a gang who participated with this group in fantastic adventures; no one had seen him with these boys. He claimed to have a girlfriend who had borne him a son several weeks before hospitalization; his family was unaware of any girlfriend. He said he was a big marijuana smoker; on the ward he seemed unable to light an ordinary cigarette. The Rorschach was presented as part of a full battery of tests. His performance on the cognitive and projective testing gave the impression he was in some sense "guessing" about his reality. On the vocabulary subtest of the WISC–R as the words got harder, the patient asked after being asked the meaning of "fable," "What if I don't know, just guess?" Later he gave perfectly coherent but inaccurate defintions to difficult words. For example, "When someone gets out of jail" to "belfry." On the Rorschach he seemed also to respond to a salient feature of the blots, but to be unable to integrate them. He would make remarks like "I hate this," and "Oh God? What does it look like . . ."

He divided the blots in the most unusual ways, perceiving a kite in the center of I, and pants (with hole) from the center of II. He responded whether his response made sense or not, often in grandiose ways. On one blot (VII) he saw an "art museum," pointing out the entrance and two statues. The data suggested that this patient felt compelled to respond whether he could respond appropriately or not, and to respond in impressive ways. We decided to turn his propensity for story telling into part of his program; as a reinforcer for appropriate behavior he was allowed to present to his class comics of his own rendition along with accompanying story. He did very well during the hospitalization. There was never any evidence of a psychotic process. As he was allowed to function within the area of his capability, his behavior became more appropriate, and outside of his story-telling sessions we did not hear his fantastic tales.

A second set of difficulties often associated with mental retardation are language disorders. Expressive language may be particularly deficient because of neurologic disorders that interfere with cognition, in general, and language functions, in particular. Even without neurologic disorders, there is a high incidence of communication problems in the mentally retarded population (see Chapter 3). In those cases in which individuals are handicapped in expressing themselves, projective techniques can be useful in understanding the person's representations of the environment. Figure drawings are obviously useful for this purpose. In addition, we have used projective techniques to rule out the diagnosis of a thought disorder by modifying the administration technique substantially. Two examples of the use of the Rorschach with language-impaired, mentally retarded individuals are presented. In both instances, projective techniques were helpful in determining that the patient's behavior problems were not manifestations of psychosis but the result of frustrations imposed on the individuals by their impairments.

An 18-year-old girl with cerebral palsy was referred for evaluation of possible psychosis. She had shown an increase of odd and compulsive behaviors (including running water and rearranging furniture), separation anxiety (sleep disturbance), and labile affect (alternating laughing and crying). We estimated her IQ in the 40s on the Peabody Picture Vocabulary and her mental age at about 7 years. This patient's motor problems interfered with many aspects of her functioning. Unfortunately, even her articulation was affected, and she was extremely difficult to understand. The psychologist who evaluated her presented the Rorschach blots, and through a process of attempting to understand and reproduce the patient's statements, (along with something that approached the process of elimination), ascertained the patient's responses, which included "hats" and "mountains." This demonstrated that the patient's percepts were simple but that she perceived reality like other people.

Another patient, 26 years old, was referred for explosive and aggressive behavior. He had a long history of mental retardation associated with severe language problems so that he could not say more than three-word sentences. A neurologic examination suggested some organic dysfunctions. The reason for his outbursts needed to be understood in order to ascertain whether they were related to his difficulties in communicating, or some serious psychopathology. On the WAIS he achieved a Full Scale IQ Score of 47, with a Verbal IQ Score of 50, and Performance IQ Score of 51. The Draw-a-Person revealed a mental age of 8-6, and the Bender-Gestalt was more like that of a boy of 5 years. Thus, we had no reason to expect a Rorschach more complex than that of a child of 5 to 8 years. The Rorschach was actually simpler than that, and quite limited. However, the patient made every attempt to communicate with the examiner. These efforts to communicate made it clear that this problem was with language specifically and not some more general interpersonal problem. He presented percepts that were appropriate to the blots, and there were no primitive intrusions so he seemed able to deal with external reality. Capitalizing on the symmetrical aspects of the cards, he saw winged percepts, butterflies and birds, in many of the blots. Unable to articulate the word "butterfly" (it came out more "bumfly") he gestured with his arms; at this point the examiner offered the word "butterfly" as a possibility, and the patient confirmed this percept. The projectives along with the other evaluations suggested that this young man was not imposing his own concerns on the world, but was actively trying to understand and deal with his environment. As a result, his treatment program emphasized helping him to relax when frustrated and angry and to verbalize his negative feelings in simple terms before he was at the point of explosion.

SPECIAL TESTING TECHNIQUES

When we give projectives to these unusual patients with multiple problems, we take the attitude that we must be flexible. We do not know before we begin whether we are going to elicit information that is useful to diagnosis or treatment. We try then not to administer the projectives in a mechanical manner, but to make interventions that will help us to unravel a multitude of intellectual, neurologic, and personality factors. We do this with patients with average as well as below average intelligence when the change in technique will provide important information.

One 17-year-old patient was tested as part of an evaluation of what was thought to be a progressive neurologic disease. Over a ten-year period his intellectual level had fallen from the average to the low average and borderline range. He was having problems with coordination and showed clear problems with perceptual–motor functioning. The Rorschach in this case was interesting and informative. The patient had great difficulty making sense of what he saw and the percepts were immature. After eight seconds he said that the first blot looked like "paint splatter." Similarly after 85 seconds he had still not made any sense of the third blot, and said, "Paint? I don't know." For the most part his responses were very inappropriate in terms of fit of percept to blot, and included "a girl" (II), "bat" (IV), a "bird" (V), a "fish" (VI), "smoke" (VII), a "fly" (VIII), a "horse" (IX), and "jelly fish" (X). However, when the examiner tested the limits to see if the patient could in fact see what others see, he responded immediately to the aid she provided in structuring the blots. When asked on I if he saw the popular butterfly, he said immediately that he did, and pointed out the parts. On III he saw the two people when they were suggested to him, and again provided the details at once. He added that they were picking up a ribbon in the middle. On VII he justified the two rabbits when they were pointed out to him. Thus, although he could not structure his own experience, he was able to recognize reality-based percepts. Further, despite difficulties in organizing his percepts and his clear cognitive confusion, there was no evidence that his thinking had been disrupted by the intrusion of primitive concerns, nor was the content of his percepts dysphoric or bizarre. In addition, he did not show the kind of logical errors associated with thought disturbance. We concluded that while the patient was suffering from some degree of confusion, it did not appear to be attributable at the time to gross emotional disturbance or thought disorder proper. Furthermore, the patient was able to use the structure provided for him over time. Wondering if a week after he was given the Rorschach he would persist in seeing nothing but paint on the first and third blots as he had during the first administration, we readministered the first four blots. After two seconds the patient saw a "bat" on one, and not the butterfly as had been suggested by the examiner. After five seconds he saw the two people on the third blot, this time picking up a "bowl." Thus, he had not simply memorized what the examiner had provided, nor had he simply remembered his own improvised response. He had in fact reintegrated the percept on the second occasion, using the first learning experience very much to his benefit. On the second blot he saw a "butterfly" rather than a girl's face, which was not a "good" response, but better than his first attempt. On the fourth, he saw a bat just as he did before. Thus, it was ascertained that whatever deficits he was suffering from, his cognitive behavior was amenable to education and change. This observation provided great impetus to attempts to train him to assess and respond to the situations he found himself in.

We routinely experiment with administration of the Rorschach with our retarded patients as well. In some cases, the Rorshach is readministered to determine whether the patient is capable of better performance with more experience with the task. In others, the inquiry may be administered immediately after the patient identifies a percept in order to minimize problems with memory and perceptual confusion. Occasionally, several Rorschachs are administered in order to document the patient's progress over time.

A 17-year-old girl was referred for a long history of cognitive and emotional problems. She was evaluated at various points during her hospitalization in order to ascertain the effect the milieu and medication on her functioning. Early in the hospitalization the patient's thinking was very disordered. While the first intellectual tests suggested cognitive functioning between three and six years, a Stanford-Binet done later in the hospitalization indicated higher intellectual functioning, more like a girl of six or seven. With time as this patient responded to treatment, her performance on the Rorschach became less subject to primitive intrusions and her responses became less fragmented. A comparison of responses to the first blot will exemplify this point. On the first Rorschach she said the first blot "looked like somebody had put splinters in a puppy dog. This looks like a heart. And somebody has long hair. And this looks like a spider and that's his wings coming out, and that is his head and that's his nose, and that's his mouth." On the second administration, she saw "a body. Two hands. It looks like she is going to fall off the airplane. And these hands are going to grab her." While her response was still anxious, it was also somewhat less fragmented and less bizarre. By the third Rorschach the response was even less subject to the patient's personal concerns. "Looks like a lady between two men. And it looks like she's pushing them away from her because she's crowded. She has long arms next to her, beside here. That's her hands." Even in the last Rorschach performance this patient's anxieties about destruction and deterioration, and the vulnerability of her thinking to disruption were evident. However, the multiple administrations showed definite gains in the clarity of her thinking.

GUIDELINES

Be flexible in the administration of the projectives, much as you would be for a young child. Do not be afraid to experiment. If on the Rorschach you think that a delayed inquiry may have created problems for an adolescent or child with memory problems, wait for a few days, and give the Rorschach over again with the inquiry following each set of responses. Then you can compare the performances and understand the impact of the individual's memory problems on his or her integration of experience.

Lower your expectations. We do not expect any more from the projective material than we would from an individual of the individual's estimated mental age. Although this method is crude, it has been useful. In using the Rorschach you can scan the norms between the individual's mental and chronological ages. From this and your experience with Rorschachs of young children, you can get an idea of whether the individual's performance might be seen at any developmental level.

Be descriptive in assessing the projectives. It is very helpful for the teachers to hear that the individual is functioning much like a younger child not just "in school," but in life. The information that the individual integrates his experience, relates to other people, and expresses his affects more like a child of his mental age than his chronological age is useful. Frequently, the information has made it possible for the caregivers to be more realistic about their expectations for the individual's behavior.

In thinking diagnostically, use what you understand about the basic features of psychopathology. Once you have accounted for the basic immaturity of the protocol by correcting for cognitive age, you can assess the features that seem unexplained: differential developmental levels of functioning, as with excessive concreteness, impulsivity, and perseveration, which might be associated with the individual's symptoms and point to possible treatments.

Of all the projectives, the Rorschach may be most useful. Particularly for individuals where you are unsure of the baseline expectations, it is helpful to have an array of behaviors to different stimuli so that you can compare better with poorer functioning, and understand and describe the factors behind this differential functioning. There are also easy ways of viewing the Rorschach material developmentally by utilizing the work done by Ames, (et al., 1952; Ames, Metraux, & Walker, 1971) and her colleagues, and by referring to the norms compiled by Exner and Weiner (1982) as part of the Comprehensive System.

In these ways the use of projectives with retarded and dual diagnosis patients can be extremely fruitful. Projective techniques can help not only to identify psychopathology beyond retardation, but also to aid in minimizing emotional disturbances in mentally retarded individuals.

REFERENCES

Ames, LB, Learned, J, Metraux, RW, & Walker, RN. (1952). *Child Rorschach responses.* New York: Paul B. Hoeber

Ames, LB, Metraux, RW, & Walker, RN. (1971). *Adolescent Rorschach responses* (rev. ed.). New York: Bruner/Mazel

Anastasi, A. (1954). *Psychological testing.* New York: MacMillan

Beck, S. (1932). The Rorschach Test as applied to the feeble-minded group. *Archives of Psychology,* 84, No. 136

Beck, S. (1945). *Rorschach's test: II. A variety of personality pictures.* New York: Grune & Stratton

Beck, S. (1952). *Rorschach's test: III. Advances in interpretation.* New York: Grune & Stratton

Beck, SJ, Beck, AG, Levitt, EL, Molish, HB. (1961). *Rorschach's test: I. Basic processes* (3rd ed.). New York: Grune & Stratton

Derevensky, JL. (1979). Children's fears: A developmental comparison of normal and exceptional children. *Journal of Genetic Psychology, 135,* 11–21

Exner, JE. (1974). *The Rorschach: A comprehensive system* (Vol. 1). New York: Wiley

Exner, JE. (1978). *The Rorschach: A comprehensive system. Current research and advanced interpretation* (Vol. 2). New York: Wiley

Exner, JE, & Weiner, IB. (1982). *The Rorschach: A comprehensive system. Assessment of children and adolescents* (Vol. 3). New York: Wiley

Hemmendinger, L. (1953). Perceptual organization and development as reflected in the structure of the Rorschach test responses. *Journal of Projective Techniques, 17,* 162–170

Hemmendinger, L. (1960). Developmental scores. In M Rickers-Ovsiankina (Ed.), *Rorschach psychology*. New York: Wiley

Jolles, I. (1947). The diagnostic implicative of Rorschach's test in case studies of mental defectives. *Genetic Psychology Monographs, 36,* 189–198

Klopfer, B. (1956). *Developments in the Rorschach technique. Fields of application* (Vol. 2). New York: World Book

Klopfer, B, Ainsworth, MD, Klopfer, W, & Holt, RR. (1954). *Developments in the Rorschach technique. Technique and theory* (Vol. 1). New York: Harcourt, Brace, & World

Klopfer, B, & Kelley, D. (1942). *The Rorschach technique.* New York: World Book

Rapaport, D, Gill, MM, & Schafer, R. (1968). *Diagnostic psychological testing.* New York: International Universities Press

Schafer, R. (1948). *The clinical application of psychological tests.* New York: International Universities Press

Ludwik S. Szymanski

12

Diagnosis of Mental Disorders in Mentally Retarded Persons

Mental health professionals have had many misconceptions about mental disorders in retarded persons. These misconceptions may form an important obstacle to the recognition and formal diagnosis of mental disorders in these individuals, even beyond the usual difficulties encountered in making such diagnosis in general. The first and most important misconception has been the view of retarded persons as a homogenous population with stereotyped features. In fact, there is a much wider gap between a mildly retarded, self-supporting adult and a profoundly retarded one, than between two randomly picked persons of normal intelligence. The spectrum of adaptation, personality patterns, communication abilities, all of which are important to consider before diagnosis is made, is very broad. Thus, even in this chapter, when a reference is made to "retarded persons," it should be seen only as an approximation and in practice individual circumstances have to be considered first.

Philips (1966) listed three common misconceptions about the behavior of retarded persons: that it is a function of retardation rather than of interpersonal relationships, that it is different in kind from that in a nonretarded child, and that it is a result of an organic brain damage. One of the results of these misconceptions had been a view that retarded persons do not suffer from mental disorders, but that their disturbed behaviors represent a simple reaction to environmental mismanagement. Another view, probably rooted in psychodynamic theory, would see retarded persons as unable to have a mental

CHILDREN WITH EMOTIONAL DISORDERS AND DEVELOPMENTAL DISABILITIES ISBN 0–8089–1700–5

disorder, because they cannot develop an internalized conflict. These views in effect denied that retarded persons experienced human emotions. The organic etiology, automatically inferred from the presence of retardation, would usually lead to a stereotyped diagnosis of some "organic" disorder and would imply incurability.

DIAGNOSTIC TERMINOLOGY

In the field of mental retardation, even more than in the field of mental health in general, there has been considerable confusion about the consistent use of terminology, such as mental disorders, mental illness, emotional disorders, and behavioral disorders. In fact, use of a particular term often has administrative connotations and denotes that one, rather than another discipline, should be in charge. The danger inherent in this changing and idiosyncratic terminology is that it is used to classify people, instead of disorders. For instance, the recently popularized term "dual diagnosis" (besides being meaningless, in the first place) has been used to denote persons who are considered too retarded for a mental health, and too disturbed for a mental retardation, facility. As the result they are either segregated as a different class of persons or receive no services at all.

The DSM III (APA, 1980) has introduced some order to this confusion, although it has its limitations. Its (relatively) specific descriptive criteria permit better focusing on clinical presentation (and its variations) as the basis for diagnosis. It also recognizes that the symptomatic expression and the meaning of a clinical feature depends on person's age. It is very relevant to retarded persons, if we consider developmental, rather than chronological age. The DSM III is more reliable in diagnosis of broader categories, than of specific disorder (Rutter & Shaffer, 1980). It is generally reliable in diagnosis of mental retardation (Cantwell, Russell, Mattison, & Will, 1979).

THE MEANING OF THE FORMAL DIAGNOSIS

That the presence of mental retardation may reduce the chances of making a correct diagnosis of mental illness, was shown experimentally (Reiss, Levitan, & Szyszko, 1982; Reiss & Szyszko, 1983). These experiments were based on presenting to a group of clinical psychologists case histories fulfilling DSM III criteria for a particular mental disorder, with half of the cases being also mentally retarded.

Not infrequently, workers in the mental retardation field express the opinion that the formal diagnosis of a mental disorder is an unnecessary "label." In fact, even Adolph Meyer had felt that formal diagnosis is unimportant and the focus should be on what the problems are and what should be done about them. The latter is certainly true. However if problems concerning a diagnostic "label" arise, they are usually the result of either a wrong diagnosis or of its misuse, not merely of it being made. The formal diagnosis has its value besides the obvious administrative/statistical one. It helps in clearing anxiety and confusion about the nature of the observed behavior, and may lead to a specific treatment. For instance, an uncooperative behavior of a retarded person in an institution, that has been seen as "attention getting" and created anger among the staff, may be a part of a major depression and may be ameliorated by an appropriate treatment. Last but not least, there may be considerable research value to valid diagnostic data.

THE DIAGNOSTIC PROCESS

The Referral

Retarded persons have contact with many caregivers: parents, teachers, various attendants, medical, and mental health professionals, each of whom may be disturbed by one facet of person's behavior and not by another. Each of these caregivers may have different expectations of the diagnostic evaluation. Some of these expectations, which we often see in our clinic, are that the diagnosis of a mental illness will justify that the individual in question has not responded to a "program" and therefore should be removed from it until cured; that a diagnosis of mental disorder will be ruled out, thus freeing a school system from the responsibility to pay for a private school for disturbed children (while the parents have the opposite expectation); that the new diagnosis will lead to something new and not tried yet.

Some of these expectations are openly stated as the reason for referral, others are not. These were termed manifest and latent expectations (Szymanski, 1980). The diagnostician has to recognize these various expectations of the different principals in the particular case and deal with them accordingly, lest "shopping" for a more favorable opinion follows the completion of the diagnostic process.

The Diagnostic Interview

An interview with a retarded person is often compared with an interview with a child of same mental age. This is not necessarily accurate, since even if there are some similarities between the two, there are considerable differences. In both cases the client is brought to the diagnostician by someone else, rather than refers self because of problems he or she wants to resolve. As the result, in both situations the client has to be prepared for the diagnostic evaluation, through explanations geared to his or her level of understanding. Optimally, the caregivers should be instructed in this respect at the time the first appointment is set. Considering the universality of retarded persons' low self-esteem, attention should be paid that the explanations do not convey the message that person's "bad" behavior is the reason for the evaluation (which could thus be seen as a punishment).

The next important similarity is the need to communicate with the client in the manner appropriate to his developmental level. However, while in the case of a child this can be generally inferred from the chronological age, with the retarded persons one has to assess the communicative abilities from a variety of sources, such as immediate personal observation, especially of the pattern of communication with the caregivers, as well as from history. In our clinic we usually first see the caregivers and the client jointly and lead them unobtrusively to enter into an interaction, would it be verbal or not. A retarded adult is not a child regardless of his mental age, has had different life experiences, and unless profoundly retarded does see himself as an adult. Thus it is necessary to communicate respectfully. Not infrequently beginning residents assume that if a person is retarded he must be approached as a child and start the interview even with mildly retarded, well-functioning and employed adults, by asking if they knew their age, or offering them toys.

Directiveness has been often mentioned as important when interviewing retarded clients (Jakab, 1970; Menolascino & Bernstein, 1970; Szymanski, 1977, 1980). It provides structure and thus support to a person who may be anxious, expects to fail in a "test," is passive and dependent, and who has difficulties in organizing his or her own communications because of language and cognitive deficits. However, retarded persons are also often suggestible and therefore directiveness should not be confused with leading questions. Optimally, in order to have the clients act spontaneously, each topic or activity should be approached first in a general way and more structure and directiveness should be applied only if necessary to help the client to respond.

If required, appropriate limits have to be set, just as with nonretarded children. If the patient is overactive, tests limits, does not cooperate, and a supportive approach is not helpful, strict verbal limits, reinforced with immediate rewards, can be helpful. The patient's response to such structure can have a considerable diagnostic and predictive value as to what approach in education and treatment will be helpful.

Nonverbal communication and behavioral observations are particularly important, since many retarded clients do not have adequate verbal language abilities (see Chapter 3). Even if they do, having had many unsatisfactory experiences with failed "tests," they may elect silence, or other uncooperative behaviors as means of avoidance. The nonverbal approaches include play and other activities as well as observations of nonverbal behavior. The manner and the degree of relatedeness, level of attention, curiosity and patterns of exploration, response to and utilization of sensory stimuli, patterns of interaction with others and in particular with the parents, are all important. In play activities the diagnostician should give the patient the opportunity for maximal spontaneity but if necessary, certain situations (e.g., in doll play) can be "staged" to explore a child's reaction.

Retarded persons are cared for and depend on many caregivers. Therefore a careful history obtained from all the caregivers is essential. In particular, there are often considerable disagreements between caregivers concerning how the patient is viewed and should be managed. These disagreements, catching the patient in the middle, may be the principal or contributing cause of the behavioral disturbance that brought the patient for the evaluation.

It has been pointed out that a diagnostic psychiatric evaluation of retarded persons should be done in a comprehensive context, not as an isolated endeavour (Menolascino & Bernstein, 1970; Szymanski, 1980). It is necessary to have a good understanding of a patient's developmental, social, and educational history and current life circumstances. Therefore a comprehensive history and review of past materials and test results is necessary. A common mistake is to accept at face value that, "there were no medical findings," or "the chromosomes were normal." The diagnostician should review the actual data from the relevant tests and examinations and then decide if they were adequate. Often, advances in medical knowledge make such past tests obsolete. For instances, until about 1980, the cell culture media used in chromosomal testing made it impossible to detect Fragile X abnormality, now considered the second most common one associated with mental retardation, after Down's syndrome. Another example may be a situation when a mother has had three children retarded for unknown reason. Only careful history and perhaps PKU testing of the mother will reveal that she has PKU, but due to early diet treatment her development was normal. However, the residual high blood level of phenylalanine was neurotoxic enough to damage the fetus (maternal PKU). Other past tests, psychological ones included, should be reviewed in a similarly critical manner.

ASSESSMENT OF CLINICAL DATA

Assessment of the meaning of the clinical material is not always easy. A number of issues should be considered.

Is the particular behavior appropriate for an earlier developmental stage and represents the patient's immaturity, or is it deviant and inappropriate in any situation? A severe self-injurious behavior or delusional system will belong to the latter, while some self-abuse in the context of a temper tantrum and preoccupation with an imaginary friend exemplify the former.

What is developmentally appropriate for the client? With nonretarded children the chronological age is a good guide to what might be expected. With retarded ones, there is often a fallacy that mental age serves the same role. However it is only an arbitrary number representing an average of diverse scores achieved on various subtests, which may be widely scattered and may be affected out of proportion by one very high or very low score. A retarded, 25-year-old person with an MA of 6 is not a child of six. One has to take into account his or her discrete cognitive, communicative, and other abilities; life experiences; educational exposure. Unfortunately it may be difficult if not impossible to arrive to a concrete formula representing all these factors, and in many cases the diagnostician's clinical experience will be called upon to provide an answer.

What is the role of the associated handicaps in the genesis of the symptom? A frequently asked question is whether aggression may be a result of an epileptic seizure. Although this may happen only rarely (Delgado-Escueta, Mattson, King, Goldensohn, Spiegel, Madsen, Crandall, Dreifuss, & Porter, 1981), appropriate neurologic evaluation including EEG telemetry with video-taping, may be necessary in some cases. Another example may be an autistic-like behavior in a blind child, related to sensory isolation, rather than representing infantile autism.

Is the particular behavior abnormal or adaptive, considering the client's life circumstances? A typical example will be an aggression or self-injurious behavior occurring in an institutionalized individual, who is ignored and understimulated until such behaviors occur. In fact they may be seen as quite "healthy," since they result in the client obtaining staff attention.

DIAGNOSTIC FORMULATIONS

The DSM III, although not a perfect instrument, is quite helpful in formulating a diagnosis in the case of retarded patient. After the importance and nature of each symptom/behavior has been assessed as described above, the next task is to correlate these with the specific diagnostic criteria as described in the DSM 3. In some situations the criteria cannot be strictly satisfied, for instance, if they call for some sort of verbalized complaint or other expression and if the patient does not have enough verbal capacities for this purpose. In fact, with the retarded persons as a group, one has to rely a great deal on nonverbal symptoms while making a diagnosis: general behavior, affect, somatic symptoms, or change in the level of functioning.

EXAMPLES OF SPECIFIC DIAGNOSTIC CATEGORIES

Organic Mental Disorders

Clinicians are often overly concerned with dividing mental disorders into organic and nonorganic (Woodward, Jaffe, & Brown, 1970). In the past and even now the term "organic" was loosely applied, often by implication. If the patient was retarded and also suffered of another disorder such as seizures, then virtually all his or her behavioral abnormalities would be seen as organic, even if similar ones could be seen in other persons, without "organicity". The DSM III is quite specific in its requirement that organic pathology and its etiologic relationship to the behavioral disturbance be clearly demonstrated. It also states that not diagnosing an organic disorder does not necessarily mean that organic factors are not present. Axis 3 is particularly helpful here for recording a coexisting neurologic or other disorder, thought relevant, but not proven as etiologically related to the mental disturbance. This issue is discussed particularly succintly by Lipowski (1980).

Psychotic Disorders

Past literature reflected confusion as to whether psychotic disorders existed in retarded persons and whether they were different in nature (Reid, 1972). More recently, Russell and Tanguay (1981) pointed out the relationship that may exist between retardation and psychosis, in that psychotic disorder may lead to the decrease in cognitive functioning.

Adaptation of the DSM III criteria to diagnosis of psychosis in retarded persons may not always be easy. For instance, to be diagnosed as having schizophrenia, the patient has to have verbal capacities sufficient to provide evidence of delusions, hallucinations, and/or incoherence. The limitations of making such a diagnosis in retarded persons have been pointed out by Reid (1972) and Heaton-Ward (1977). Thus one may have to make a more general diagnosis of a psychotic disorder (rather than of a more specific category), such as of atypical psychosis. In these cases one has often to rely on clinical presentation, such as grossly disorganized behavior and inappropriate affect.

Affective Disorders

These have been rarely recognized in retarded persons, although the literature, particularly older studies based on case reports, had mentioned their existence (review by Sovner & Hurley, 1983). In fact in earlier years it had been questioned whether nonpsychotic depression could exist in retarded persons, since they were seen as unable to appreciate society's expectations and thus experience guilt and a sense of unworthiness (Gardner, 1967). Most of the existing literature focused on "psychotic depression" and some cases of manic-depressive illness were described as well (Reid, 1972; Reid & Naylor, 1976; Rivinus & Harmatz, 1979). Reid (1972) pointed out that retarded persons may rarely complain of feeling depressed. The actual clinical picture may vary according to the verbal–conceptual level. In more retarded persons, increase in dependency, apathy, withdrawal, and somatic symptoms may predominate, while the higher-functioning ones may voice verbal complaints, particularly of feeling "bad" or "sick." Our study (currently in progress) points to a not infrequent existence of nonpsychotic depression in retarded persons, which is often undiagnosed, since these patients, while disturbed, are not disturbing to their caregivers. However, making an accurate diagnosis in them is obviously very important, as it will lead to specific and usually effective treatment with antidepressants.

Two disorders are important to consider in the differential diagnosis of depression in retarded persons. In persons with Down's syndrome one should consider Alzheimer's disease, since its neuropathology has been found in most of these individuals who reach middle age (Burger & Vogel, 1973; Gath, 1981 Malamud, 1972; Olsen & Shaw, 1969) . Its clinical expression is still debated, but it appears that it may be associated with loss of certain functions (Miniszek, 1983). An accurate history focusing particularly on loss of memory and of concrete skills (vs. loss of motivation only) and comprehensive neurologic assessment may be helpful in establishing the diagnosis. The other condition has been described as "relocation syndrome" in institutionalized older persons as well as in retarded persons, who are moved abruptly to a new locale (Carsrud, Carsrud, Henderson, Alisch, & Fowler, 1979; Cochran, Sran, & Varano, 1977). The symptoms may include weight loss, confusion, withdrawal, and in some cases may represent true depression.

RECOMMENDATIONS FOR MANAGEMENT

The diagnostic assessment, to be useful to the referring person and to the patient, should result in management recommendations. The specific treatment modalities are discussed elsewhere in this book, therefore only general remarks about the form of the recommendations will be made.

Unfortunately many mental health professionals conclude an otherwise excellent diagnostic assessment with a vague summary, often rooted in obscure theoretical discussion of presumed psychopathology and with unnecessary minute details of the findings, but fail to give a clear statement of the diagnosis and the recommendations. This is particularly important with retarded persons who are often referred by relatively untrained caregivers who expect results understandable to them.

To be effective, the diagnostic summary should be brief, but clear and focused on important issues. It should restate the reasons for the referral, describe the salient points in the history and the concrete observations of visible behaviors and other symptoms that lead the clinician to the diagnosis. These findings should be discussed in light of other knowledge about the individual (e.g., their relationship with other handicaps he or she might have, environmental factors, etc). Thus the findings should be presented not as isolated items but integrated with the total knowledge about the patient. The management plan should be concrete and "generic," stating first the elements of the recommended intervention (such as the required features of the educational or other placement, or the specific approaches to be used in psychotherapy). Although the recommendations should be realistic in light of available resources, the optimal intervention should be described as well, leaving the caregivers to make the final decision as to what will be realistic for them.

Last but not least, the informing conference, particularly if the family of the retarded person is involved, is most important. Their feelings should be recognized and respected. The recommended treatment should be clearly relevant to the complaints the family has and to the specific findings. While being supportive, one should not be condescending and should not treat the family as "patients," but as allies.

REFERENCES

Burger, PC, & Vogel, FS. (1973). The development of the pathologic changes of Alzheimer's disease and senile dementia in patients with Down's syndrome. *American Journal of Pathology, 73,* 457–468

Cantwell, DP, Russell, AT, Mattison, R, & Will, L. (1979). A comparison of DSM-II and DSM-III in the diagnosis of childhood psychiatric disorders. *Archives of General Psychiatry, 36,* 1208–1213

Carsrud, AL, Carsrud, KB, Henderson, DP, Alisch, CJ, & Fowler, AV. (1979). Effects of social and environmental change on institutionalized mentally retarded persons: The relocation syndrome reconsidered. *American Journal of Mental Deficiency, 84,* 266–272

Cochran, WE, Sran, PK, & Varano, GA. (1977). The relocation syndrome in mentally retarded individuals. *Mental Retardation, 15,* 10–12

Delgado-Escueta, AV, Mattson, RH, King, L, Goldensohn, ES, Spiegel, H, Madsen, J, Crandall, P, Dreifuss, F, & Porter, R. (1981). The nature of aggression during epileptic seizures. Special Report. *New England Journal of Medicine, 305,* 711

Diagnostic and Statistical Manual of Mental Disorders (DSM III). (1980). Washington, DC: American Psychiatric Association

Gardner, WI. (1967). Occurrence of severe depressive reactions in the mentally retarded. *American Journal of Psychiatry, 124,* 142–144

Gath, A. (1981). Cerebral degeneration in Down's syndrome. *Developmental Medicine and Child Neurology, 23,* 814–817

Heaton-Ward, A. (1977). Psychosis in mental handicap. *British Journal of Psychiatry, 130,* 525–533

Jakab, I. (1970). Psychotherapy of the mentally retarded child. In NR Bernstein (Ed.), *Diminished people.* Boston, MA: Little, Brown

Lipowski, ZJ. (1980). A new look at organic brain syndromes. *American Journal of Psychiatry, 137,* 674–678

Malamud, N. (1972). Neuropathology of organic brain syndromes associated with aging. In CM Gaitz (Ed.), *Aging and the brain.* New York: Plenum

Menolascino, FJ, & Bernstein, NR. (1970). Psychiatric assessment of the mentally retarded child. In NR Bernstein (Ed.), *Diminished people.* Boston, MA: Little, Brown

Miniszek, NA. (1983). Development of Alzheimer disease in Down syndrome individuals. *American Journal of Mental Deficiency, 87,* 377–385

Olsen, MI, & Shaw, CM. (1969). Presenile dementia and Alzheimer's disease in mongolism. *Brain, 92,* 147–156

Philips, I. (1966). Children, mental retardation and emotional disorder. In I Philips (Ed.), *Prevention and treatment of mental retardation.* New York: Basic Books

Reid, AH. (1972). Psychosis in adult mental defectives. *British Journal of Psychiatry, 120,* 205–212

Reid, AH, & Naylor, GJ. (1976). Short cycle manic depressive psychosis in mental defectives: A clinical and physiological study. *Journal of Mental Deficiency Research, 20,* 67–76

Reiss, S, Levitan, GW, & Szyszko, J. (1982). Emotional disturbance and mental retardation: Diagnostic overshadowing. *American Journal of Mental Deficiency 86,* 567–574

Reiss, S, & Szyszko, J. (1983). Diagnostic overshadowing and professional experience with mentally retarded persons. *American Journal of Mental Deficiency, 87,* 396–402

Rivinus, TM, & Harmatz, JS. (1979). Diagnosis and lithium treatment of affective disorder in the retarded: Five case studies. *American Journal of Psychiatry, 136,* 551–554

Russell, AT, & Tanguay, PE. (1981). Mental illness and mental retardation: Cause or coincidence? *American Journal of Mental Deficiency, 85,* 570–574

Rutter, M, & Shaffer, D. (1980). DSM-III, A step forward or back in terms of the classification of child psychiatric disorders? *Journal of the American Academy of Child Psychiatry, 19,* 371–394

Sovner, R, & Hurley, A. (1983). Do the mentally retarded suffer from affective illness? *Archives of General Psychiatry, 40,* 61–67

Szymanski, LS. (1977). Psychiatric diagnostic evaluation of mentally retarded individuals. *Journal of the American Academy of Child Psychiatry, 16,* 67–87

Szymanski, LS. (1980). Psychiatric diagnosis of retarded persons. In LS Szymanski & PE Tanguay (Eds.), *Emotional disorders of mentally retarded persons.* Baltimore, MD: University Park Press

Woodward, KF, Jaffe, N, & Brown, D. (1970). Early psychiatric intervention for young mentally retarded children. In FJ Menolascino, (Ed.), *Psychiatric approaches to mental retardation.* New York: Basic Books

Marian Sigman

13

Individual and Group Psychotherapy with Mentally Retarded Adolescents

Psychotherapy is a treatment procedure that involves the use of an interpersonal relationship between a mental health professional and a patient or client with the goal of ameliorating emotional problems and improving the patient's coping abilities (Bialer, 1967; Syzmanski, 1980). Psychotherapy is an important method of treatment for emotional disorders in children with normal intelligence. However, psychotherapy is only rarely employed with mentally retarded children and adolescents.

This is partly due to the lack of recognition that emotional problems are often independent from cognitive deficits in the mentally retarded. In recent years, however, there has been an increase in the awareness that some mentally retarded individuals suffer from emotional and behavioral problems that primarily have a psychological basis and that psychological interventions can be useful for ameliorating these disturbances. This increased awareness is partly a consequence of the movement towards deinstitutionalization and normalization. As mentally retarded children and adults attempt to adjust to regular school and vocational environments, their adaptive skills and emotional strengths become critical. There is some disagreement whether deinstitutionalization results in less maladaptive behaviors (Eyman & Call, 1977) or an increase in adjustment disorders due to stress (Coffman & Harris, 1980). Whatever the overall effects of deinstitutionalization, coping with normal work

---

Portions of this chapter appeared in Welch, VO, & Sigman, M. (1980). Group psychotherapy with mentally retarded, emotionally disturbed adolescents. *Journal of Clinical Child Psychology, 9,* 209–213. With permission.

CHILDREN WITH EMOTIONAL DISORDERS AND DEVELOPMENTAL DISABILITIES ISBN 0–8089–1700–5

and living conditions places a greater focus on emotional strengths and weaknesses than adaptation to institutional settings.

While there is more widespread attention given to the emotional and behavioral problems of mentally retarded individuals, the use of psychotherapy with these individuals remains controversial. Evidence of this controversy can be seen in the treatment of the subject by two volumes devoted to the topic of emotional disorders in mentally retarded individuals published in the last few years. The volume edited by Syzmanski and Tanguay (1980) contains two chapters discussing the use of individual and group psychotherapy with mentally retarded individuals. On the other hand, only about two pages are spent on the subject in the book edited by Matson and Barrett (1982), where psychotherapy is referred to as "an endangered species among currently available habilitative procedures." In contrast, thoughtful reviews of the uses of pharmacotherapy and behavioral therapy comprise the two chapters on treatment.

The basis for the criticism of psychotherapy in the mentally retarded is two-fold. First, critics point to the lack of empirical evidence of the efficacy of psychotherapy in general and of applications to mentally retarded individuals specifically. While it is true that the results of some outcome studies have been contradictory (Albini & Dinitz, 1965; Jakab, 1970; Lott, 1970; Sternlicht, 1965, 1966), most studies conclude that psychotherapy can be useful with mentally retarded individuals (Bozarth & Roberts, 1970; Chess, 1962; Humes, Adamcyzk, & Myco, 1969; Mann, Beaber, & Jacobson, 1969; Silvestri, 1977). On the other hand, much of the evidence is marred by the methodological problems characteristic of studies of psychotherapy in general. These methodological problems include the use of raters familiar with the group assignment of subjects, use of subjective outcome measures, and nonrandom assignment of subjects to treatments.

The second set of criticisms of the use of psychotherapy focuses on the limitations of the mentally retarded in using verbal mediators (Borokowski & Johnson, 1968) or symbolic representational systems. Psychotherapy is considered inappropriate for the mentally retarded individual because of its reliance on the patient's capacity to reflect on his own experience, a capacity that the mentally retarded individual is considered to lack. This line of argument is faulty for two reasons; first because the delineation of psychotherapy is too narrow and, second, because the description of the abilities of mentally retarded individuals is oversimplified.

The process of psychotherapy varies a great deal across groups of patients. To focus on just one dimension, psychotherapy can vary a great deal in terms of the directiveness of the therapist. In those approaches that are most like counseling, the therapist attempts to clarify current feelings and reactions of the patient and makes suggestions of alternative forms of action. In more intensive, less directive forms of therapy, the patient develops insights into his own reactions and behaviors with the help of the therapist's reflections and interpretation. The approaches differ in terms of the level of activity of the therapist as well as the degree of focus on current situations as opposed to more formative events in the patient's past experiences. The approaches also differ in terms of the use of transference. In more traditional forms of therapy, the transference of feelings by the patient onto the therapist is often discussed explicitly in order to help the patient understand his own perceptions and reactions. While transference occurs in all forms of therapy and the therapist is aware of its manifestations, the material may be explored less directly in some situations. The approach that the therapist uses varies along these dimensions and most therapists shape their approach in accordance with the individual characteristics of the patient. Psychotherapy with children and with adults who have poorly integrated personalities is usually more directive, and less emphasis is placed on the patient's development of insight. Thus, even with many patients of normal intelligence, less reliance is placed on the patient's abilities for self-awareness.

Similar adjustments in psychotherapeutic approaches and techniques can be made with mentally retarded patients. As in people of normal intelligence, there is wide variability in the abilities of retarded people to reflect about themselves. These abilities differ as a function of the level of retardation, the age of the individual, and the particular individual characteristics of the mentally retarded person. Moderately retarded individuals and mildly retarded children have very limited abilities to use verbal mediators and to understand their own behaviors or those of others. On the other hand, mildly retarded adolescents and young adults can understand social situations to a considerable degree. Thus, there are significant numbers of mildly retarded adolescents and adults who can benefit from less directive, more traditional forms of psychotherapy. In summary, the argument that psychotherapy is inappropriate for the mentally retarded is based on oversimplified assumptions about the process of psychotherapy and the abilities of mentally retarded individuals.

The focus of this chapter will be on psychotherapy with adolescents and adults, rather than with children. An eight- or ten-year-old child with an IQ in the 60–70 range has limited capacities for using verbal interventions. For this reason, behavioral techniques are more useful. We have also employed play therapy as one would with a child of 4–6 years of age. Play therapy has also been used to develop symbolic, language, motor, and social skills (Leland & Smith, 1965; Morrison & Newcomber, 1975) and can be useful in helping the child adjust to new or difficult social situations. As with moderately retarded adolescents and adults, the child's capacity for self-awareness is limited. In the following discussion, the focus will be on more verbal forms of therapy suitable for mildly retarded adolescents and adults.

The efficacy of the psychotherapeutic approach with mildly retarded adolescents became evident to us at UCLA only gradually over a number of years. Because of the efforts of George Tarjan, MD and James Simmons, MD, two inpatient psychiatric wards and an outpatient clinic were established to care for dual-diagnosis children and adolescents, along with other emotionally disturbed patients. The staff on the inpatient wards use behavioral principles, with token economies and a focus on positive reinforcement. Principles of behavior modification, and individualized behavioral programs are designed for each adolescent. Behavioral principles are also employed in the special school setting, occupational therapy, and recreational therapy.

In working with these adolescents over time, it became increasingly clear that even sophisticated forms of behavior modification would not deal with some of the problems experienced by our mentally retarded patients, such as their poor self-esteem. Furthermore, psychotherapy was used as matter of course by psychiatry and psychology trainees with adolescents of normal intelligence, many of whom had more severe behavior and emotional problems than their retarded peers. Since the patients with mild retardation and borderline intelligence were often indistinguishable from the adolescents with low-normal and average intelligence, some trainees began to use individual psychotherapy with the retarded adolescents when it seemed applicable. We gradually realized that the psychotherapeutic intervention, even of short duration, was an effective treatment technique with our mildly retarded patients.

THE GOALS AND STAGES OF PSYCHOTHERAPY

The goals of psychotherapy with retarded individuals are similar to those with nonretarded persons. The aims of psychotherapy are to alleviate psychopathological symptoms, improve socially acceptable behavior, and to enable the individual to function better, develop according to his or her potential and accept and like himself or herself more (Smith, McKinnon, & Kessler, 1976). In Jakab's words, the aim is for a "more integrated, interactional development of the total personality toward emotional and intellectual maturity," (1970, p. 225).

The process of psychotherapy is similar for retarded and nonretarded patients (Chess, 1962). Several authors have outlined the stages of psychotherapy (Jakab, 1970; Syzmanski, 1980). In the first stage, the therapist builds a relationship with a patient. In some cases, and this has been true for two psychotic, mentally retarded young women in our service, the formation of a relationship is the *only* work completed during therapy. For these two patients, the development of their capacity to trust another individual was a major accomplishment. For many of the other retarded patients, the therapeutic relationships is often the first sustained interpersonal interaction in which they have felt a sense of safety and acceptance.

In the second stage, the patient has the opportunity to express feelings of anxiety and aggression in a safe environment. For many retarded children and adolescents, this relationship may be their first opportunity to express and explore their ambivalent feelings. Some of our adolescents are deeply troubled by their own strongly negative feelings toward teachers, peers, and parents, and have never realized that the experience of ambivalence is shared by others. For these adolescents, a great deal of energy has been invested in blocking their negative feelings. The consequences range from inattention and hyperactivity to sudden explosive temper tantrums at school and at home.

Most therapists who work with retarded individuals stress the advantages of the therapeutic situation for helping the individual to understand his own behaviors and motives and those of others. As pointed out in a recent study of adults who are adjusting well in the community (Zeitlin & Turner, 1984), many retarded individuals do not seem to have developed the capacity to distinguish between their own emotional states, and respond to all arousing situations in an undifferentiated manner. Psychotherapy can be very useful in helping the patient to understand and accept his own reactions and generate strategies for expressing his feelings in a constructive manner.

The transference relationship that influences every stage of therapy, is, of course, a very useful place to explore these issues. In our experience, we have often had to begin the exploration of negative feelings with reactions to peers, staff, or teachers since the adolescent did not feel secure enough to express negative, angry feelings toward the therapist. After there was more comfort in exploring these feelings, the therapist could begin to point out similarities in the adolescent's reaction to the therapist and, finally, to other people in his life. The generalization to family relations has been made easier in our setting by the involvement of most adolescents in family therapy concurrently with their individual psychotherapy.

In the final phase, the transference relationship has to be resolved so that the patient has somewhat more realistic expectations of the therapist. The adolescent is encouraged in his increased capacity to understand and express feelings and behaviors. However, usually with retarded adolescents there is less emphasis placed on self-reliance than may be true for termination of therapy with children and adolescents of normal intelligence. The stresses suffered by mentally retarded individuals are so significant that these individuals may require counseling at various points in their lives. Furthermore, the evidence is that well-functioning mentally retarded adults maintain their successful adaptations to the environment by learning when and how to rely on social service workers (Zeitlin & Turner, 1982). Thus, there may be less emphasis placed on the adolescent's development of independence and self-reliance in the final phase of psychotherapy with the mentally retarded individual than with the individual of normal intelligence.

SPECIAL ISSUES RELATED TO PSYCHOTHERAPY WITH MENTALLY RETARDED ADOLESCENTS

Certain issues arise in psychotherapy with the mentally retarded adolescent. Like other adolescents, the mentally retarded individual faces expectations from family, peers, and self due to age and physical maturity. The transition from elementary school to the larger, more impersonal setting of a junior high school and, then, to high school may be particularly difficult for a mentally retarded child who has functioned well in the more protected elementary school environment.

In a recent study, a group of mentally retarded adults who are living independently in the community were asked about their experiences as adolescents (Zeitlin & Turner, 1982). These interviews were carried out as part of a study investigating intensive interactions over a prolonged period of time by field workers who saw the individuals regularly in many settings and, therefore, developed close relationships with them. Family members were also interviewed whenever possible. For 28 of the 46 individuals, adolescence was remembered as a time of acute stress. The nature of the problems was similar to that of many adolescents (Erikson, 1968; Offer, Marcus, & Offer, 1970) but with some differences in emphasis. As for the adolescent of normal intelligence, the parent–child relationship was a central area of tension for these individuals because of their increased desires for independence. However, the issue of independence was more complex for these adolescents because of their families' concerns about their competence to function in a wider world. Most of the adults in this sample recollected that they consciously wished to have more independence than was allowed by families and schools.

A second issue for all adolescents is the need to establish a sense of identity. For the mentally retarded adolescent, the sense of self must incorporate the individual's definition of his own handicap. Adolescence was a particularly trying period for these mentally retarded individuals because they really recognized their own limitations for the first time. Furthermore, this recognition emerged in a period when the individual felt a need to make choices and function somewhat independently.

Another major area of focus that these adults recollected as important during adolescence was their relationships with peers and siblings. During adolescence, some individuals were rejected more openly by schoolmates and felt themselves to be falling behind siblings in terms of achievements and independence. They often found themselves to have fewer friends in this period of time. Emotional control, a problem for all adolescents, was particularly difficult for these individuals. As mentioned above, some mentally retarded adolescents have not learned to distinguish their own affects or to express them in effective, self-regulated ways. Thus, emotional overresponsivity may be manifested in a variety of settings. Sexuality is, of course, an important issue for all adolescents. Given the absence of normative expectations, the lack of a peer network, and emotional overresponsivity, sexual feelings and behaviors raised serious concerns for these mentally retarded adolescents and their parents. In summary, during these interviews, mentally retarded adults and their families recollected the usual problems of this period exacerbated by a limited set of normative expectations and the absence of the peer support system available to many adolescents of normal intelligence.

These difficulties were reported by mentally retarded adults with little history of emotional disturbance. However, the mentally retarded adolescent whose adjustment has been less satisfactory is even more limited in the resources available for dealing with the pressures of adolescence. Frequently, these teenagers are attempting to deal with perceived needs for independence without having initially developed trusting relationships with their parents. Thus, the problems that appear to arise from issues of independence may actually reflect earlier needs for separation and individuation. Peer relationships may never have been satisfactory so that the therapist has to encourage more elementary forms of contact with peers. In other words, the dual-diagnosis adolescent is often struggling with difficulties unresolved from earlier periods and therapy must focus on these issues instead of the more usual problems of adolescence. Of course, this is true as well for emotionally disturbed adolescents of normal intelligence.

REVIEW OF CASES

Much of the material in this chapter is based on the author's clinical experiences as a supervisor of psychology interns on an inpatient ward for emotionally disturbed adolescents, many of whom were mentally retarded. As a basis for the discussion, it may be of use to describe a sample of 10 individuals seen over a five year period. This selection from all the cases supervised is not random. I have chosen cases to represent varying intellectual abilities, chronological ages, symptomatology, and some degree of successful outcome. The purpose of this description of a sample of cases is to allow the reader to judge the extent to which the principles elucidated in the chapter are germane for various clinical populations.

The 10 selected patients ranged in age from 12 to 22 years with a mean age of 16.1 years. Their intelligence quotients on the WISC-R varied from 45 to 77 with a mean IQ of 64. Five lived with both parents while the other five lived with either a single parent or a foster family. There were 6 females and 4 males in the group, two of the young women were Black, and all were from English-speaking families. Many of their problems centered around difficulties in getting along with peers. In fact, none of these adolescents could be said to have had positive relationships with peers and, in many cases, they had either no friendships or very destructive relationships. In some cases, the adolescents had been out of school for a number of months or years because of school phobias, incidences of running away, psychosomatic problems, or aggressive behavior. Hyperactivity was reported as a previous problem in three cases but attention problems in school persisted into adolescence for many children. Family relations were extremely strained in all cases. In some instances, these adolescents had been abused physically or sexually. Some family interactions were marked by angry interchanges while, in other cases, the family system was enmeshed and parents and siblings were manipulated by the adolescent. None of these 10 adolescents showed evidence of psychosis while in the inpatient service, although several occasionally displayed confused thinking and loose associations. On the other hand, several adolescents were originally referred because of the possibility of psychosis. In two cases, we concluded that the patient had a cognitive or language disorder rather than a thought disorder. In two other cases, it seemed likely that the adolescents occasionally lost the capacity to perceive reality accurately when at home because of their extremely chaotic family environments and limited cognitive skills.

The 10 cases were seen by 10 psychology trainees, most of whom were postdoctoral fellows. They were seen two to three times a week for 40 minute sessions on the inpatient service for periods ranging from 4 to 10 months. Four were followed with outpatient therapy for periods ranging from 4 months to two years.

In terms of the major issues in treatment, three overall patterns emerged. One group of adolescents, who were in the younger age group and had IQs in the borderline range, had functioned fairly well throughout elementary school. These adolescents came from very protective families who attempted to shelter their children from cognitive or social challenges. Consequently, the adolescents had limited peer contacts and, in some cases, were almost phobic in their reaction to others in their age range. The overall treatment in these cases was aimed toward helping them individuate from their families and develop some sense of competence and self-reliance. During treatment these teenagers did develop greater understanding of themselves and their families and began to feel some ability to regulate their own lives. While peer relationships remained an uncomfortable area for them, they were able to form a small number of close relationships.

A second group of teenagers, who were somewhat older and had intelligence quotients in the 60–72 range, came from very disorganized families who were often abusive as well. They were more able to form social relationships with others but often these relationships were self-destructive. Their social skills and understanding appeared to be better on the surface than was actually true and they covered their gaps in comprehension of others by a facade of social sophistication. Furthermore, their capacity to tolerate frustration and their emotional control was very limited. Here the aim of therapy was to help them develop greater impulse control. A number of these individuals were in psychotherapy for fairly extended periods and showed definite improvement. While there were periods of regression, these teenagers became better able to modulate their responses, to tolerate frustration, and to plan for the future. Furthermore, they developed some ability to differentiate between peer relationships that were helpful and those that were more exploitative. It is expected that these individuals will require counseling at other periods in their lives.

A third group of patients were between 16–22 years of age and had intelligence quotients in the range from 45 to 65. These individuals had always been in protected environments and had functioned fairly well. However, they began to be increasingly rebellious in their late teenage years and manifested more frequent temper tantrums and an increase in running away from school or home. Peer relationships were often surprisingly good, although there were limitations in the level of verbal communication. The overall focus of treatment was three-fold in these cases. First, it was clear that these adolescents needed to separate from their families and move into more independent living situations, although they were quite frightened about this change. Besides helping these adolescents to make this transition, they needed to learn to recognize their own emotional states and respond more appropriately. Finally, some of the adolescents needed support in coming to terms with the frustrations of their own limitations. It is of interest to note that one young man returned to the clinic as an outpatient after several years. At this point, the nature of his problems had matured. During his initial, brief treatment period, the focus was on helping him to move out of his home and regulate and express his angry feelings more appropriately. When he returned to the outpatient clinic after several years, his major concern was about a sexual relationship with a young woman in his semi-independent living situation. Thus, this third group of patients was dealing with adaptations to the vocational, social, and sexual issues of young adulthood (See Chapter 4).

It should be noted that we have also worked with a number of chronic psychotic, mentally retarded adolescents. In my opinion, they have shown little sustained improvement. In the two cases in which the adolescents seemed better organized, the major improvement derived from the children's increased capacity to trust the therapist. The families were extremely supportive to their children and mostly needed help in choosing appropriate activities for them. In other cases, there were small gains made but the emotional and behavioral strengths of these adolescents tended to fluctuate widely and erratically. Chess (1962) has also reported that psychotic, mentally retarded children seem least treatable with psychotherapy.

CONSIDERATIONS BASED ON VARYING DEVELOPMENTAL LEVELS

The major principle in all clinical work with the mentally retarded individual is that treatment must be shaped by the varying levels of development within the individual. While this is true for therapy with individuals of normal intelligence whose emotional strengths are frequently more compromised than their intellectual competence, the variations between these domains are even broader for the mentally retarded individual. In assessment and treatment, three individual characteristics must be considered: developmental level, level of psychological differentiation, and chronological age.

Developmental level is most simply defined as mental age. Although adaptive skills may alter overall functioning, we find it useful to have some approximation of the intellectual competence of the child. By establishing that the child with whom we are working has the cognitive skills of a particular age group, we are able to tailor our expectations and verbalizations more appropriately. For example, if an adolescent of 15 years has an overall IQ in the 60–70 range, it is helpful to realize that the adolescent has cognitive strategies more like those of a 8–9-year-old child. Generally, the basis for this estimation of developmental level is broader than simply an intelligence quotient. On our service, we tend to use evaluations of school achievements and assessments of language skills in addition to intelligence test scores to formulate an approximate developmental level for the individual in treatment.

Psychological differentiation reflects the nature of the emotional and social concerns as well as the behavioral, adaptive, and social skills manifested by the child. In our experience, level of psychological differentiation for the mentally retarded child is a function of both developmental level and chronological age. Generally, the child's real issues and strengths are congruent with developmental level so that the 15-year-old adolescent with a mental age of 8–9 years will be more concerned with peer interactions and school achievement than with independence from parents. However, the expression of these issues may be in adolescent terms. As an example, 15-year-old mentally retarded adolescents may want to date and listen to rock music, although they are not really concerned with the sexual and social issues typically associated with these activities. Of course, psychological differentiation may be far below developmental level in the very disturbed or deprived mentally retarded child. Given the nature of the cognitive deficit, it is unlikely that a mentally retarded individual could function at a psychological level higher than the developmental level.

Finally, the therapist must take into account the child's chronological age. The drives and needs of the child may be a function of physical maturity, which is directly related to chronological age. Even more important, many of the child's experiences will be determined by his chronological age. Our society defines expectations and roles for all individuals in terms of chronological age. The mentally retarded child and adolescent cannot escape from these definitions. Thus, chronological age is an important consideration in the assessment and treatment process. In summary, the therapist must consider developmental level, psychological differentiation, and chronological age in formulating the overall approach to psychotherapy.

MODIFICATIONS IN PSYCHOTHERAPEUTIC TECHNIQUES

Certain specific modifications in the therapeutic process are usually required. The mentally retarded individual frequently has language comprehension skills that are particularly impaired (See Chapter 3). For this reason, verbalizations should be briefer and more explicit than those employed with nonretarded children, even of the same developmental level. In general, it is useful to focus on contemporaneous events rather than those in the past. The mentally retarded child may have more limited capacity to remember past events and to generalize from the past to the present. Finally, self-disclosure is appropriate in treatment of the retarded child and adolescent. This individual may have more difficulties in distinguishing between fantasy and reality. While it is useful to understand projections of fantasy material onto the therapist, the mentally retarded patient needs explicit assistance in establishing reality. The use of self-disclosure by the therapist can be an important aid in this regard.

The therapeutic process must also be altered for mentally retarded individuals because they have often experienced so many failures and are particularly sensitive to criticism. As Smith, McKinnon, and Kessler (1976) point out, interpretations are often misperceived as criticisms in therapy, hence mentally retarded individuals may require reassurances that other people share their feelings. Retarded children and adolescents need positive social reinforcement because of their multiple experiences of rejection and limited sense of competence. They may not be able to internalize a feeling of competence without having their achievements noted and praised by another person. One of the advantages of individual psychotherapy, even of short duration, is that the child can be provided with the opportunity to incorporate discrete experiences of success into an image of the self as competent.

A final modification in therapy with mentally retarded children and adolescents is that the therapist may have to incorporate a range of concrete activities into the therapeutic process. This may be particularly true for younger or more impaired children. These children may be less able to interact verbally in a sustained fashion. Various play activities, such as board games, doll play, drawing, cooking, and physical activities can be interspersed with more verbal interactions. These activities can be used to explore the child's experiences, such as feelings of failure, hostility, and fearfulness. The child may learn more about his reactions in the concrete situation than would be possible in the more symbolic, verbal domain.

THE IMPORTANCE OF A MULTIFACETED TREATMENT APPROACH

Psychotherapy is best combined with other interventions if it is to have a strong impact on the mentally retarded child. As mentioned previously, mentally retarded children and adolescents with emotional problems frequently function poorly in school and in recreational settings. For this reason, more structured, individualized school programs and recreational activities may be needed. Family therapy may be an important component of treatment to help the child and family adjust to each other in a more appropriate fashion. Group therapy is also often useful for mentally retarded adolescents. In fact, if the therapist combines group and individual therapy, material from the group experience can be a crucial part of the individual casework. The therapist must be aware of the interventions occurring in other domains. In the optimal situation, specific aims can be made congruent from one setting to another. This is particularly important for the mentally retarded child who has difficulty in generalizing what has been learned. It also affords the child with more opportunities and modalities for growth in any direction. At the very least, the therapist must communicate with teachers and parents. The mentally retarded child may be less able to represent occurrences in his life accurately. For this reason, the therapist must monitor these occurrences more than would be necessary with a child of normal intelligence.

GROUP THERAPY WITH ADOLESCENTS

Along with other clinicians, we have found group therapy to be very useful with mentally retarded adolescents (Fine & Dawson, 1967; Gottwald, 1964; Miezio, 1967; Rosen & Rosen, 1969; Rotman & Golburgh, 1967). Our groups have consisted of 6–8 patients and two leaders at any one time with most patients remaining in the groups for about 4 months (Welch & Sigman, 1980). We have generally used a somewhat structured, more behavioral approach to group therapy.

Group psychotherapy with retarded adolescents shares some of the advantages of group work with adolescents of normal intellect. The group process facilitates work on the developmental tasks of adolescence discussed previously. Another advantage of this mode of treatment is its general acceptability to adolescents who may feel more comfortable with peers than adults and who may feel that a group is less associated with being ill than is individual treatment. A group can also foster increased social interaction, increased self-esteem, and decreased feelings of isolation.

In conducting a therapy group for the retarded, several treatment problems appear to be unique to this population. As discussed above, a major factor is the discrepancy between chronological age and developmental age, which by definition is not found in adolescents of normal intellect. In group psychotherapy, the therapist must simultaneously note the developmental age–chronological age asynchrony not just for one but for several patients and adjust the content and level of group interaction accordingly.

In addition to asynchronies in development, many groups of retarded adolescents present with multileveled problems of a greater variety than is typical in an adolescent group of normal intellect. For example, many retarded individuals have physical problems such as epilepsy (Cytryn & Lourie, 1967). Some authors point to this variability in group composition as detrimental to group process. Criticizing groups for the retarded as often assembled on the basis of a single criterion—the label "mentally retarded"—Berkovitz and Sugar

(1975) argue for groups gathered by consideration of type of disturbance as is typically done for other types of patients. However, because of the mutiproblem nature of the population, more diversity may have to be tolerated. In fact, the range of problems in such groups is often beneficial. In our groups, presenting problems ranged from acting-out or running away to withdrawal or depression, less than average to poor social skills, and a variety of physical problems from epilepsy to kidney failure. Patients appeared to learn from this amalgam that there are numerous ways in which one can be "handicapped" and, conversely, that each of them had different areas of competence.

We have also found, in agreement with others (Berkovitz & Sugar, 1975; Sternlicht, 1965), that the therapist working with a retarded group must be a very active leader. For each patient, the therapist must attend to developmental levels, psychological levels, and chronological age, to physical as well as emotional problems, and to variable verbal and social skills. It is the therapist who must provide structure and maintain movement in the group. For example, the therapist may have to aid in the generation of a topic of discussion, tie in related experiences, or prompt members to contribute. Where social skills are reduced, the therapist must facilitate process as well as content. Individuals may have to be reminded to listen and helped to acknowledge the feelings of others. The reduced verbal skills of these patients make it necessary for the therapist to monitor verbal exchange, simplifying it as needed. The therapist must periodically check for the group's understanding of not only the therapist's language but of the communication among group members. It is important to communicate clearly, repeatedly, and consistently, in order to maximize correct perceptions. Sentences should be short; questions should be asked one at a time; and directions should be simple and concrete. Patients are often unable to bridge material from one session to the next or even within session. Thus, the therapist must point out connections between statements and events. Connecting experiences and/or information helps the patients draw conclusions and generalize learning.

Because of the greater need for concreteness and explicitness and because of reduced verbal skills in such patient groups as compared to groups of normal intelligence, it is often necessary to supplement talk therapy with additional forms of therapy, both verbal and nonverbal. We would agree with Sternlicht (1965) that there are a variety of nonverbal techniques that can be successfully applied to conduct psychotherapy with the retarded just as one might use nonverbal techniques in the treatment of a young child. We have used play techniques, games, role play, music, and drawings. In one self-revealing game, each member of the group was asked to take turns responding to questions such as, "If you were a car, what car would you be?" or "If you were an animal, what animal would you be?" At times we have utilized experiential learning through group activities such as picnics, trips to town and to the movies, and roller skating. The aim was to provide a positive shared experience that enhanced the use of social skills and increased peer interaction and group cohesiveness.

Despite the necessary specialized considerations outlined above, there are particular advantages to group treatment with retarded adolescents. Contact with peers and a sense of belonging to a peer group may be, in itself, beneficial to these adolescents who often grew up misfits in groups composed of age mates of normal intellect. Even if these adolescents have been in classrooms with other mentally retarded children, they have rarely developed an awareness of other children or a sense of group cohesion in the classroom. From the research on the contribution of peer interaction to social–emotional development, Hartup (1979) points out that children lacking in peer interaction either due to social withdrawal or social rejection were likely to experience discomfort, anxiety, and a general unwillingness to engage the environment. He also suggests that mastery of aggressive impulses and sexual socialization take place in the context of peer relations and may not be possible without it. Thus, the group experience appears beneficial in decreasing feelings of inadequacy and anxiety and in providing a context for social–emotional development.

One frequently commented upon advantage of the group treatment approach for many populations is that it provides the patient with numerous behavioral models (Berkovitz & Sugar, 1975; Jakab, 1970). This is especially an advantage for retarded populations. In the group treatment situation, behaviors of peers observed to receive praise and support from the therapist or other patients will be more likely to be adopted, while behaviors observed to be ignored or reap disapproval will infrequently be adopted. Similarly, behaviors of the therapist who has status and who is valued will be more likely to be emulated. Modeling can be a more rapid means of learning because the patient does not have to experience each behavior and its consequences personally. Also, unlike individual treatment, the group offers more types of models, introducing the patient to more behavioral alternatives.

In a similar manner, there is more opportunity for feedback in group treatment. The patient's own behaviors are responded to not just by an adult therapist but by peers. This provides the individual with varied feedback that may be more meaningful and produce results that are more generalizable than feedback from a single adult. This is as true for the retarded population as for any other population.

The demands for communication produced by the group process seem to increase or augment the verbal skills of retarded adolescents. Even the least verbal of adolescents in our groups showed increased attempts to verbalize, though the group offered both nonverbal as well as verbal means of communication. This may have occurred because adolescents are particularly motivated to relate to their peers. The group as a whole appears to enhance the skill of those of lesser verbal ability rather than reduce the level of the more skilled.

While we have not formally assessed outcome for our groups, some subjective impressions of the unique contribution of groups can be presented.

In general, there has been an increase in social awareness among group members with a concomitant decrease in egocentricity or narcissism as noted in their verbal exchange. They express more statements indicating awareness of the needs and feelings of others. There is an increase in the use of social skills such as listening skills and an improvement in the ability to sit still, attend to others, and reflect before acting. We especially observe a change in the direction of more open expression of affect. This appeared to come about as patients became more aware of their feelings and as they became more able to express affect verbally rather than solely through physical acting-out. During the course of the treatment, some groups of adolescents have shown the ability and willingness to discuss not just temporary day-to-day problems but issues of significant concern. At times they revealed insights into their limitations. Perhaps one of the most poignant discussions was centered around the meaning of the term "handicapped" and what it feels like to be "handicapped." These issues were often not discussed with their individual therapists, but in the safety of similar others, many of our adolescents opened up. Our adolescents were also able to reflect on what they had learned in the group and on the importance of the group to them.

Given these benefits, it seems that group psychotherapy is underutilized. Those groups that are formed tend to be found in inpatient settings. Group treatment should be used with outpatients as well. Because of efforts at mainstreaming, there may, in fact, be an increased need for such treatment for retarded adolescents. While there is some evidence that outpatient groups for the retarded are feasible and successful (Pikey, Goldman, & Kleinman, 1961), several issues in addition to those presented for inpatient groups must be considered.

First, there is a question of segregated group treatment of the retarded versus a mixed group of adolescents whose intellect varies from the retarded to the normal level. In this regard, it should be noted that adolescents whose IQs fell within the normal range occasionally were placed in our inpatient groups. This integration was successful because the emotional problems of the nonretarded adolescents were similar to some of the problems of the retarded adolescents. We believe that the added IQ variability can be accommodated if the adolescents share similar emotional experiences and problems. If not, too much variance may be introduced and communication within the group may break down. Similarity in personal interests and issues also contributes to a sense of group support and enhances self-esteem. This is a factor in the success of homogeneous groups such as women's groups, divorced persons' groups, or groups for alcoholics. In addition, in a mixed group, it may take the retarded participants longer to develop a sense of safety and trust so that they then can reveal their feelings. The retarded adolescents may also be made more aware of their verbal limitations in comparison to the other adolescents and this may inhibit their full participation.

Integrated groups are likely to be viewed favorably in those outpatient settings where efforts toward mainstreaming in retarded individuals are being implemented. On the other hand, in outpatient settings, particularly in school settings, there is greater diversity in both emotional problems and intelligence. In designing outpatient groups, the need for balancing the interests and abilities of group participants may be more critical than in inpatient settings where more homogeneity is usual. The inpatient group may also progress more quickly because the participants are exposed to an entire milieu that encourages the relaxation of defenses and increased self-expression. The group members are likely to know each other well and to share common experiences. In addition, specific shared experiences can be referred to as concrete examples, a helpful technique in working with retarded adolescents. To the extent that the members of the outpatient group share experiences or that experiences are created by group participation, the progress of the group may be accelerated.

PROBLEMS IN TREATING RETARDED CHILDREN AND ADOLESCENTS

Therapists who work with mentally retarded children and adolescents may have certain emotional reactions that hinder treatment. The major difficulty is that the potential level of achievement for the retarded child or adolescent is limited. At best, the patient, therapist, and family will see growth and improvement. However, the rate of change may be slow and the retarded person's accomplishments may not be appreciable. The therapist may wonder if the outcome is worth the expenditure of time and emotional involvement.

A countertransference problem that is particularly germane to retarded child populations is the fantasy of saving the child. The therapist may wish to save the child not only from parents, teachers, and peers but also from the society at large, which scorns them. When a therapist holds this attitude, the result may be overinvolvement, which may undermine the patient's competence and alienate significant others in the child's life. In line with this fantasy, the therapist must guard against the expectation in himself, the child, and the child's family that therapy will "cure" the retardation.

Despite the challenges presented by psychotherapy with retarded children and adolescents, their needs for such help are enormous and the effects are substantial. Some of the adolescents we have worked with have never talked to anyone in their lives about their feelings and perceptions. The improvement they experience and show after psychotherapy is dramatic. We are not advocating individual and group psychotherapy as the exclusive means of intervention. Certainly, most retarded children and adolescents benefit from educational, recreational, and occupational therapies, and behavioral paradigms are frequently useful in structuring their environments. However, individual and group psychotherapy can make unique contributions to the treatment of retarded individuals. While there are difficulties in using these techniques with this population, the difficulties are not so great as to be prohibitive. The rewards of seeing growth and change in a retarded adolescent more than compensates for the extended efforts.

Acknowledgment

The material in this chapter was gathered through the professional efforts of the psychology trainees who worked on the inpatient ward for developmentally disabled adolescents from June 1977 to September 1982. Ellen Nahknikian, Ph.D. and Veronica Ortega-Welch, Ph.D. contributed particularly. I am grateful to the interdisciplinary staff who worked with me during that period. Martha Jura, Ph.D., Klaus K. Minde, M.D., and Mary O'Connor, Ph.D. made helpful comments on an earlier version of this chapter.

REFERENCES

Albini, JL, & Dinitz, S. (1965). Psychotherapy with disturbed and defective children: An evaluation of changes in behavior and attitudes. *American Journal of Mental Deficiency, 69,* 560–567

Berkovitz, IH, & Sugar, M. (1975). Indications and contraindications for young psychotherapy. In M Sugar (Ed.), *The adolescent in group and family therapy* (pp. 3–26). New York: Brunner/Mazel

Bialer, I. (1967). Psychotherapy and other adjustment techniques with the mentally retarded. In AA Baumeister (Ed.), *Mental retardation: Appraisal, education and rehabilitation* (pp. 138–180). Chicago: Aldine Publishing

Borokowski, JG, & Johnson, LO. (1968). Mediation and the paired-associate learning of normals and retardates. *American Journal of Mental Deficiency, 72,* 610–613

Bozarth, JD, & Roberts, RR. (1970). Effectiveness of counselor-trainees with mentally retarded sheltered workshop clients. *Training School Bulletin, 67,* 119–122

Chess, S. (1962). Psychiatric treatment of the mentally retarded child with behavior problems. *American Journal of Orthopsychiatry, 32,* 863–869

Coffman, TL, & Harris, MC. (1980). Transition shock and adjustment of mentally retarded persons. *Mental Retardation, 18,* 3–9

Cytryn, L, & Lourie, RS. (1967). Mental retardation. In AM Freedman & HK Kaplan (Eds.), *Comprehensive textbook of psychiatry* (pp. 817–856). Baltimore, MD: Williams and Wilkins

Erikson, EH. (1968). *Identity: Youth and crisis.* New York: Norton

Eyman, RK, & Call, T. (1977). Maladaptive behavior and community placement of mentally retarded persons. *American Journal of Mental Deficiency, 82,* 137–144

Fine, R, & Dawson, JC. (1967). A therapy program for the mildly retarded adolescent. *American Journal of Mental Deficiency, 69,* 23–30

Gottwald, HL. (1964). A special program for educable-emotionally disturbed retarded. *Mental Retardation, 2,* 353–359

Hartup, WW. (1979). Peer relations and the growth of social competence. In MW Kent & JE Rolf (Eds.), *Primary prevention of psychopathology: Social competence in children* (Vol. 3) (pp. 150–170). Hanover, NH: University Press of New England

Humes, C, Adamcyzk, J, & Myco, R. (1969). A school study of group counselling with educable retarded adolescents. *American Journal of Mental Deficiency, 74,* 191–195

Jakab, I. (1970). Psychotherapy of the mentally retarded child. In NR Berstein (Ed.), *Diminished people: Problems and care of the mentally retarded.* Boston, MA: Little, Brown

Leland, H, & Smith, DI. (1965). *Play therapy with mentally subnormal children.* New York: Grune & Stratton

Lott, G. (1970). Psychotherapy of the mentally retarded: Values and cautions. In FJ Menaloscino (Ed.), *Psychiatric approaches to mental retardation* (pp. 227–250). New York: Basic Books

Mann, PH, Beaber, JO, & Jacobson, MD. (1969). The effect of group counseling on educable mentally retarded boys' self-concepts. *Exceptional Children, 35,* 359–366

Matson, TL, & Barrett RP. (1982). *Psychopathology in the mentally retarded.* New York: Grune & Stratton

Miezio, S. (1967). Group therapy with mentally retarded adolescents in institutional settings. *International Journal of Group Psychotherapy, 17,* 321–327

Morrison, TL, & Newcomber, BL. (1975). Effects of directive vs. nondirective play therapy with institutionalized mentally retarded children. *American Journal of Mental Deficiency, 79,* 666–669

Offer, D, Marcus, D, & Offer, JL. (1970). A longitudinal study of normal adolescent boys. *American Journal of Psychiatry, 126,* 917–924

Pikey, L, Goldman, M, & Kleinman, B. (1961). Psychodrama and empathic ability in mentally retarded. *American Journal of Mental Deficiency, 65,* 595–605

Rosen, HG, & Rosen, S. (1969). Group therapy as an instrument to develop a concept of self-worth in the adolescent and young adult mentally retarded. *Mental Retardation, 7,* 52–55

Rotman, CB, & Golburgh, SJ. (1967). Group counseling mentally retarded adolescents. *Mental Retardation, 5,* 13–16

Silvestri, R. (1977). Implosive therapy treatment of emotionally disturbed retardates. *Journal of Consulting and Clinical Psychology, 45,* 14–22

Smith, E, McKinnon, R, & Kessler, JW. (1976). Psychotherapy with mentally retarded children. *Psychoanalytic Study of the Child, 31,* 493–514

Sternlicht, M. (1965). Psychotherapeutic techniques useful with the mentally retarded: A review and critique. *Psychiatric Quarterly, 39,* 84–90

Sternlicht, M. (1966). Psychotherapeutic procedures with the retarded. In NR Ellis (Ed.), *International review of research in mental retardation.* New York: Academic Press

Sternlicht, M. (1977). Issues in counselling and psychotherapy with mentally retarded individuals. In I Bialer & M Sternlicht (Eds.), *The psychology of mental retardation: Issues and approaches.* New York: Psychological Dimensions

Syzmanski, LS. (1980). Individual psychotherapy with retarded persons. In LS Syzmanski & PE Tanguay (Eds.), *Emotional disorders of mentally retarded persons* (pp. 131–149). Baltimore, MD: University Park Press

Syzmanski, LS, & Tanguay, PE. (Eds.). (1980). *Emotional disorders of mentally retarded persons.* Baltimore, MD: University Park Press

Welch, VO, & Sigman, M. (1980). Group psychotherapy with mentally retarded, emotionally disturbed adolescents. *Journal of Clinical Child Psychology, 9,* 209–210

Zeitlin, AG, & Turner, JL. (1982, March). *Coping with adolescence: Perspectives of retarded individuals and their families.* Paper presented at the Gatlinberg Conference on Research in Mental Retardation, Gatlinburg, TN

Zeitlin, AG, & Turner, JL. (1984). Self-perspectives on being handicapped: Stigma and adjustment. In RB Edgerton (Ed.), Lives in process: Mentally retarded adults in a large city. *AAMD Monograph, No. 6, pp. 93–120*

Frederick Frankel
Steven R. Forness

14

Educational and Clinical Behavioral Approaches to the Child and Adolescent with Dual Disabilities

The client with dual disabilities is a child or adolescent with delayed cognitive and adaptive development and some other pathological condition. The classification of pathology is taken to mean a condition significantly more intense (either in frequency or severity) than that occurring in the general population of same-aged peers, which is significantly more prolonged than would be expected in normal development and, which causes significant distress to either the client, his family, or the community (Rutter, 1975). The most frequent pathological conditions accompanying symptoms of delayed cognitive development are behavior problems (aggression, noncompliance, tantrums, and self-injurious behavior), emotional problems (depression, anxiety), problems in socialization (withdrawal, deficiencies in social skills, attachment, assertiveness), and certain conditions that can be classified as involving generalized impairments in information processing (attention deficits, psychosis).

The service needs called into play by the problems posed by clients with dual disabilities may often be large as compared with clients with a single disability. Particularly important, and we believe central to these service needs, is the need for special educational services as well as an overall habilitation plan. Behavioral techniques can and usually have played an integral role in the fulfillment of both of these needs.

The problems posed by the client with dual disabilities have been different for educators and clinical behaviorists. The structure of the educational service delivery system has been by diagnostic category and has not been devised to accomodate individuals who straddle these categories. In devising clinical treatment, the contributions of factors associated with each diagnostic category

CHILDREN WITH EMOTIONAL DISORDERS AND DEVELOPMENTAL DISABILITIES ISBN 0–8089–1700–5

that the client manifests is more than the simple sum. Thus, the present authors have divided this chapter into two major sections, concerned with educational and behavioral approaches. In making this division, it is acknowledged that there is much overlap between the two approaches; behavioral approaches are commonly used in the classroom, and educational interventions play a central role in the overall habilitation plan. The division into two major sections is meant to highlight factors that exemplify each approach.

EDUCATIONAL APPROACHES

The education of mentally retarded or developmentally disabled children has been a problem of increasing concern to school personnel. Generally, special education has been organized around a diagnostic-categorical approach in which separate programs are devised for the mentally retarded, the emotionally disturbed, the learning disabled, and other categories of children with sensory or physical handicaps. The difficulty with such programs is that certain assumptions underlie the grouping of each category, i.e., that mentally retarded children have primarily a learning problem, that emotionally disturbed children have primarily a behavior problem, and so forth. However, there are mentally retarded pupils whose principal difficulty is problems in classroom behavior as well as emotionally disturbed students who function at such low levels of adaptation that their basic problem is a developmental one. A recent study of more than 2000 school children referred for evaluation to interdisciplinary developmental disability clinics across the country suggests that more than one fourth had serious behavioral problems (Forness, Urbano, Rotberg, Bender, Gardner, Lynch, & Zemanek, 1980). Direct observation of over 600 pupils in EMR and TMR classrooms also confirms a wide range of disruptive classroom behaviors (Russell & Forness, 1985), and examination of EMR classrooms reveals children with a range of physical and behavioral disorders (MacMillan & Barthwick, 1980).

Educators have therefore recognized that a more individualized approach to programming is needed; and indeed Public Law 94-142, the Right to Education For All Handicapped Act, now requires more flexibility in designing programs for children who do not fit readily into traditional diagnostic categories (Forness, 1981). The remainder of this section will describe the present state of school programs for children with developmental and behavioral disorders.

Special Education Classification of Disability

Children served in special education are defined by the types of difficulties they present in the classroom. Thus, children with behavior problems or emotional disorders are defined as children whose deviation from age-appropriate social or emotional behavior significantly interferes either with their ability to profit from regular classroom instruction or instruction with other children in the class (Hewett & Taylor, 1980). Autistic children, who represent the extremes of this category, require very specialized programs (Forness, 1974a). Learning disabled children are children who display an educationally significant discrepancy between their intellectual potential and actual school performance that cannot be explained in terms of intellectual, experiential, sensory, or physical problems (Bryan & Bryan, 1975; Tarjan & Forness, 1979). Hyperactivity may also be present in learning-disabled children and require special management (Forness, 1975). Mentally retarded children are classified into three groups (Forness, 1974b, Tarjan & Forness, 1979). Educable mentally retarded (EMR) children are defined as those who cannot adapt or respond to the normal instruction in regular elementary grades because of subaverage intellectual functioning (generally in the 50–70 or 75 IQ range) but who have the potential for learning basic academic skills at the second to seventh grade level. Trainable mentally retarded (TMR) are those who do not have the intellectual potential (generally in the 30 to 50 IQ range) for academic achievement beyond the first or second grade level but who can profit from instruction in skills designed to give them a measure of independence in adult life. Profoundly mentally retarded children (PMR) are those whose intellectual potential (below 30 IQ) is so limited that they will probably function only at the preschool academic level and will need continued, intense care and supervision.

There are also categories for children with speech, language, physical, or sensory handicaps who require physical modifications of the school environment or special instructional aides or training in order to make acceptable school progress. These include children with aphasia, crippling or chronically debilitating conditions, the deaf or hard of hearing, and the blind or partially sighted. Also included in these categories are children with seizure disorders and multiply handicapped individuals.

The term "special education" implies that these children will either need to be segregated from the regular classroom and placed in special classes, where their needs may be more easily met, or will at least need some form of sustained special assistance not ordinarily provided to nonhandicapped children in regular classrooms.

US Department of Education surveys estimate that approximately 10 to 11 percent of all school children are receiving special education. Of these, the largest groups are the speech handicapped and the learning disabled at 3 to 4 percent each, the mentally retarded at slightly less than 2 percent, the emotionally disturbed or behavior disordered at around one percent, and the remaining categories at well under one percent each.

Development of Current Special Education Programs

During the past ten years, special education has been undergoing a great deal of change and experiencing considerable controversy. This process still continues. Until a few years ago special education was equated with special classes. Handicapped children were taken out of their communities, or at least out of their regular classrooms, and placed in special classes where they received "special education." It was not until the late 1950s that significant attention was paid to the effectiveness of this "special class model." A number of subsequent studies indicated that mildly retarded children left in regular classrooms achieved academically at a higher level than comparable retarded children assigned to special classes, but the evidence has never been viewed as conclusive (Carlberg & Kavale, 1980). Not only was effectiveness of the special class model questioned, but in the past two decades, a large body of research has emerged (see Hewett & Forness, 1984; MacMillan, 1982; or Mercer & Snell, 1977 for reviews) that questions the basic concept of "the mentally retarded student" and, by implication, the learning of other types of handicapped children as well. Before this point, there had existed a rather traditional tendency to think of mental retardation as a lack of intelligent behavior and to ascribe less intelligent behavior to a lack of intelligence. Thanks to studies in such areas as discrimination learning, metamemory, social motivation, labeling, and behavior modification, intelligence is no longer seen as an all-encompassing, general commodity but appears to depend on a host of motivational and situational variables. These variables greatly determine whether or not a teacher elicits "intelligent" behavior from a so-called retarded child, or for that matter, any handicapped child, as we shall see in the second section of this chapter.

The above evidence began to appear in the special education literature in the form of serious criticism about the practice of special education (Dunn, 1968; Forness, 1972; President's Committee on Mental Retardation, 1969). More significantly at this juncture, parents of handicapped children began to make their own dissatisfaction heard in the form of various class-action lawsuits, which challenged various procedures related to the testing of minority children, placement in special education classes, exclusion of some children from special education and countless other procedures (see reviews by Burt, 1975; Cohen & DeYoung, 1973). The resolution of these issues, as described above, was in fact the passage in 1976 of a federal law: Public Law 94-142, "Right to Education for the Handicapped." It not only provides federal money to mandate special education programs across the nation; but, perhaps, more importantly, it provides several protections for handicapped children and their families, as we shall see below.

Educational Evaluation and Assessment

Mildly handicapped children, i.e., those with behavior disorders, learning disabilities, speech problems, mild retardation, and mild physical or sensory impairments, are usually identified by different mechanisms than the severely handicapped, i.e., those with serious emotional problems, autism, aphasia, severe or profound retardation, cerebral palsy, and the blind or the deaf. Mildly handicapped children are often not identified as such before reaching school age. Although a potentially mildly retarded or behavior disordered child may have problems in communication, physical development, and socialization during the preschool years, differences tend to be moderate and may not cause undue concern until after the child begins formal schooling. At that point, the teacher seeks help, and the child usually is referred for evaluation by a school psychologist or other members of a special education evaluation team.

Severely handicapped children, on the other hand, are often identified before reaching school age. Children who appear listless, fail to smile or babble, or are unable to sit up, walk, or talk within a normal length of time are all suspect. A pediatrician is usually the first person to whom concerned parents come for advice. Most pediatricians are not experts in mental retardation, and will often refer parents to clinics, other agencies that specialize in developmental disabilities, or school programs, which are now available for severely handicapped children as young as three years. Children with a potential dual disability, i.e., also involving a behavior problem, are often identified rather quickly, because of the obviously disruptive nature of their difficulty.

The first step in any case involving a dual diagnostic child is to review developmental or school records to determine what difficulties the child has experienced related to learning or adjustment. Such information should be analyzed for any significant trends and should be supplemented by extensive interviews of parents, the child, and even the teacher if the child is in school. Questions to be pursued include the following. When did the problem first seem to occur? Does it seem to be a behavior problem, a learning problem or both? If it is both, did one seem to cause or at least precede the other? Did the problem seem to be linked to some significant event occurring at home? How did the problem first come to the attention of parents? If a behavior problem, under what conditions does it seem to occur? What are the events that seem to precede an occurrence of the problem? What seem to be the consequences from teacher, from peers? What attempts have been made in the past to manage the behavior by school personnel, by parents? How successful have they been? If a learning problem, does it involve just reading skills or other areas as well? Was the problem noticeable from before the child began to attend school, the very beginning of school, or subsequently? Do siblings have similar problems? Is the child in a preschool, a regular class or is he receiving some form of special education? Has the child repeated any grades? Were there problems prior to school entrance that might be related to the present problem? What is the child's perception of his problem? What are the parents' expectations for the child?

A clinical or school psychologist should then be contacted to arrange for psychological evaluation. In addition to a standardized individual intelligence test such as the WISC–R or the Stanford-Binet, other tests of social or developmental functioning may be necessary. These tests and others mentioned herein are discussed in some detail in other chapters, along with some of their disadvantages in the testing of minority children. A "school" version of the AAMD adaptive behavior scale is also available if mental retardation is suspected (Lambert & Nicholl, 1976). A speech or hearing specialist should also be consulted when the presence of a speech, language, or hearing impairment is suspected. Vision screening or pediatric examination may also be warranted. Other tests of perceptual motor functioning, linguistic impairment, or a variety of individual tests in reading or other areas of academic functioning or readiness may be used to analyze specific types of learning difficulties. Sometimes a more careful examination of subtest scores on the WISC–R can also provide indications of a learning disability (Smith, Coleman, Dokecki, & Davis, 1977).

For children of school age, school history and related reports are essential, but standardized achievement tests must be administered to determine the child's academic progress, independently of teacher assessment (for detailed review of specific educational testing see Howell, Kaplan, and O'Connell, 1979, or Sinclair, 1983). This testing may often be performed by a school psychologist or a special education resource specialist who may even attempt "diagnostic teaching" with the child. An example of this is presented in the case of RJ below. The PIAT (Peabody Individual Achievement Test) is commonly used (Dunn & Markwardt, 1970; Wilson & Spangler, 1974), since it is particularly appropriate when language problems are suspected, i.e., the child responds to questions by pointing to one of four answer panels or by answering in relatively short answers. Results provide grade-level scores based on standardized performance for children at each age. One should also not forget other areas of school achievement, as well as the child's functioning in physical education and recreation. A specialist in adaptive P.E. or an occupational therapist may also be called upon to assess the child's potential in these areas as well. For adolescents, assessment of prevocational skills may also be warranted (Forness, Thornton, & Horton, 1981).

The final step in the evaluation process is a tentative formulation of a diagnosis of the child's educational problems. This proceeds along the lines of the general criteria listed for each category of exceptionality listed at the beginning of this chapter. Bear in mind, however, that educational diagnoses are made only in reference to the types of programs or interventions the child needs in school. In a sense, diagnosis here is a determination of the child's eligibility for special education. For the child with dual disabilities, additional considerations are specific suggestions to the child's teacher for handling learning or behavior problems in the classroom; recommendation for placement in some form of modified special education or related services (or recommendation for a regular classroom if conditions warrant it); or recommendation for residential schooling. Common types of special education programs will be listed in following sections, in the context of developing the child's individual educational plan.

Individual Educational Planning: The IEP

The individual educational plan or IEP is a written document that is the basis of the child's schooling (Forness, 1979b; Torres, 1977; Turnbull, Strickland, & Hammer, 1978a, 1978b). It is developed in one or a series of meetings with all significant people involved: the parents, the child's current teacher, and a special education specialist or administrator. Some cases may require the additional presence of a school psychologist, the school principal, a physician, the school nurse or social worker, a speech therapist, and the physical education teacher or therapist. There are four sections to the IEP that are developed in the meeting(s). The first section usually contains a detailed description of the child's present level of functioning. It may include the state of the child's physical health and any physical abnormalities or problems; results of screening tests in hearing and vision; the child's developmental history; results of all psychological, perceptual, and educational testing; results of a mental status examination, in cases where serious emotional problems may be present; the child's adaptive behavior or a description of his or her adjustment to home and neighborhood life; the child's adjustment to classroom and school life, as measured by rating scales or reports of direct observation of the child in the classroom or in play situations; results of assessments of physical fitness or motor dexterity; and assessment of vocational or career status. Note that only three or four of the above items may be sufficient in cases where the child's problem is relatively circumscribed.

The second section of the plan contains the goals and short-term objectives for the child's school program, based on the assessment of the child's strengths and weaknesses, just described. Goals are referenced to expected progress for the child by the end of the school year. Separate goals may be written for all academic areas (language, reading, mathematics, etc.) and for physical, social, emotional, and vocational skills. The third section contains the types of services and programs the child needs to receive, when these should begin, how long they should last, and which professionals will be responsible for each of them. In this section, then, are the means whereby goals and objectives are to be accomplished. In a complex case, for example, of a severely retarded youngster with multiple handicaps and for whom several goals have been stated in different areas, many statements might have to be made describing the child's special school placement, length of school day, behavioral approaches needed, related medications and how these will be prescribed and administered, speech therapy, parent training, and coordination of services. The fifth section contains the evaluation scheme for the child's program, including techniques or tests will be used to measure the child's progress, which criteria will determine success in each area, and who will decide if each criterion has been met. Thus, the IEP is an attempt at a more comprehensive view of habilitation of the child, albeit focusing on the educational contribution.

Behavioral measurement, interventions and terminology have been especially useful in the development of the IEP.

The IEP should be a team effort with parents and school district personnel participating equally, although initial results suggest that parents have less influence (Gilliam & Coleman, 1981; Goldstein, Strickland, Turnbull, & Curry, 1980). Certain timetables are built into Public Law 94–142 to insure that children are served quickly and efficiently. When disagreements arise, the parents have a right to request an impartial fair hearing before a person who is not employed by the school district and whose judgment is binding. The fair hearing process includes various rights of appeal, prior examination of evidence, and other legal protections. In some cases, hearings may result in funding of school or related services by private agencies. The law also provides for a "surrogate" parent, for those children who need it, to insure that their rights are protected.

Special Education Programs

Special education for children with dual disabilities can be described by grouping programs into two areas: special classes or schools and mainstreaming arrangements. Special class or special school approaches are generally as follows: a residential institution for long-term custodial care, an acute psychiatric hospital for short-term treatment, a special teacher to tutor the child at home on a daily basis, a residential school, a special day school, or placement in a special classroom in a regular school, either for the entire day or the better part of it. Although mainstreaming means different things to various professionals, there is some agreement that it is defined by two criteria: the mainstreamed child spends more than half the time in the regular classroom and the regular classroom teacher has the primary responsibility for the child's progress (MacMillan, Jones, & Meyers, 1976). It implies that the child's learning handicaps or behavior problems are not so severe as to preclude their effective remediation in a regular classroom setting.

Criteria for considering whether or not to mainstream a particular child relate to such factors as the age of the child, the pervasiveness and degree of handicap, the curriculum modifications that might be needed, the child's peer relationships and social skills, the number of children in the regular classroom, teacher competency, and family resources (Forness, 1979a). There are generally two approaches to helping mainstreamed children: the "special education teacher consultant" who assists the regular classroom teacher (Miller & Sabatino, 1978) and the "resource room" in which the child is given special help for one or two periods each day (Sindelar & Deno, 1978).

For mildly mentally retarded children (IQ 50 to 70 or 75), special classes are often designated as EMR (educable mentally retarded) classrooms. Other classes may be designated as "educationally handicapped" or "learning disability" classes and contain learning-disabled or behavior-disordered children as well as some retarded children. Preschool levels of these classes (ages three to six years) are available in increasing numbers and provide experiences for children to improve their school readiness as much as normal preschools do for younger children, but at a slower pace. Special education classes at the primary level (ages six to nine years) provide experiences in oral language and speech development, sensorimotor development, self-awareness, group membership and social adjustment, self-care, safety, manipulation of materials, work habits, following directions, and reading readiness. At this level, academic tasks may not be generally emphasized for mentally retarded children except for beginning instruction in counting and recognition of letters or words. By the elementary level (ages eight to thirteen years), EMR children will have begun to learn tool-skill subjects such as reading, writing, spelling, and math. The secondary level provides consolidation in the use of basic-skill subjects learned earlier, but with increasing emphasis on preparation for work and home-living, especially with the mildly retarded. Toward the end of their formal school careers, mildly retarded youths will often be assigned to a work-study program, a vocational training program run by an agency other than the school, or even a trial job on a part-time basis.

Moderately and severely mentally retarded children (IQ 30 to 50) are placed in TMR (trainable mentally retarded) classrooms. Other special day-classes for children with severe handicaps may include "seriously emotionally disturbed" or "autistic" classes. In most cases, young TMR children are placed in nursery schools or development centers that provide habit-training and language-development programs. Special education is typically provided for elementary and secondary TMR children in special day-schools.

It is clear, however, that educational settings for severely and moderately handicapped children can and should range from residential school placement up to and including integration into regular classroom settings, depending on the particular strengths and weaknesses of the individual child (Burton & Hirshoren, 1979). Emphasis should generally be on language development, self-help skills, socialization, and preparation for daily living. With increasing emphasis as the child grows older, special education programs are generally geared to prepare the child to function optimally at home or in community residential settings and to work in sheltered workshops or other work situations where special supervision is available.

The profoundly mentally retarded, those that fall at the lower end of the severely handicapped category (below IQ 30), as well as those severely mentally retarded who have multihandicapping conditions, tend to present unique problems in medical and behavioral management. These children generally have special needs for continuing supervision or custodial care. It has been suggested that their educational goals emphasize skills that will maximize their happiness within the environment rather than unrealistic expectations for a future role in everyday society (Rago & Cleland, 1978).

In order to provide a more practical illustration of these concepts, the following case of an adolescent with a dual diagnosis will be presented. The case was selected because it best illustrates several of the special educational issues discussed thus far.

RG was a 13-year-old black youngster who was first seen for interdisciplinary evaluation at a University hospital outpatient psychiatric clinic. He was brought to the clinic at the urging of school personnel who were unable to maintain him in his public school EMR classroom because of his behavior. He was reportedly involved in fights with peers, in "running loose" on the school campus, in physical aggression toward his teachers, and in a variety of other disruptive behaviors. His tested IQ had been reportedly too low for him to be placed in a program for educationally handicapped (EH) youngsters, which only accepted children of normal intelligence with learning disabilities and/or conduct-disordered children without severe learning difficulty.

The school was apparently at a loss. They could not continue him in his present EMR placement because his behavior problems seemed impossible to manage in a junior high EMR classroom of 15 pupils. On the other hand, the smaller EH classroom, which might have been an appropriate setting for a child with conduct problems, was not appropriate for a mentally retarded youngster who might easily have been taken advantage of and/or socially rejected by children with near normal intelligence. The upset in his school routine was apparently making RG more anxious, agitated, and less manageable during after-school hours.

RG was the third child in a family of four boys. Pregnancy and delivery were complicated by an attempt at self-induced abortion, in the fourth month, resulting in an emergency room visit with premature contractions and considerable bleeding but no actual expulsion of the fetus. At delivery, labor was prolonged; and RG was described as a sometimes listless, sometimes agitated infant who appeared slow in development compared to his two older brothers.

RG was recognized as a problem child almost as soon as he entered kindergarten and was referred for evaluation. The school psychologist's report described RG as hyperactive and difficult to manage in the testing situation and suggested that his obtained IQ scores may not have been valid. IQ was reported as 58 with considerably more impairment on language items. Achievement and other developmental testing suggested virtually no letter or number skills and subsequent language testing placed his expressive language age at about two years. RG was placed on a "waiting list" for EMR placement for the remainder of the school year, and his attendance in the regular kindergarten program for the remainder of the year was sporadic at best.

RG entered the EMR class the following year and apparently made some progress in this class, though he continued to be a behavior problem; and his classroom management was mainly effected by having the classroom aide in his class spend large amounts of her time providing individual instruction for RG, who seemed to require it.

RG was subsequently hospitalized on an inpatient ward for developmentally-disabled children. Achievement testing during the first two days of inpatient school showed his achievement close to the middle third-grade level in most subjects. The reason for the discrepancy with previous testing was that the Peabody Individual Test of Achievement (PIAT) was used. The PIAT is a test that is generally more conducive to determining achievement in minority or language-delayed children, because it mainly requires the child to point to one of four pictures illustrating the possible correct answer.

RG was first placed in the inpatient elementary classroom with seven other children who were also functioning at third- to seventh-grade levels. The approach in this classroom was to individualize instruction so that each of the three or four periods of the daily school program was tailored specifically to each child's level of functioning in reading, math, and language arts. Thus a weekly schedule was laid out in advance on each child's desk, indicating the page numbers of the books, worksheets, or lessons that the child would be expected to complete for each period. At the end of each completed task or lesson the teacher corrected the child's work and gave feedback and praise to the child on what he or she had completed. Thus RG could see progress and know what to expect next.

For behavior management, "group" points were administered during a formal five-minute period at the end of each hour in school. Each child was asked in turn, by a child designated as "point monitor," to specify the number of points, on a scale of five, which the class earned for that hour. Criteria were specified in advance, and reviewed with the class periodically, in such areas as raising one's hand before talking, minding one's business, being in one's assigned area when designated, sharing and cooperating with classmates. If a child's estimation of the group's behavior varied significantly from that of his or her classmates, the teacher asked the child to give the reasons for his decision, and children were allowed to discuss pros and cons of the validity of the rating. The teacher retained ultimate approval of the final numerical rating in case of unresolved disagreement. Group points were accumulated toward a classroom treat or outing at the end of the week. The rationale for this system had to do with the pervasiveness of peer influences on socialization at this age and on the importance of a child's perceptions of appropriate behavior in a social context.

If serious aggression or disruptive outbursts occurred, the child was placed for a brief period (usually five to ten minutes) in a "time-out room" adjacent to the classroom. For subsequent episodes, the child was allowed to go to the time-out room unassisted, if he or she could do so with a brief prompt, in order to give increasingly more responsibility for his or her own behavior. Some children were also given simultaneous instruction in learning how to approach tasks and to "talk themselves through" their lessons as general strategies to give them more verbal control over their own impulsive or inattentive behavior. Thus antecedent events such as level of curriculum, types of materials, and choice of learning strategies were emphasized, as well as consequences for good and bad behavior.

RG responded very well to this program. In four months, he gained more than one-year in reading and seven months in math. His classroom behavior improved to the point that only occasional prompts were needed to help him maintain good classroom deportment. However, since certain issues in RG's family situation were still unresolved and therapeutic progress on the ward was still limited, RG was transferred to an adolescent ward where he could continue a similar therapeutic milieu but do so with adolescents closer to his chronological age and interests, as he was now 13 years old. At this point, he was also transferred to the lower secondary classroom program in the inpatient school.

This classroom had some 12 to 14 pupils with a much broader span of achievement levels (fourth through ninth grade). The class had programs in which somewhat more emphasis was placed on individual instruction, with a more immediate reinforcement system in which individually earned points could be exchanged directly for certain privileges in the hospital or accumulated for tangible items such as record albums, clothes, and the like. An additional rationale for this particular change for RG was that his rate of academic progress was so rapid that a more individualized program might be considered more useful in determining just how far he could go in terms of academic potential. Indeed IQ testing completed at about this point indicated an IQ of 68, or some ten points higher than his previously reported IQ. There was also considerably less imbalance between verbal and performance items. When the SOMPA correction for minority student performance was employed (see chapter on psychological tests), RG's IQ was actually estimated to be in the low 70s. He also attended a vocational shop program once each week where he worked on a variety of typical shop projects designed to help him become familiar with such a setting and to apply his newly acquired academic skills in a more practical situation. RG continued to make good academic and behavioral progress in his school program; and, at the time of discharge three months later, was achieving at the middle to upper fourth grade in reading and at the beginning fourth-grade level in math skills. He was, moreover, relatively consistent in being able to meet the social demands of classroom situations.

RG's family situation, while not completely resolved, was such that he could be discharged to his grandmother's care with a relatively good prognosis for continued social adjustment. His academic progress, coupled with what could be considered a more valid estimate of his IQ, also meant that he could now be placed in a program for educationally handicapped youngsters. Though he could technically continue to be considered "mentally retarded" under the existing AAMD definition, his conduct and behavior problems were much improved; and his potential for continued academic prgress was soundly demonstrated by his performance in the hospital school prior to discharge. An IEP meeting was held with public school personnel, RGs grandmother, and his NPI teacher some two weeks prior to discharge. His level of functioning was reviewed and goals in academic subjects were formulated based on his predicted level of performance, at least partly determined by previous rate of progress in the hospital school. Goals in socialization stressed expected progress in peer relationships and in dealing with aduit authority. He was recommended for the junior high school educationally handicapped program with mainstreaming in physical education and in beginning vocational shop classes. At last follow-up, he was making satisfactory progress in these situations.

The case described above illustrates several concepts discussed in the first part of this chapter. For example, public school special education classrooms are not always organized in such a way that a dual diagnostic child "fits" the system. The only way in which RG could be accommodated was by nearly "disenfranchising" himself from the EMR category. This was possible because of careful assessment of intellectual potential, under optimum conditions and using pluralistic norms for minority children, and by strong evidence that RG's attainment under the best of conditions was probably far better than might be predicted based on his existing IQ. An interdisciplinary approach, where several aspects of RG's social and developmental functioning could be approached in concert, was also necessary.

It is not at all clear that even a careful meeting of RG's school needs alone could have produced the progress seen. Individual therapy, a therapeutic and structured milieu, and ongoing attention to RG's eventual home situation were also necessary and had to be carefully coordinated across all settings in the hospital. That a productive IEP meeting with a good outcome was possible for such a complicated case was in no small measure due to the carefully documented testing and observation of RG's school progress, which was possible over a period of months. This included a broad assessment not only of academic and classroom management needs but of cognitive strategies to insure that RG could "internalize" approaches to problem solving in both social and academic areas.

Mainstreaming was not yet a consideration for RG, except in limited fashion, because of the complicated nature of his problems. Despite its appeal, mainstreaming might have undermined RG's progress at this point because the gap between his successful hospital school experience and the academic demands of a regular classroom was far too wide for effective generalization of skills from one setting to the next. The beginnings of a vocational program to meet RG's needs for ultimate self-sufficiency at a realistic level was also important and would no doubt become increasingly more so as time went on. RG's case illustrates not only the potential problems and pitfalls of caring for the child with dual disabilities but also the extraordinary effort needed to overcome both the child's school disorders as well as the defects in the educational system that often hinder this effective treatment.

It is clear that special education is still in a state of transition. The historical trends discussed earlier continue to drive the field in sometimes opposing directions. For more detailed descriptions of issues, programs, and methods, the reader is referred to representative texts by Bryan and Bryan (1975) on the learning-disabled; Hewett and Taylor (1980) on the emotionally disturbed; Payne, Palloway, Smith and Payne (1977) on the mildly retarded; Sontag (1977) on the severely and profoundly handicapped; Bender and Valletutti (1976) on the severely handicapped; and to Hewett and Forness (1984) or Kirk and Gallagher (1979) for a comparative description of programs for all types of handicapped children. For the child with behavioral problems, however, the success of his or her school program and related treatment may often depend quite heavily on the particular motivation and management strategies used in that setting. Behavioral approaches have been possibly the most significant development in the education and training of the developmentally disabled in recent decades (Forness, 1976; Forness & MacMillan, 1970). We now turn to the contributions that clinical behaviorists have had in this area.

THE CLINICAL BEHAVIORAL APPROACH

Behavioral technology has been shown to be effective in controlling behavioral disorders occurring in a milieu in which highly structured contingencies are applied to both desirable and undesirable behaviors. Examples of this are the token economy applied in the psychiatric inpatient ward milieu

(Ayllon & Azrin, 1968), the special education classroom employing social consequences supplemented by tangible rewards when necessary (Forness, Frankel, & Landman, 1976; Frankel & Graham, 1976), and approaches that train parents to provide predictable and consistent consequences for the desirable and undesirable behavior of their children (Patterson & Reid, 1973).

The clinical behavioral approach evolved from a much larger tradition of experimentation that was conducted in the operant rat labs of the mid-1960s. The operant approach was selected over other extant empirical approaches (e.g., cognitive or developmental) because of the emphasis placed on the behavior of individual organisms, rather than the average results from groups of subjects. This approach was characterized by three basic tenets, which were adopted pragmatically by its clinically oriented disciples. These were objectivity in defining behavior, examination of the relationships between successive microbehavioral events, and the use of measurement of overt behaviors for fine tuning of the parameters of the treatment approach. Each one of these tenets will be discussed presently.

An objectively defined observable behavioral event served as the basic datum of this new form of applied behavioral science. Human interactions were broken down into discrete microbehavioral units although they occurred in streams of events. Each behavioral event in this stream was worthy of consideration in its own right (especially if it required augmentation or diminution). For example, having a meal was not considered as one behavior, but perhaps as the stream of successive events: sitting in a seat in front of a plate of food, putting a napkin on the lap, picking up a fork, jabbing a small piece of food, etc. If a deficiency in a client's eating could be localized to any one of these behaviors, further division into component behaviors would become necessary. For instance, baseline observation of a client might indicate that he has difficulty in holding a fork. In this case, the behaviors would be divided into the following microbehavioral sequence: extending the hand towards the fork, opening the hand with palm facing down, touching the fork concurrently with the finger tips of the thumb, first and second fingers, or firming the grip.

Objectivity in this context implies that independent observers are likely to agree that each behavior has or has not occurred. This is attained by the nature of descriptions, which rely upon what is overt and easily observable. Microbehaviors are inherently more objective than gross behavioral categories such as "appropriate eating." On the other hand, mentalistic events, such as thoughts, feelings, and motives, have inherently little reliability.

Conceptualizing behavioral events as a stream anticipates the importance of the relationship between successive behavioral events, i.e., antecedents and consequences of particular behaviors of interest (target behaviors). This often involves preliminary observation or educated guesses as to behavioral events that might typically occur before or after the target behavior. The basic assumption for this endeavor is that target behaviors can be brought under control by controlling the events that typically happen close to them in time. For example, a child's tantrums might be followed by attempts at soothing by his parents. Eliminating this parental response to this situation might then eliminate the tantrums. Another example is when a child fails to eat his meal. Eating behavior can only occur after the child is sitting down at the table. This suggests that a necessary precondition to eating is sitting at the table in front of a plate of food. Under special circumstances, the antecedents and consequences earn names for themselves, such as positive reinforcers, negative reinforcers, punishers, or discriminative stimuli, depending upon the relationship between these events and the target behavior. The reader wishing to obtain more familiarity with this terminology may consult Reynolds (1968).

The third basic tenet was that measurement of behaviors of interest serve as a cornerstone of this approach. The use of this measurement dictates the course of treatment. At the outset, taking baseline measurement establishes the magnitude of the problem and the necessity for change. For instance, a child may be referred for treatment of aggressive behavior in a classroom setting. Baseline measurements indicate that he or she hits his or her classmates 3 times per hour, while his or her classmates each hit one another 6 times per hour. This suggests that intervention may be aimed at the wrong child and the intervention should be modified accordingly.

Taking measurement at the outset of treatment is also necessary to document the relationships between the target behavior, and hypothesized antecedents and consequences. For example, a parent may feel that whenever her son becomes agitated (i.e., hyperventilates) he eventually hits someone. It is usually informative to document this hypothesized relationship. Behaviors such as hyperventilation seem to have obvious predictive validity for eventual aggression. In practice, measurement of the frequency that hyperventilation and aggression co-occur for different individuals have yielded different results. In some cases hyperventilation has predicted aggression, while in other cases the child almost never aggressed after he or she was able to take deep breaths. This underscores the importance of discovery of the laws of behavior for each individual through behavioral assessment.

Taking continuous measurement during treatment can be a source of immediate feedback as to the success of treatment. For instance, a teacher wants to increase a child's prosocial interactions to acceptible levels within 7 weeks (e.g., to 15 per hour in a crowded playdeck). If preliminary observations indicate a rate of 1 per hour, the teacher can be assured that he or she is headed toward this objective if the mean rate of prosocial interactions increases an average of just 2 per week. If the observed mean weekly increase falls short of this figure, the teacher can either revise the goals of the IEP, or "fine tune" the intervention. A clinical example of this fine tuning is the case of MS, which has been discussed in more detail elsewhere (study following is from Frankel, Moss, Schofield, & Simmons, 1976; with permission).

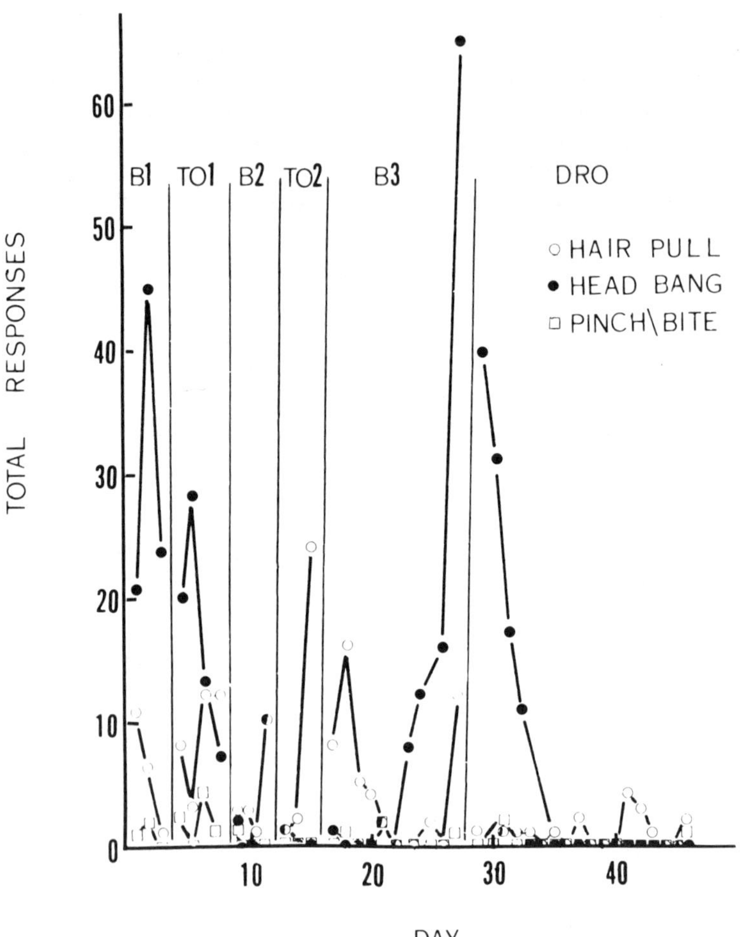

Fig. 14-1. Total number of incidents of pulling teacher's hair (hair pulls), head bangs, and pinching or biting (pinch/bite) for each day of Baselines (B1, B2, B3), chair restriction time out (TO1), seclusion room time out (TO2), and differential reinforcement (DRO) programs. [Reprinted from Frankel, F, Moss, D, Schofield, S, & Simmons, JQ. (1976). Case study: Use of differential reinforcement to suppress self-injurious and aggressive behavior. *Psychological Reports, 39,* 843–849. With permission.]

MS was a 6 year, 8 month old profoundly retarded child who was also diagnosed as schizophrenic.* She was hospitalized for an evaluation and short-term behavioral work-up. She displayed numerous autistic features including hand-flapping, rocking, staring at lights, lack of social or play interactions, and lack of communicative speech. Intervention was instituted for aggression (biting, pinching and hair-pulling), and headbanging.

* This child may not have received the same diagnosis if seen today.

Figure 14-1 depicts the results of measurement taken concurrently with treatment. Baseline observations revealed a rate of 30 headbangs per day and a rate of 6 aggressive acts per day. Two attempts were made to consequate behaviors with restriction to a seclusion room (time-out programs). Both programs resulted in the decrease in one of these behaviors and the increase in the other. Finally, on day 23 a DRO program was instituted (this program will be discussed in more detail in a later part of this chapter), which was eventually successful in reducing both behaviors to very low rates. (Frankel et al., 1976)

It is evident from Figure 14-1 that there was sufficient evidence for the effectiveness of the DRO program by the third day of this program, as the rate had been steadily decreasing. Without concurrent measurement throughout treatment, it would have been impossible to discern this. We have discussed by example some types of measurement systems employed by clinical behaviorists. Readers seeking a more detailed treatment of this are advised to consult Kazdin (1980).

Viewpoints Shared by Clinical Behaviorists

Clinical Behaviorism has changed over the years, to the point where there are currently several different directions which the field has been taking. Nevertheless, most current adherents share several viewpoints. These views will be referred to as the orientation towards the present, the mechanistic conceptualization of mental activity, environmental determinism, and therapeutic responsibility.

Clinical behaviorists cling fast to the view that it is necessary only to look at present relationships in the stream of behavior in order to see the roots of change. The focus on the present is shared with other approaches, e.g., the Gestalt approach of Perls (1969) and the communication approach to family therapy (Goldenberg & Goldenberg, 1980). While it is certainly true that history cannot be changed, sometimes the mistakes of the past can avoid repetition. Clinical behaviorists of today usually look at the origin of target behaviors, as well as previous attempts at treatment. This assessment frequently suggests underlying motivation and reinforcers currently maintaining target behaviors.

The mechanistic conceptualization of mental activity still has some strict adherents among clinical behaviorists. The primary assumption is that it is unnecessary to consider thoughts and feelings, only to look at overt behavior. Recent extensions of the behavioral approach address such covert responses as self-instruction and coping statements. This approach has combined the rich traditions of operant and cognitive psychology. Reviews of this approach (Kendall & Hollon, 1979) devote much discussion to the findings of basic cognitive research as support for these new interventions. Modifications of this approach have proven useful for children as young as 4 years old (Spivak, Platt, & Shure, 1976). Therefore at least some clinical behaviorists no longer try to intervene exclusively upon overt behavior.

Initial resounding successes with severely regressed clients (Ullman & Krasner, 1965) made it appear that there were virtually no limitations to the changes that could be made upon behavior. The doctrine used to support this early position will be referred to as Environmental Determinism; all problems have their roots in environmental events and relations between behavior and consequences (Ferster, 1961). However, after 18 years of efforts, it seems as if the limitations of the approach have been encountered. The behavioral approach has proven useful in optimizing gains made by mentally retarded, organically impaired, and psychotic individuals, but it has not completely reversed processes underlying these conditions. Behavioral techniques have not decreased the necessity for using medications (Falloon, Boyd, & McGill, 1980). Rather than being an approach that would eliminate the use of medication, the technology of behavioral measurement can increase the sensitivity of clinicians to their effects. The two cases presented below will exemplify this point.

Implicit in clinical behaviorist doctrine from the very earliest, was the degree of responsibility that the therapist and client assume for behavior change. The early 1960s brought challenges to the "medical model" of psychiatric treatment (Szasz, 1961). The client was cast as a helpless and passive recipient of psychiatric treatment. If he failed to improve, then either the diagnosis or the treatment was incorrect. The central issue then, was who was responsible for client motivation. Clinical behaviorists accepted some of this responsibility. First, they accepted responsibility to find ways to augment client motivation through their search, discovery, and use of effective reinforcers. Second, they accepted responsibility for shortfalls in results by assessing them and modifying their interventions accordingly.

Special Problems of Clients with Dual Disabilities

Behavioral treatment plans consist of increasing adaptive behaviors in areas of deficiency and decreasing behavioral excesses, or undesired behaviors. As with many multifactorial processes, the treatment plan aimed at clients having a combination of delayed cognitive development and some other pathological condition would be somewhat more complex than would be the treatment plan developed for either condition alone. On the one hand, the presence of delayed cognitive development implies a slower learning rate (Estes, 1970). As mentioned in the first section, slower learning rates may depend upon motivational and situational variables rather than an all-encompassing quality of the individual. Nevertheless, decreases in learning rates may serve to prolong the time necessary for the effects of interventions to be noticeable. In some cases, e.g., severe self-injurious behavior, this might serve to modify the nature of the approach taken. For instance, more aversive measures may need to be employed to avoid serious health hazards that would be posed by the longer course of treatment with milder interventions (Schreibman, Frankel, & LaVigna, 1977).

Furthermore, learning studies of the mentally retarded show a production deficiency in the use of strategies (Bray, 1979). Demonstration of benefits from specific training in strategic behavior have been equivocal for the mentally retarded (for reviews of boths sides of this controversy see Brown, 1978; Borkowski & Cavanaugh, 1979). This strongly suggests that training in cognitive techniques such as self-control, and more advanced problem-solving techniques may be too ambitious an undertaking for clients with dual disabilities. However, the downward extension of this approach by Spivak, et al. (1976) may have some utility.

Delay in social functioning usually manifests itself not only in production of desirable social behaviors but also in development of moral concepts (Sigman, Ungerer, & Russell, 1983). This means that the dual diagnostic client will have a more limited understanding of social interactions and will be at earlier levels of moral development. Social reinforcers aimed at these clients will have to be geared down accordingly. For instance, peer acceptance may not motivate change in some clients who are functioning at lower levels of social development, but rather gaining adult attention and tangible rewards (as in a system of token reward) may be more effective. MacMillan & Forness (1973) have suggested a reinforcement hierarchy, corresponding to the needs of clients at different stages of moral development. Development occurs as the child moves up this hierarchy in the subtlety and complexity of potential reinforcers.

The combination of cognitive delay and either psychotic or organically-based etiology complicates treatment considerably more. Current theory posits that the schizophrenic decompensation represents an unusual stress reaction in a biologically predisposed individual (Falloon, et al., 1980). Thus there are inherent vulnerabilities in these clients that are not presently well understood. Also, with autistic clients, one cannot assume that stimuli are effective in the same ways as with more intact clients. For example, there is much research indicating that autistic children do not process more than one stimulus at a time (Frankel, Simmons, Fichter, & Freeman, 1984; Lovaas, Koegel, Schreibman, & Rehm, 1971), and that they do not profit as much from being told they are incorrect as do mentally retarded children of the same IQ and mental age (Frankel, 1981). Thus, the highly idiosynchratic nature of stimulus effects upon clients may further complicate treatment attempts.

Some degree of probing and experimentation must be done to determine the precise nature and effects of stressors upon the psychotic client or the particular stereotypic response patterns of autistic individuals (Frankel, Freeman, Ritvo, & Pardo, 1978). For autistic individuals, different motivators have been discovered (Frankel, Freeman, Ritvo, Chikami, & Carr, 1976). Therefore one must be prepared to see different modes of emotional expression in these individuals. Our research has shown that autistic children, thought to be devoid of social responsivity to adults, nevertheless show deterioration in behavior when deprived of their favorite teachers (Frankel, Simmons, & Olson, 1977). A clinical case exemplifies this point.

JR was a 13-year-old caucasian male admitted to a child inpatient unit by hi parents after he could no longer be managed in his latest special-class setting. Over th past two years, his behavior became increasingly aggressive. Prior to admission, he ha been throwing tables and chairs at people in school. According to the special educato these instances were unpredictable and quite alarming. His father also reported that h was unable to control JR at times and that punishment seemed to make matters worse He appeared to the professionals working with him to have a conduct disorder.

JR was given a complete diagnostic workup. On the WISC–R, his performanc score was 67 and his verbal score was 74, yielding a full scale IQ of 70. However, psychiatric interview and projective testing indicated that JR had auditory hallucinations and disordered thinking. Observations early in his hospitalization indicated that JR' disturbance in conduct was mediated by deterioration in thinking consequent t anxiety-producing events.

JR's rate of aggression was initially moderately high while on the living un (interestingly, aggression was not a problem for JR during school times). Nursin records showed that he had to be placed in brief seclusion consequent to aggressio more than 15 times during the first week, but this was steadily decreasing each week. B the third week, there were no instances of aggression. However, on week 4, JR wa informed by his father that his grandfather had died. Interviews with JR indicated that h became quite confused soon after hearing this, his gait became more "floppy", hi speech became more slurred and tangential. Instances of aggression had to b consequated on 3–4 occasions over the next 3 days. JR was eventually able to verbaliz that he was quite confused and upset. With guidance of his therapist, he eventuall understood that this reaction was due to his fear of losing his father, and, perhaps mor importantly, he realized that when he was afraid, he became confused and upset (an vice versa). No recurrence of aggression or of hallucinations was noted throughout 5 subsequent months of hospitalization.

A less severe instance of this apparent deterioration in thinking occurred when J was reunited with his father on weekly visits. At these times, he would become extremel inattentive and be "floppy" in his gait. When asked what he was thinking of, he said tha he was glad to see his father and was nervous about this meeting.

Clinical observations indicated that anxiety had unusual effects upon thi child. In order for treatment to be completely effective, the effects of anxiety ha to be assessed and treated. What seemed like a case of conduct disorder turne out to be the results of a psychotic reaction. This anxiety was treated in differen ways in the different situations. The special educator working with JR afte admission noted that JR would become uncomfortable when asked to go at a fast pace in his learning or when forced to speak before the class. Her respons was to allow JR to go at his own pace in both of these matters. On the living unit the approach was to increase the understanding of both JR and those aroun him with respect to the effects of anxiety. Rather than take more sever measures after anxiety-precipitating events, ward staff maintained his curren behavioral program. JR no doubt found it helpful to be reminded of why he wa having difficulty in thinking, and was comforted at being reminded, since h reported feeling quite poorly. Steadfast maintenance of his behavioral progran was a dependable feature of his life. Helping him understand his reactions helped him to "bounce back" more quickly from them.

The next sections of this chapter will consider contributions that the behavioral approach can make to different aspects of the treatment of the client with dual disabilities. It will be evident from this discussion that the behavioral approach can influence all aspects of the diagnostic and treatment process. Examples of treatment approaches are intended only to exemplify the contributions of this approach in this area and are not meant to be comprehensive.

CONTRIBUTIONS OF BEHAVIORAL TECHNOLOGY TO PSYCHODIAGNOSTIC TESTING

The behavioral approach to assessment has contributed to the diagnostic process in several ways. The most obvious way has been to control behaviors that interfere with testing (and usually also with achievement in the classroom). Another way is by suggesting behavioral correlates to poor performance, which may subsequently be subject to modification. In this way, target behaviors may be selected for augmentation or diminution.

Behavioral techniques can be employed during the course of psychological testing and have resulted in fewer children being labeled as "untestable" (Freeman & Ritvo, 1976). The case of ES typifies how an increasingly richer schedule of behavioral consequences for compliance (defined as attempts to perform the tasks composing the intelligence test) resulted in a more detailed assessment of a seriously emotionally disturbed boy.

ES was a caucasian male who was physically abused by his alcoholic biological mother. He had his first psychiatric hospitalization at age 5 years. Intellectual testing at this time yielded a Full Scale IQ of 70 on the WPPSI. At this time, he was also showing slow language development, temper tantrums, and destructiveness. His second hospitalization at age 8 years resulted after unsuccessful placements in 14 different foster homes. Psychological testing attempted to determine if ES's behavior problems were in part due to an underlying cognitive defect.

Clinical observations suggested that ES had difficulty in understanding interpersonal interactions and was under poor verbal control. In addition, he would tantrum when he saw that he was not mastering a task. His attempts at controlling the testing situation ranged from insisting upon choosing the next task, to trying to get the examiner to repeat his inappropriate verbalizations. In order to get him to perform the tasks involved in the WISC–R, it was necessary to structure reward contingencies to an extreme degree. At first, ES was offered a reward of his choice, to be given at the end of the session. Constant reminders of this reward were not sufficient to motivate compliance. The second attempt was more successful. A grid of 20 boxes was drawn on a card. He was told that for doing what the examiner said, a check would be made by the examiner in one of these boxes. When all of the boxes had checks in them, he would get a reward of his choice. He was then asked what this might be (e.g., a candy bar, a soda pop, or an inexpensive toy). A check was immediately entered in a box for ES's first compliance, and thereafter compliance was randomly reinforced with check entries immediately after they occurred (ES did not need to be correct in his attempts). Prompts consisted of the examiner saying "Do———, so that I can give you another check. I really want you to get all of these boxes checked." In response to compliance, the examiner continued to give praise on every occasion and would sometimes say, "Good, now I can give you another check." The power struggle ceased during the remaining testing sessions.

The increased structure of reward provided by the examiner during the course of psychodiagnostic testing made a more accurate assessment of the child's potential level of functioning possible, and suggested a particular intervention that would aid with this child's noncompliance. Behavioral techniques turned a very difficult testing situation into one that was more easily manageable for the examiner and also more enjoyable for the client.

In addition to manipulation of consequences for compliance, behavioral techniques include a descriptive approach to code observations made of test-taking behavior. This can also enhance the utility of information obtained from psychological testing. This is especially helpful for areas of skill weakness observed in intelligence testing. Sometimes changing a behavior associated with poor performance can itself improve performance despite the contributions of organismic factors. The case of GJ exemplifies this point.

GJ was a 15-year-old black male who was the product of an abnormal pregnancy (his mother reported having gestational diabetes and gaining 20 lbs). His birthweight was in the third percentile and he had to be incubated for 2–3 weeks to allow full development of his lungs. At the time of testing, GJ was somewhat unusual in appearance, as his head circumference was in the 75th percentile for his age, while his height was in the 3rd percentile and his weight in the 25th percentile. His gait was also awkward. He demonstrated some articulation problems and he evidenced pronounced pauses in mid-sentence.

GJ was referred because of problems in short attention span, visuo–motor delays that included reading and writing skills and failure to progress in academics for 2 years previous to the evaluation. Problems at home were fighting with peers, defiance of authority, temper outbursts, and impulsively talking-out. GJ was attending junior high school in an eighth-grade class for the educationally handicapped.

Results of psychological testing showed GJ to have vastly discrepant abilities. On the WISC–R his Verbal IQ was 82, and his Performance IQ was 48. GJ's most pronounced deficits were found in the Picture Arrangement subtest, a test in which GJ had to arrange a series of pictures in sequence to tell a story. His original attempt yielded a scaled score of 1. Behavioral observations indicated that GJ showed much the same difficulty in keeping his attention on this task as he evidenced in school. He would begin to work on an arrangement, then talk about something irrelevant to the task (usually an interest of his). The question arose as to whether he could not perform the task, causing his attention to wander (e.g., a defense mechanism preventing him from experiencing failure), or if his wandering attention prevented him from completing a task he could potentially accomplish. This attention and irrelevant conversation problem occurred on many of the performance subtests of the WISC–R, so that establishing the cause of poor performance for this test could have implications for GJ's overall performance abilities.

To test these alternatives, the subtest was readministered with the words, "Work as carefully as you can," repeated constantly. This simultaneously eliminated his tendency to talk about topics irrelevant to the task and increased his scale score on this subtest to 5.

Although it was realized that GJ had profound neuropsychological deficits, a prosthesis was proposed as a result of behavioral observations and subsequent testing. A suggestion was made that a tape loop (with the same reminder recorded) be played for GJ when he was working on tasks requiring sustained attention.

The case of GJ demonstrates that clear organically-based impairment may have expressions in overt behavior, which may be subject to modification. Behavioral observation can suggest target behaviors hypothesized to affect performance. Subsequent small changes in the task demand characteristics, governed by such hypotheses, can confirm the relationship between the overt behaviors and performance, and in so doing, suggest treatment techniques.

Behavioral Assessment of the Effects of Medication

Use of medication for clients with dual disabilities has been useful in some respects and detrimental in others (Breuning & Polling, 1982). Clearly for clients with "organic involvement", such as psychotic, mood disordered, and attention deficit disorders, treatment very often cannot proceed until the organic factor is addressed with appropriate medication. However, the use of medication may have two undesirable effects.

A frequent assumption (or perhaps a hope) entertained by treatment staff and parents is that medication alone will completely remediate all of the symptoms involved in a disorder. One can hope that this may happen, but this hope should be entertained with open eyes. A more reasonable expectation is that medication will at best affect some of the symptoms composing a disorder, but may sometimes have side-effects. A second undesirable effect is related to the first, that any symptomatic improvement occurring at or after the time that medication has been introduced is solely attributable to medication. In clinical observations during behavioral consultations to inpatient wards for developmentally-disabled children and adolescents, these two undesirable effects of medication programs have frequently been observed to occur.

Clearly it is difficult for people to be objective in relating improvement to medication. Perhaps this is because medication comes in a form and is administered under such circumstances as to optimize placebo effects (Ullman & Krasner, 1965). Behavioral measurement can thus play an important role in determining which effects can be attributable to medication, and which are not. Two different approaches have proven valuable in this regard. In one approach, a "checklist" of carefully worded target symptoms is given to caretakers to fill out on a daily basis. Such checklists have been instrumental in the diagnosis and treatment of attention deficit disorder (Connors, 1972). However, there has been some concern over whether "treating the checklist" has validity for treating the disorder. Case examples of each of these approaches follow.

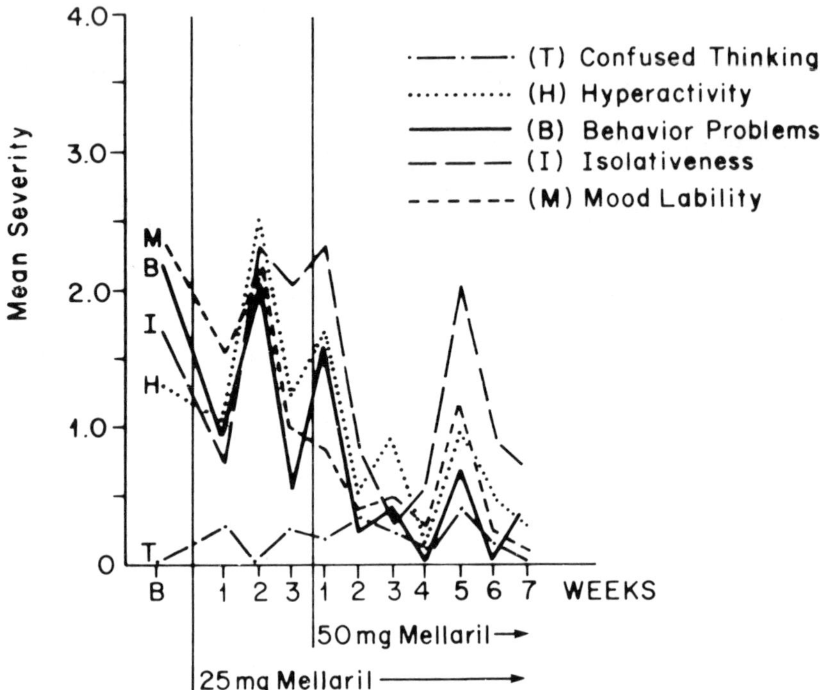

Fig. 14-2. Mean parental checklist ratings for each week of Baseline (B) and medication trials for the 5 different categories of behaviors.

One case was a 13-year-old caucasian male who was seen in outpatient systems-oriented family therapy for over a year. A complete diagnostic workup indicated that he was not in the mentally retarded range of intelligence but was diagnosed as having schizotypal personality disorder. Symptoms evident upon interview and part of the criteria for this disorder were poor face-to-face rapport with the interviewer, social isolation, his reports of his thoughts "talking" to him, and catastrophic reactions out of proportion to the precipitants. During several weeks in which he was particularly problematic in all areas of his functioning, his parents requested medication. LK was referred to a Child Psychiatrist for evaluation and Mellaril (25 mg per day) was prescribed. A 25-item checklist was developed from a larger pool of items (Lesser, 1981) in conjunction with the Child Psychiatrist and the parents. Items of this resulting checklist were grouped into five categories designed to assess all relevant areas of his functioning: Mood lability (e.g., cries often), Confused thinking (e.g., talks of seeing things that aren't there), Hyperactivity (e.g., finds it hard to sit still), Behavior problems (e.g., aggression) and Isolativeness (e.g., prefers to be alone). Each item was rated by both parents as either frequent, very often, occasionally, rarely, or never occurring during each day.

The parents agreed to a one week baseline measurement on this checklist to be able to tell if the medication was effective, and test the appropriateness of the items selected. Figure 14-2 shows the results of baseline and 10 weeks of medication trials.

From the figure, it was evident that the initial dosage of Mellaril had little, if any lasting effects. These initial results prompted an increase in the dosage to 50 mg per day. This resulted in decreased ratings of severity in most checklist categories. Confused thinking increased slightly in severity, no doubt a side-effect of the medication. Isolativeness was not affected, when compared with baseline. This was probably because items in this category reflected a social skill deficit. He was subsequently enrolled in a behavioral treatment group in which modeling and immediate reinforcement were used to train social skills. Follow-up reports indicated that isolativeness decreased substantially.

It was clear from the measurements taken by the parents that medication was of benefit, but was not the "silver bullet" that would give them an unproblematic child. As a result of the feedback provided by the measurement system, the therapist, parents, and Child Psychiatrist were effective allies in the treatment process.

Subsequent efforts at replicating this procedure on an inpatient ward have not met with similar success. Effects generally noted have not been as convincing. There are many differences between the two situations which may be responsible for these differing results. First, many different raters are used on the inpatient ward, whereas only the parents are used (and only in concert to form one set of agreed-upon ratings). The variability may be greater on the inpatient wards, possibly obscuring the effects of medication. Second, ratings tend to decrease in severity during the first two weeks of hospitalization (perhaps a "honeymoon" effect). This may be the effect of increased structure and/or other nonspecific effects of the milieu. Therefore the contribution of medication may be somewhat diminished in comparison to this large initial effect. Clearly, future research should suggest useful means of measurement of medication effects on inpatient wards that can be performed with efficacy.

Another approach to assessment can be considered as less direct. Instead of assessment of medication effects upon symptoms related to psychiatric disturbance, the effects of medication upon the client's habilitation program is measured. Such assessment may have much validity, since remediation of symptoms may have no effects on the acquisition of adaptive behavior, as noted in the case of LK. In an inpatient setting, habilitation programs leave behind various permanent products. Examples of this are the number of points the client earned per week on his token economy program (clients tend to carefully keep these records in order to exchange them for rewards) and the number of times per week that the client had to be secluded (staff must document each instance for compliance with JCAH standards). The case of AW exemplifies the assessment of the effects of medication with the use of permanent products.

AW was a 13-year-old caucasian male admitted for hospitalization after 4 months of steadily deteriorating behavior in the home and disruptive behavior in his class for educationally handicapped students. He would scratch his Mother and sister and at one point threatened his sister with a kitchen knife. Previously AW had a long history of isolativeness and behavior problems. He was diagnosed at age 6 years as hyperactive and more recently as schizophrenic, although his diagnostic picture was much more

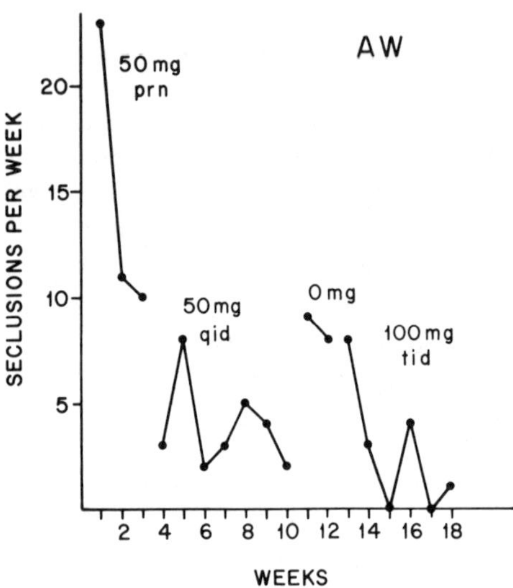

Fig. 14-3. Mean number of seclusion time outs per week as a function of different doses and schedules of medication.

complex. AW had tremendous social anxiety: after some of his actions, he would ruminate for hours with self-deprecating criticism.

Initially AW was extremely aggressive, characterized both in the rate of his aggression and in the tenacity with which he would pursue his victims. He would typically plan his attacks and then follow through with these plans some time removed from their inception. Suspiciousness of "shrinks," as he called them, initially prohibited the psychologist from giving any kind of testing. Immediately upon hospitalization, AW was placed on a trial of thorazine. Figure 14-3 shows the number of times per week that AW was sufficiently aggressive to be placed in seclusion over 18 weeks of hospitalization. From the figure it is apparent that the number of seclusions decreased steadily during this time. Three different levels of medication were applied by the ward Psychiatrist. The effects of medication are partially confounded with the effects of milieu, as client's aggressiveness typically decreases over time with hospitalization on this particular ward. Thus the decreases noted when medication regimen was changed from 50 mg as needed (weeks 1–3) to 50 mg qid (weeks 4–10) could not be clearly attributed to medication. What was convincing were the effects of withdrawal of medication (weeks 12 and 13) and reinstatement (weeks 14–18). This demonstrates clearly that medication contributed to the decreases in seclusions for this client.

However, to attribute all gains to medication is a serious error. Notice that the rates during weeks 11 and 12 were still far less than during week 1.

The case of AW exemplifies three major considerations in the measurement of medication effects. First, the data for this client seems to have less variability than the data for LK. This may be idiosyncratic to these cases, but it may also be characteristic of the different data systems. Although both curves were averaged over similar time periods (i.e., each data point represented one week) LK's data represent a single judgment by parents at the end of the day while AW's data represents the permanent products of each 24-hour day of staff documentation.

The second consideration is related to attributions that professionals and paraprofessionals make with regard to medication. Before Figure 14-3 was presented to ward staff, they believed that the medication, and not their treatment milieu was responsible for improvement in AW's behavior. They also erroneously thought that AW's behavior during weeks 11 and 12 reverted completely back to that of week 1. Attributions changed considerably after presentation of Figure 14-3 to staff. In general, staff have to fight the tendency to overattribute client improvement to medications and underattribute to ward milieu.

A third consideration is not evident in the data presented in Figure 14-3, and for this reason is quite important. So-called side-effects of medication, were not indicated. Apart from physiologic side-effects, a general concern to assess in this regard is whether medication interferes with adaptive behavior. Decreases observed in aggressive behavior noted in AW's seclusion data might have been the result of more general suppression of all behaviors. Clearly AW appeared medicated at times, but special educators working with him reported no change in his educational progress and ward staff reported slight increases in his ability to earn points on his tokens economy program through week 10.

Some Examples of Behavioral Treatment Techniques

As mentioned in the beginning of this section, the earliest behavioral approaches were drawn directly from the operant experimental literature. Operant laboratories gave us four techniques for decreasing behaviors: extinction, time out, differential reinforcement of other behavior (DRO), and punishment. This technology also provided us with four techniques for increasing behaviors: shaping, the errorless technique, partial reinforcement, and token reinforcement. Several other techniques have been developed by clinical behaviorists from these more basic techniques (e.g., the token economy, social skills or assertive training, and overcorrection). These basic techniques have continued to be among the most effective treatments for decreasing undesirable behaviors (Frankel & Simmons, 1976, in press). Several cases will serve to exemplify problems and outcomes of these procedures with clients having dual disabilities. The reader seeking more extensive reviews of outcome may consult Kazdin (1980).

Extinction is a technique whereby the events reinforcing a behavior are removed and the behavior is allowed to run its natural course. In some cases, the reinforcement is not clear, but removal of considerable stimulation decreases the behavior. The case of EA exemplifies this form of extinction program. This case has been reported previously (Jones, Simmons, & Frankel, 1974) and is summarized briefly.

EA was a 9-year-old severely retarded autistic girl. Her speech was composed primarily of echolalia. She showed several stereotyped behaviors (spinning a ring from

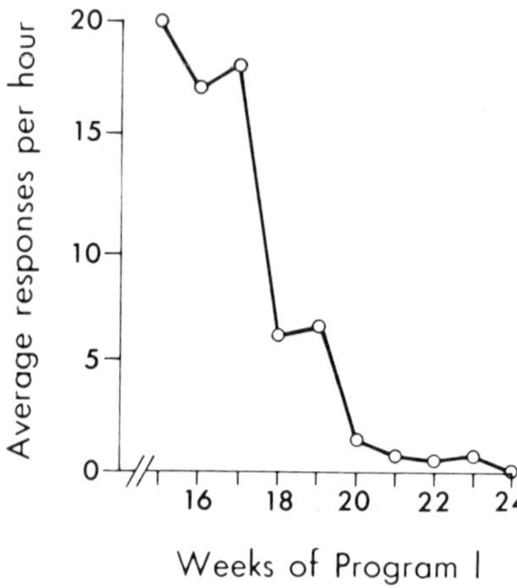

Fig. 14-4. Mean number of self-injurious behaviors per hour observed in the day room during the last 10 weeks of the initial extinction intervention.

a ring-toss game, and twirling numerous other objects). When left to herself, she would spend most of her time engaged in these behaviors. Her self-help skills were also minimal. She was toilet trained, would eat with a spoon or fork and could dress herself (but not tie her shoes). Social skills were also minimal. She could bounce a ball back to another person and would sing along to music.

Since the age of 5 years old, EA had exhibited self-injurious behavior consisting of hitting the dorsum of her hand or wrist against her front teeth. During the course of the present treatment another self-injurious behavior emerged: jabbing her abdomen with her index finger. Several programs over 4 years were unsuccessful in eliminating her self-injury. The extinction program reported here took place during her second hospitalization. It consisted of placing her in a 8 foot by 10 foot room alone for 4 hours per day without restraints (she was in tubular restraints during the remainder of the day).

The extinction procedure resulted in a decrease in all forms of self-injury from an initial rate of 34,000 per week to 0 per week by the 17th week. This rate remained at 0 over the next 6 weeks. More importantly, this decrease generalized to the ward day room at an unexpected pace. Figure 14-4 presents EA's rate of self-injury in the ward day room (where there were usually several other clients present), from week 15 to week 24 of the program. As shown in the Figure, this rate dropped from 20 per hour to 0 by week 21.

EA has been followed for almost 10 years. During this time, self-injurious behaviors returned on several occasions. The social isolation program was instituted each time the behavior returned and resulted in complete cessation of the behavior within 3 weeks.

This program resulted serendipitously from the collection of baseline data for EA. The subsequent success of the program very likely resulted from the spontaneous generalization this client made from the isolation room to the ward. Although such generalization has been noted in several case studies (Frankel & Simmons, 1976), it may not occur for most clients. This was probably because the reinforcers maintaining EA' s self-injury were atypical. For instance, highly controlled comparisons of her rate of self-injury suggested no effects of the presence of adults (see Fig. 14-5). Reports from staff at EA's

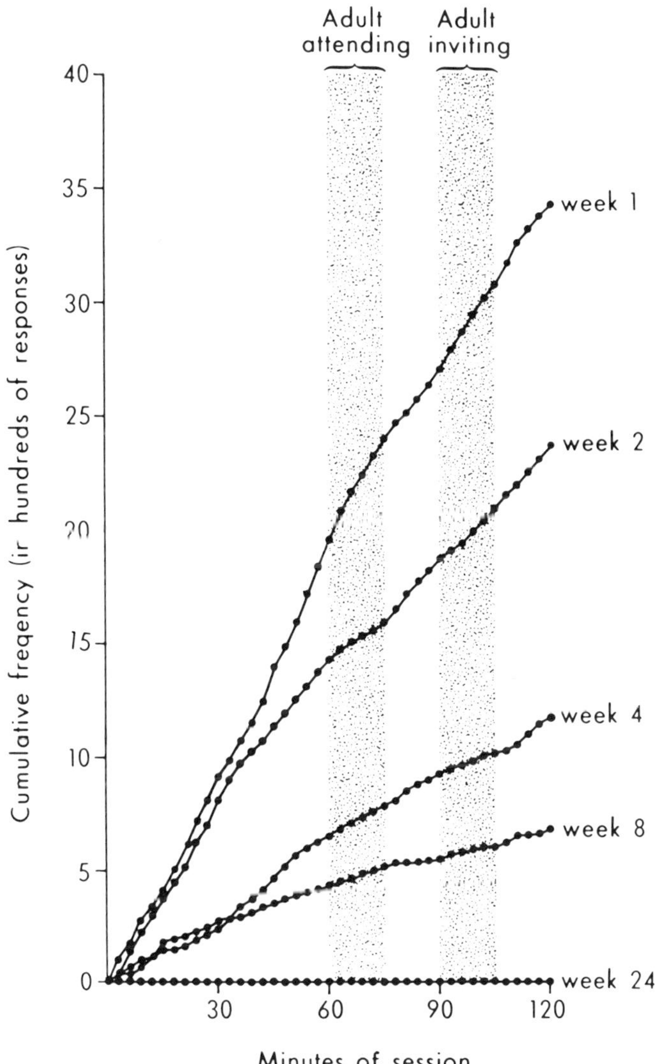

Fig. 14-5. Cumulative frequency of self-injurious behaviors as a function of adult attending, adult inviting to play and adult ignoring (white background).

subsequent placement indicated that the isolation program was reinstituted because of its simplicity and effectiveness.

In contrast, most extinction programs involve the withholding of an identified consequent event. This event has obvious reinforcing effects upon a target behavior. Severely and profoundly mentally retarded clients typically find pleasant interactions with an adult caretaker reinforcing. A more typically designed extinction program involves the use of ignoring the target behavior, both actively (i.e., turning away during unstructured times when the target behavior begins) and passively (i.e., pretending the target behavior did not occur after a command was made and repeating the command or prompting compliance). The usual result of these types of programs upon young developmentally-disabled clients is that self-injury and tantrums decrease over the course of several weeks.

Sometimes the application of reinforcement can have powerful suppressive effects upon an undesired behavior when the timing is optimal. Such a program is called a DRO intervention. The description of the case MS was presented at the beginning of this section. The DRO intervention is now described in more detail.

Baseline observations made during days 23 and 24 revealed that MS's rate of self-injurious behavior was much lower during play time than during structured teaching sessions. The time between successive deviant behaviors was frequently as long as 1 minute for play and 5 seconds for teaching sessions. This led to the following initial program designed to differentially reinforce behaviors other than maladaptives. During play sessions, each time a kitchen timer set to l minute was allowed to lapse without deviant behavior, a candy (which MS liked) was placed in her mouth and she was praised. If a deviant behavior occurred before 1 minute elapsed, the timer was reset to 1 minute.

The 5-second interval required for teaching sessions required more elaborate arrangements. For these sessions, an observer sat behind a one-way mirror with a stop watch and spoke into a transmitter after each 5 seconds in which no maladaptives occurred. The teacher heard these markers on an earphone receiver and delivered praise and tangible reward. In both situations, when MS decreased her rate of maladaptives sufficiently to allow 50 percent of the timed intervals to fully elapse, the lengths of the intervals were increased. By the fifth teaching and play sessions, the intervals had both been lengthened to 10 minutes during play and 15 seconds during teaching sessions. Figure 14-l shows the effects of the DRO program upon rates of both types of deviant behaviors. From the figure it is apparent that this program had immediate and dramatic effects upon suppression of deviant behavior.

The last example of operant techniques that will be presented here is that of behavioral shaping. The shaping technique can be used for a variety of objectives, which range from training self-help skills to mentally retarded children (Baker, Heifetz, & Murphy, 1980) to training discriminations by autistic children (e.g., the "errorless" technique, cf., Schreibman, 1975). The case of TT exemplifies this.

TT was a 15-year-old Philipino-American male attending eighth-grade classes for the educationally handicapped. He was admitted to an inpatient ward for adolescents because of an inability of parents and teachers to control aggression towards peers over the course of 4 months after the divorce of the biological parents. According to the parents and the client, aggressive incidents were precipitated around incidents where other males would attempt to become friendly with his girlfriend.

Psychological testing at admission revealed that TT was functioning in the mildly mentally retarded range of intelligence. On the WISC–R, he obtained a Verbal IQ of 78, and a Performance IQ of 46 which yielded a Full Scale IQ of 60. Particularly important for behavioral intervention were relative strengths, which TT displayed in rote memory of isolated facts and his ability to plan. Aggression was not observed in the hospital situation although his interpersonal skills were noted to be severely limited. His conversational skills were limited to confabulation of grandiose tales to peers, beginning to speak while someone was in the middle of a sentence, "leering" at and invading personal space of female clients in apparent attempts to engage them, and constantly repeating the same request to staff.

The interactive behaviors noted by ward staff could all be accounted for by deficits in his verbal and nonverbal abilities concerned with initiating a verbal interaction. Intelligence testing indicated that he could potentially learn these (i.e., his verbal abilities were much higher than were apparent from his behavior) and that a rote learning approach (a relative strength of his) would probably be the best means of training. A combination of role-playing and shaping techniques were therefore used by his ward staff in individual sessions to accomplish this. During these sessions, one staff (the peer model) played a peer and reacted as a typical peer might to TT's statements. This staff also praised attempts of TT at appropriate interaction. Another staff served as a coach, whispering suggestions for conversation in TT's ear and helping TT maintain a comfortable distance from the peer model.

TT viewed these sessions as extremely enjoyable, responding readily to suggestions by his coach for topics of conversation and eliciting suggestions whenever necessary by cupping his hand over one ear and bending towards his coach. At first it was necessary for the coach to give TT specific things to say each time his turn came to talk and to prompt TT to keep his distance by gently pushing him back. The peer model would praise the successful performance of any part of the coach's suggestions. As the sessions continued TT was shaped into originating more of the conversation by gradually decreasing the amount of information conveyed on each suggestion or prompt. One session was devoted to training TT to enter a conversation appropriately. Two peer models talking to one another were used. The coach trained TT to wait for pauses in the conversation before he began talking. The peer models would then praise TT's appropriate entry into the conversation. Generalization to the ward was accomplished by having staff remind TT with minimal prompts before he attempted to enter conversations of peers. Considerable decreases in TT's repetitious requests, confabulations, leering at female clients and interrupting conversations were noted and TT was observed to initiate more conversations appropriately.

The most outstanding feature of this program was the client's receptivity to being coached and his willingness to follow the direction and use suggestions in later conversation. Behavioral interventions that use modeling, role-playing, teaching self-monitoring, or self-instruction techniques depend heavily upon the motivation and compliance of the client. They should be couched within an activity that the client enjoys, and where the therapeutic aspects of the activity may even seem secondary to the therapeutic benefits to the client. Very often specific interventions such as those described can show considerable benefits within several sessions.

Behavioral Interventions Involving Significant Others

Behavioral techniques will readily generalize to new situations if the behavior of persons in the new situation is supportive of the changes brought about by intervention. From a cost-effectiveness point of view, it is well to include these persons in the original behavioral intervention as much as possible. Sometimes from a therapeutic viewpoint, the inclusion of significant others in behavioral programming is the only way to change behaviors. The case of MG illustrates this point.

MG was a 26-year-old caucasian male who was living with his mother (his father had died 2 years earlier). He had extreme difficulty in verbal expression as his articulation was poor, his verbal output was slow and contained few words. Conversations were held with MG because he usually was able to express key words, having those around him fill in the rest. Intelligence testing with the WAIS revealed that he was functioning in the moderately mentally retarded range. He obtained a Verbal IQ of 50 and a Performance IQ of 51, yielding a Full Scale IQ of 47. He was admitted to an inpatient adolescent ward serving developmentally disabled clients because of loss of temper and destructive behaviors in the home, such as tearing his clothes, and aggression against others.

Two months of hospitalization resulted in elimination of MG's aggressive behavior, but his clothes-tearing remained unchanged. Also during this time, his mother, with the help and support of ward staff, decided to place MG in a group home. However, he still would see his mother on weekends and would call her daily.

Behavioral consultation was sought after clothes-tearing continued for 2.5 years after discharge. An interview was held that included MG, his mother and the referring social worker. From the interview, it was evident that part of the relationship between MG and his mother appeared to maintain clothes-tearing. Mrs G reported that MG would always talk to her first about the clothes that he had recently torn and would always bring these clothes home with him on weekends for his mother to mend. Mrs. G's reaction was to scold MG for tearing his clothes and then to mend them and give them back to him to wear or buy him new clothes. MG reported that he tore his clothes out of anger, but reports from the group home parents indicated some planning in his actions, as he would sometimes delay a long period of time after a provocative incident. Mrs G also indicated that after she would scold MG, she would eventually discuss with him why he tore his clothes and what made him angry.

It was hypothesized that clothes tearing was maintained by Mrs. G's increased attention and her willingness to hear what made MG angry. Mrs G was instructed to ignore MG's requests to mend his clothes, not to talk about torn clothes with MG, and to routinely go over his day with him when he called and to discuss with him the incidents that made him angry. This program reduced the necessity for MG to tear his clothes in order to express his anger. He was also subsequently encouraged to talk to the group home parents about things that made him angry. Measurement of success was made by having either the group home parent or the social worker check MG's closet (where he always left torn clothes) on a weekly basis to count the number of items torn. Six month follow-up indicated no evidence of torn clothes. MG continued to discuss things that angered him with his mother and house parents.

In the case of MG, Mrs. G unwittingly played a crucial part in maintaining clothes-tearing for her son. Through this behavior, MG was able to gain nurturance from Mrs. G (by her mending his clothes) and also was able to express his anger in response to specific questions from Mrs. G. In this way, clothes-tearing became a setting event enabling MG to get his mother to produce another setting event, cross-examination by Mrs. G, which enabled MG to express his anger. Behavioral intervention was not intended to reduce the need MG had to express his anger or to seek reassurance or nurturance from his mother. Intervention was intended to reduce the necessity of the undesired behavior in fulfilling these needs by providing more appropriate behaviors to replace them.

In general, the parent–child relationship is a setting in which undesirable behaviors may be learned in order to help an individual satisfy needs. The needs may be fulfilled with these behaviors but a price is paid: the behaviors are distressful to one or both parties. In the past two decades, many behavioral programs have been developed that focus upon the parent–child relationship. In families with younger children and developmentally-delayed adolescents, an approach employing the parent as a therapeutic ally in much the same manner as the case of MG is often successful (e.g., Wiltz & Patterson, 1974). In families with higher-functioning adolescents, training communication skills of both parents and adolescents has proven more successful (Alexander & Parsons, 1973; Kifer, Lewis, Green, & Phillips, 1974).

SUMMARY AND DISCUSSION

The client with dual disabilities has cognitive delays and other pathological conditions that have the net effect of reducing his or her repertoire of skills. Significant advances in educational and therapeutic approaches over the past two decades have enabled professionals to provide specialized, fine-tuned environments for these clients to facilitate their acquisition of these skills. Special education programs have had a potent effect upon the prognosis of many clients with dual disabilities (e.g., Rutter, Greenfield, & Lockyer, 1967). Behavioral techniques have been a great aid in the delivery of special educational programs, as well as the overall habilitation of the client with dual disabilities.

The success of both behavioral techniques and special education has in the past been attributable to basic research, which has eventually led to improvement in techniques. From basic research on basic discrimination learning and memory processes, management programs have developed. Recently, research on cognitive processes have been incorporated by clinical behaviorists into treatment techniques. Currently these techniques are not readily applicable to the habilitation of most clients with dual disabilities because they have been developed from studies of children of average abilities. More research is needed on the learning characteristics of developmentally-delayed and emotionally disturbed children in order for continued advances in this area.

Readers wishing a survey of research in these areas that have been applied to the developmentally-disabled should consult Ellis (1979).

Acknowledgments

The successful implementation of a behavioral program requires the cooperation and dedication of many professionals. The authors gratefully acknowledge the indispensable contributions of the following people for the cases presented in this paper: "RG"—Staff of the Interim classroom, NPI School, UCLA; "MS"—Staff of the Early Childhood Learning Program, NPI School; "JR"—Nursing staff, inpatient ward A-West, NPI, UCLA; "GJ"—Robert Asarnow, PhD, Neuropsychologist, and Lillian Lesser, MD, consulting Child Psychiatrist; "AW"—staff of inpatient ward 6-West, NPI; "EA"—nursing staff of inpatient ward 5-West, NPI; "PJ"—Steven Funderburk, MD, Pediatric Neurologist; "TT"—Linda Saddlemyre, RN, and Charles Fields, RN; "MG"—Linda Andron, MSW.

REFERENCES

Alexander, J, & Parsons, B. (1973). Short-term behavioral intervention with delinquent families. Impact on family process and recidivism. *Journal of Abnormal Psychology, 81,* 219–225

Ayllon, T, & Azrin, N. (1968). *The token economy: A motivational system for therapy and rehabilitation.* New York: Appleton-Century-Crofts

Baker, B, Heifetz, L, & Murphy, D. (1980). Behavioral training for parents of mentally retarded children. *American Journal of Mental Deficiency, 85,* 31–38

Bender, M, & Valletutti, PJ. (1976). *Teaching the moderately and severely handicapped: Curriculum objectives, strategies, and activities* (Vols. 1–3). Baltimore, MD: University Park Press

Borkowski, J, & Cavanaugh, J. (1979). Maintenance and generalization of skills and strategies by the retarded. In N Ellis (Ed.), *Handbook of mental deficiency. Psychological theory and research.* Hillsdale, NJ: Erlbaum

Bray, N. (1979). Strategy production in the retarded. In NR Ellis (Ed.), *Handbook of mental deficiency. Psychological theory and research.* Hillsdale, NJ: Erlbaum

Breuning, S, & Poling, A. (1982). Pharmacotherapy. In JL Matson & RP Barett (Eds.), *Psychopathology in the mentally retarded.* New York: Grune & Stratton

Brown, A. (1978). Knowing when, where and how to remember: A problem of metacognition. In R Glaser (Ed.), *Advances in instructional psychology* (Vol. 1). Hillsdale, NJ: Erlbaum

Bryan, TH, & Bryan JH. (1975). *Understanding learning disabilities.* Port Washington, NY: Alfred Publishing

Burt, RA. (1975). Judicial action to aid the retarded. In N Hobbs (Ed.), *Issues in the classification of children* (Vol. 2) (pp. 293–318). San Francisco: Jossey-Bass

Burton TA, & Hirshoren, A. (1979). The education of severely and profoundly retarded children: Are we sacrificing the child to the concept? *Exceptional Children, 45,* 598–602

Carlberg, C, & Kavale, K. (1980). The efficiency of special versus regular class placement for exceptional children: A meta-analysis. *Journal of Special Education, 14,* 294–309

Cohen, JS, & DeYoung, H. (1973). The role of litigation in the improvement of programming for the handicapped. In L Mann & D Sabatino (Eds.), *The first review of special education* (Vol. 2) (pp. 261–286). Philadelphia, PA: Journal of Special Education Press

Connors, CK. (1972). Pharmacotherapy of psychopathology. In H Quay & JS Werry (Eds.), *Psychological disorders in childhood.* New York: Wiley

Dunn, LM. (1968). Special education for the mildly retarded: Is much of it justifiable? *Exceptional Children, 35,* 5–22

Dunn, L, & Markwardt, C. (1970). *Peabody individual achievement test.* Circle Pines, MN: American Guidance Service

Ellis, NR. (1979). *Handbook of mental deficiency, psychological theory and research.* Hillsdale, NJ: Erlbaum

Estes, WK. (1970). *Learning theory and mental development.* New York: Academic Press

Falloon, I, Boyd, JL, & McGill, C. (1980). *Behavioral family therapy for schizophrenia.* Paper presented at the Symposium, "Social Competence and Psychiatric Disorder: Theory and Practice," Brown University, Providence, RI

Ferster, CB. (1961). Positive reinforcement and behavioral deficits of autistic children. *Child Development, 32,* 437–456

Forness, SR. (1972). The mildly retarded as casualties of the educational system. *Journal of School Psychology, 10,* 117–126

Forness, SR. (1974a). Educational approaches to autism. *Training School Bulletin, 71,* 167–173

Forness, SR. (1974b). Education of retarded children: A review for physicians. *American Journal of Diseases of Children, 126,* 237–242

Forness, SR. (1975). Educational approaches to hyperactive children. In D Cantwell (Ed.), *The hyperactive child: Diagnosis, management and current research* (pp. 159–172). New York: Spectrum

Forness, SR. (1976). Behavioristic orientation to categorical labels. *Journal of School Psychology, 14,* 90–96

Forness, SR. (1979a). Clinical criteria for mainstreaming mildly handicapped children. *Psychology in the Schools, 16,* 508–514

Forness, SR. (1979b). Developing the individual educational plan: Process and perspectives. *Education and Treatment of Children, 2,* 43–54

Forness, SR. (1981). Concepts of children with learning and behavior disorders: Implications for research and practice. *Exceptional Children, 48,* 56–64

Forness, S, Frankel, F, & Landman, R. (1976). Use of different types of classroom punishment by preschool teachers. *Psychological Record, 26,* 263–268

Forness, SR, & MacMillan, D. (1970). The origins of behavior modification with exceptional children. *Exceptional Children, 37,* 93–100

Forness, SR, Thornton, RL, & Horton, A. (1981). Assessment of applied academic and social skills. *Education and Training of the Mentally Retarded, 16,* 104–109

Forness, SR, Urbano, R, Rotberg, J, Bender, M, Gardner, T, Lynch, E, & Zemanek, D. (1980). Identifying children with school learning and behavior problems served by interdisciplinary hospitals and clinics. *Child Psychiatry and Human Development, 11,* 67–78

Frankel, F. (1981, July). *Problem solving behavior of autistic, retarded and normal children.* Paper presented at the Annual International Research Conference of the National Society for Autistic Children, Boston, MA

Frankel, F, Freeman, BJ, Ritvo, E, Chikami, B, & Carr, E. (1976). Effects of frequency of photic stimulation upon autistic and retarded children. *American Journal of Mental Deficiency, 81,* 32–40

Frankel, F, Freeman, BJ, Ritvo E, & Pardo, R. (1978). The effect of environmental stimulation upon the stereotyped behavior of autistic children. *Journal of Autism and Childhood Schizophrenia, 8,* 389–394

Frankel, F, & Graham, V. (1976). Systematic observation of classroom behavior of retarded and autistic preschool children. *American Journal of Mental Deficiency, 81,* 73–84

Frankel, F, Moss, D, Schofield, S, & Simmons, JQ. (1976). Case study: Use of differential reinforcement to suppress self-injurious and aggressive behavior. *Psychological Reports, 39,* 843–849

Frankel, F, & Simmons, JQ. (1976). Self-injurious behavior in schizophrenic and retarded children. *American Journal of Mental Deficiency, 80,* 512–522

Frankel, F, & Simmons, JQ. (in press). *Behavioral treatment approaches to pathological unsocialized physical aggression in young children. Journal of Child Psychology and Psychiatry*

Frankel, F, Simmons, JQ, Fichter, M, & Freeman, BJ. (1984). Stimulus overselectivity in autistic and mentally retarded children—A research note. *Journal of Child Psychology and Psychiatry, 25,* 147–155

Frankel, F, Simmons, JQ, & Olson, S. (1977). Effects of social deprivation upon operant behavior in mentally retarded and autistic children. *Journal of Pediatric Psychology, 2,* 172–175

Freeman, BJ, & Ritvo, E. (1976). Cognitive assessment. In E Ritvo, BJ Freeman, E Ornitz, & P Tanguay (Eds.), *Autism: Diagnosis, current research and management.* New York: Spectrum

Gilliam, JE, & Coleman, M. (1981). Who influences IEP committee decisions? *Exceptional Children, 47,* 642–644

Goldenberg, I, & Goldenberg, H. (1980). *Family therapy: An overview.* Monterey, CA: Brooks/Cole

Goldstein, S, Strickland, B, Turnbull, A, & Curry, L. (1980). An observational analysis of the IEP conference. *Exceptional Children, 46,* 278–286

Hewett, F, & Forness, S. (1984). *Education of exceptional learners* (3rd ed.). Boston, MA: Allyn & Bacon

Hewett, F, & Taylor, F. (1980). *Emotionally disturbed child in the classroom* (2nd ed.). Boston, MA: Allyn & Bacon

Howell, K, Kaplan, J, & O'Connell, C. (1979). *Evaluating handicapped children.* Columbus, OH: Charles Merrill

Jones, F, Simmons, JQ, & Frankel, F. (1974). Case study: An extinction procedure for eliminating self-destructive behavior in a 9-year-old autistic girl. *Journal of Autism and Childhood Schizophrenia, 4,* 241–250

Kazdin, A. (1980). *Behavior modification in applied settings.* Homewood, IL: Dorsey Press

Kendall, PC, & Hollon, SD. (1979). *Cognitive-behavioral interventions: Theory, research and procedures.* New York: Academic Press

Kifer, R, Lewis, M, Green, D, & Phillips, E. (1974). Training predelinquent youths and their parents to negotiate conflict situations. *Journal of Applied Behavior Analysis, 7,* 357–364

Kirk, SA, & Gallagher, JJ. (1979). *Educating exceptional children* (3rd ed.). Boston, MA: Houghton Mifflin

Lambert, NM, & Nicholl, RC. (1976). Dimensions of adaptive behavior of retarded and nonretarded public-school children. *American Journal of Mental Deficiency, 81,* 135–146

Lesser, L. (1981, October). *Neuroendocrine and behavioral responses in 6 child psychiatric patients.* Paper presented at the Annual Conference of the American Academy of Child Psychiatry, Dallas, TX

Lovaas, OI, Koegel, R, Schreibman, L, & Rehm, R. (1971). Selective responding of autistic children to multiple sensory input. *Journal of Abnormal Psychology, 77,* 211–222

MacMillan, DL. (1982). *Mental retardation in school and society* (2nd ed.). Boston, MA: Little, Brown

MacMillan, DL, & Barthwick, J. (1980). The new educable mentally retarded population: Can they be mainstreamed? *Mental Retardation, 18,* 155–158

MacMillan, D, & Forness, S. (1973). Behavior modification: Savior or savant? *American Journal of Mental Deficiency Monograph series 1,* 197–210

MacMillan, DL, Jones, R, & Meyers, CE. (1976). Mainstreaming the mentally retarded: Questions, cautions, and guidelines. *Mental Retardation, 14,* 3–10

Mercer, CD, & Snell, ME. (1977). *Learning theory research in mental retardation: Implications for teaching.* Columbus, OH: Charles Merrill

Miller, TL, & Sabatino, DA. (1978). An evaluation of the teacher consultant model as an approach to mainstreaming. *Exceptional Children, 45,* 86–91

Patterson, G, & Reid, JB. (1973). Intervention for families of aggressive boys: A replication study. *Behavior Research & Therapy, 11,* 383–394

Payne, JS, Palloway, EA, Smith, JE, Jr, & Payne RA. (1977). *Strategies for teaching the mentally retarded.* Columbus, OH: Charles E. Merrill

Perls, F. (1969). *Gestalt therapy verbatim.* Moab, UT: Real People Press

President's Committee on Mental Retardation and Bureau of Education of the Handicapped. (1969). *The six-hour retarded child.* Washington, DC: US Government Printing Office

Rago, WV, & Cleland, CC. (1978). Future directions in the education of the profoundly retarded. *Education and Training of the Mentally Retarded, 13,* 184–186

Reynolds, GS. (1968). *A primer of operant conditioning.* Palo Alto, CA: Scott, Foresman

Russell, A, & Forness, S. (1985). Behavioral disturbance in mentally retarded children in TMR and EMR classrooms. *American Journal of Mental Deficiency, 89,* 338–344

Rutter, M. (1975). *Helping troubled children.* New York: Plenum

Rutter, M, Greenfield, D, & Lockyer, L. (1967). A five to fifteen-year follow-up study of infantile psychosis: II. Social and behavioral outcome. *British Journal of Psychiatry, 113,* 1183–1199

Schreibman, L. (1975). Effects of within-stimulus and extra-stimulus prompting on discrimination learning in autistic children. *Journal of Applied Behavior Analysis, 8,* 91–112

Schreibman, L, Frankel, F, & LaVigna, G. (1977). *Guidelines for the use of aversive procedures in community care and health facilities for developmentally and mentally disabled children.* Sacramento, CA: California Department of Health

Sigman, M, Ungerer, J, & Russell, A. (1983). Moral judgement in relation to behavioral and cognitive disorders in adolescents. *Journal of Abnormal Child Psychology, 11,* 503–511

Sinclair, E. (1983). Educational assessment. In J Matson & J Mulick (Eds.), *Comprehensive handbook of mental retardation.* New York: Pergammon

Sindelar, P, & Deno, S. (1978). The effectiveness of resource programming. *Journal of Special Education, 12,* 17–28

Smith, MP, Coleman, M, Dokecki, P, & Davis, E. (1977). Recategorizing WISC-R scores of learning disabled children. *Journal of Learning Disabilities, 10,* 437–443

Sontag, E. (Ed.). (1977). *Educational programming for the severely and profoundly handicapped.* Reston, VA: Council for Exceptional Children

Spivak, G, Platt, J, & Shure, M. (1976). *The problem-solving approach to adjustment.* San Francisco, CA: Josey-Bass

Szasz, T. (1961). *The myth of mental illness: Foundations of a theory of personal conduct.* New York: Harper-Hoeber

Tarjan, G, & Forness, S. (1979). Disturbances of intellectual functioning. In G Usdin & J Lewis (Eds.), *Psychiatry in general practice* (pp. 498–517). New York: McGraw-Hill

Torres, S. (Ed.). (1977). *A primer on individualized educational programs for handicapped children.* Reston, VA: Foundation for Exceptional Children

Turnbull, A, Strickland, B, & Hammer, S. (1978a). The individualized educational program—Part 1: Procedural guidelines. *Journal of Learning Disabilities, 11,* 40–46

Turnbull, A, Strickland, B, & Hammer, S. (1978b). The individualized educational program—Part 2: Translating law into practice. *Journal of Learning Disabilities, 11,* 67–72

Ullman, L, & Krasner, L. (Eds.). (1965). *Case studies in behavior modification.* New York: Holt, Rinehart & Winston

Wilson, JD, & Spangler, PF. (1974). The Peabody Individual Achievement Test as a clinical tool. *Journal of Learning Disabilities, 7,* 384–387

Wiltz, N, & Patterson, G. (1974). An evaluation of parent training procedures designed to alter inappropriate aggressive behavior of boys. *Behavior Therapy, 5,* 215–221

Irene Goldenberg

15

Family Therapy with the Dual Disability Client

In the previous chapters in this volume, the association between mental retardation and emotional disorders has been discussed from both developmental and clinical perspectives. The first section of the volume reviewed the course of social, emotional, and communicative development in light of the challenges faced by the mentally retarded adult. The influence of the family in promoting or failing to promote developmental progress was frequently mentioned. In the second section of the volume, in which clinical manifestations of emotional disorders were discussed, there were references to the possible role of the family in the etiology of some of these disorders. Finally, the chapters on assessment and remediation have used as examples several interventions undertaken with or by family members of the mentally retarded individuals. While it has become clear throughout the volume that the family has a very powerful influence on the development and treatment of the mentally retarded child, the issue of the family's role has not been addressed directly.

The aim of this chapter is to discuss in broad terms those family issues that arise in relation to mental retardation. Furthermore, I will suggest that interventions with the family can play an important part in two different ways: first, in enhancing the family's adaptive response to their child and, thereby, preventing emotional disorders from arising (or, at least, minimizing their severity); and second, in treating those emotional disturbances that have developed in the mentally retarded individual whatever the etiologies of these disorders.

The adjustment of the family to the problems of the mentally retarded child is frequently critical for aiding the child's development in the social, emotional,

CHILDREN WITH EMOTIONAL DISORDERS AND DEVELOPMENTAL DISABILITIES ISBN 0–8089–1700–5

and communication spheres. The acceptance of the problems faced by the mentally retarded child, the support provided, and the encouragement of self-reliant behavior can be crucial for facilitating optimal development. In ideal situations, the family may help the child to feel adequate, to develop appropriate sources of control and gratification, and to be as self-reliant as possible. The family may grow in its ability to cooperate, support, and sustain one another. However, all too frequently, the family reaction to mental retardation does not enhance development but, in fact, exacerbates the problems of the mentally retarded child and destroys the confidence of the family members. In order to understand this response, we must first consider the kinds of issues that are faced by family members in their adjustment to the mentally retarded child.

FAMILY ISSUES AND MENTAL RETARDATION

The impact of a mentally retarded child on the family's coping ability, similar to other major stresses such as chronic illness or death of a family member, is to strain and often to disorganize its previous functioning level. Although the effect is by no means uniform, many families are overwhelmed as their usual task of trying to rear, protect, socialize, and dedicate their energies to the child's welfare is made more difficult by their child's lack of competence. As Hagamen (1980) points out, whatever a parent's personal level of adaptation, socioeconomic status, education background, general health, marital status, or geographic location, raising a mentally retarded child is associated with considerable prolonged stress. Parents appropriately are disturbed upon discovering that their much anticipated infant will be a person of limited competence. Payne and Patton (1981) have provided a useful set of questions (see Table 15-1) commonly asked by parents who learn their newborn is severely handicapped, as they try to gain some meaning from a confusing situation and begin making decisions that will impact on the lives of all family members.

Distress has a reverberating effect on the family, as well as a specific effect on each member, depending to some extent on family role. Wolfensberger (1972, p. 330), in an earlier review of published studies, found the following extensive, although certainly not exhaustive, list of early parental reactions to a mentally retarded child:

> alarm, ambivalence, anger, anguish, anxiety, avoidance, bewilderment, bitterness, catastrophic reaction, confusion, death wishes, denial, depression, despair, disappointment, disbelief, disassociation, embarrassment, envy, fear, financial worries, frustration, grief, guilt, helplessness, hopelessness, identifications, immobility, impulses to destroy the child, lethargy, mourning, overidentification, pain, projection, puzzlement, regret, rejection, remorse, self-blame, self-pity, shame, shock, sorrow, suicidal impulses, trauma, etc.

Table 15-1
Typical Questions Asked By Parents of a Severely Handicapped Newborn Infant

Will our child always be sickly?
What can be done to optimize our child's abilities?
Will our child ever talk?
What should we tell our child about being different?
Why did this happen to us?
Where can we get help and information?
What alternative placements are available, and should we consider them?
How will our child be different from other children?
Will our child always need constant care?
What foods will our child eat?
Is there any chance that our normal children's offspring might similarly be affected?
Is there anything we can do to make our child smarter?
What do most people decide to do about placement?
Whose fault is it?
Can our child be cured?
What will happen when our child grows up?
Will the child look funny?
What will the child be able to do developmentally?
Will our child be in pain?
How should we treat our child?
Will our child need special medical care?
Will our child progressively get worse?
How long will our child live?
Will we be able to love our child?
Does anything exist that can help?
Is it safe to have other children? (Will it happen again?)
Is there an operation that might help?
What will happen to our child when we die?
Are there any parent organizations that we can contact?
How should we explain this child to our family, friends, and neighbors?
Will the child be able to go to school?
Will our child ever be independent?
What is the cause of the problem? (How did it happen?)
Should we institutionalize our child?
What will the effects of this child be on our family?

From Payne, JS, & Patton, Jr. (1981). *Mental retardation* (p. 355). Columbus, OH: Charles C. Merrill. With permission.

According to Wolfensberger's survey, parental guilt is the most frequently cited reaction. Such a response may be particularly disturbing to parents if the retardation could have resulted from their deliberate behavior (e.g., a failed abortion attempt, heavy use of alcohol or other drugs during pregnancy). Hagamen (1980) notes also that a particularly important factor in parental reactions is the shattering of their prenatal fantasies, especially if the retarded infant is their firstborn child; in many cases, especially if the mother is older and the handicap severe, the parents may decide not to have more children (Barsch, 1968). Denial of the diagnosis, particularly of more mildly retarded children, is a common defensive reaction, according to Roos (1975). In many cases, distressed parents may prefer to believe their handicapped offspring is brain-damaged or autistic, perhaps less painful and less stigmatizing diagnostic labels (Wolfensberger, 1972). Finally, Olshansky (1970) cautions mental health workers to be aware that chronic sorrow may persist throughout the lives of these parents, whether the child is kept at home or institutionalized.

Since the mother so frequently bears the major responsibility for child-rearing, her distress is likely to be most apparent; indeed, she may appear to be the person with the core problem, although in reality her disturbances are more likely to represent the disarray in the family system. Fathers may withdraw emotionally from the handicapped child or perhaps the entire family, although some may feel overprotective. However, increased withdrawal by the father alongside increased overattachment by the mother is the most probable pattern (Hagamen, 1980). When Cummings (1976) compared a group of fathers of mentally retarded with a matched control group of fathers of nonretarded youngsters, he found the former more depressed and preoccupied with their handicapped child. These fathers tended to interact less with the child than did the mothers and felt less adequate as parents. Greater interaction between mother and handicapped child, while it is often frustrating and anger-producing, nevertheless apparently allows her an opportunity to feel more competent and useful.

Siblings demonstrate a wide range of responses and need not necessarily be damaged by the experience (Cleveland & Miller, 1977). Some learn to be protective and parentified particularly if the handicapped child is younger. Others, often given responsibilities before they are ready to accept them, may feel resentful over lost childhood care themselves. In some cases, a sibling may feel the additional pressure to achieve in order to compensate their parents for having a retarded child. In the case of severe retardation, as the handicapped child requires the most care and attention, siblings may feel jealous of attention directed elsewhere, resentful, angry, and perhaps guilty that they are more fortunate.

A number of factors affecting parental reactions have been catalogued by Hagamen (1980): the level of retardation (mild to profound), the age at which the retardation is recognized and by whom, the sophistication of the available health and educational services, the resources available to meet the child and family's specific needs, the personalities and social class of the parents, as well as the size and structure of the family. Very likely, it is the parents' level of adaptation—a close relationship, open communication encouraged throughout the family—that sets the family tone and helps determine how families adapt to a mentally retarded child.

In order to enhance this level of adaptation, family interventions can be very useful and may be imperative. From the moment that the parents find that their child is disabled (sometimes even before birth due to amniocentesis), the family is involved and emotional stress has an impact on the family's lifestyle, decision-making, time, finances, mobility, and problem-solving effectiveness. The problems are not likely to disappear during the life cycle of the family (O'Hara, Chaiklin, Mosher, 1980) although they may wax and wane at various times. Especially today, as the principle of "normalization" (Wolfensberger

1972) has taken hold, and the mentally retarded are "mainstreamed" into the regular classroom, work place, and community, it is more and more the family that must develop mutually satisfying ways of dealing with this challenge. Thus, the strengths of the family are particularly crucial for the lifelong adaptation of the child. Both the strengths and weaknesses of the family reside in the relationships and transactions between its members.

FAMILY THERAPY AS A PREVENTION TECHNIQUE

In recent, years, family therapy has become an increasingly popular and effective therapeutic technique (Goldenberg & Goldenberg, 1985). Begun approximately 30 years ago, and originally intended as a device to treat schizophrenics and their families, family therapy has increasingly become the treatment of choice for a wide variety of psychological and behavioral difficulties. Basic to this approach is the systems viewpoint that a family is a natural social organization, with properties all its own, that has evolved a set of rules, roles, a power structure and ways of communicating that allow various tasks to be performed effectively. When a family is stressed to the point where its customary coping devices are overloaded, as, for example, in adapting to a mentally retarded child, certain changes within the system take place as the members strive to deal with the crisis. Dysfunctional behaviors are thought to arise from the family's disequilibrium rather than from a single source, such as the mentally retarded child. Family therapy, then, is a therapeutic procedure for exploring and attempting to alleviate the ongoing interlocking emotional problems within a family system by helping its members change the family's dysfunctional transactional patterns together (Goldenberg & Goldenberg, 1985). When family therapy is used as a prevention technique, the emphasis is often on maintaining or strengthening transactional patterns that were formerly effective but have been disrupted by the new stressful situation that the family faces in relation to the problems of the mentally retarded member.

It is often the pediatrician or other physician who first informs the parents of their child's retardation. If they are informed in an insensitive manner, parents may be severely affected, although any manner of informing them will be distressing. Since the physician's contact is likely to be with the mother, her ensuing distress may lead to a recommendation of counseling or psychotherapy for her. Unfortunately, this approach only serves to emphasize the mother as the "identified patient," failing to take into account the reactions of all the family members (especially the father). More realistically, referral for family-focused sessions is more apt to deal with the emerging problems and prepare the family to respond more adaptively to forthcoming problems. A clearer understanding of the child's condition, its treatment, anticipated family responses, and prognosis can provide some orientation for the family as they continue to work out their fears and concerns. The expert system (hospitals, clinics, schools) often becomes for the family members both a support and a source of enduring frustration. While separating out the realities and the fantasies of this aid and frustration, it is frequently useful for the family therapist to help the family sort out their feelings of dependency, anger, mistrust, and confusion in reference to the various intervention systems.

Family therapy can be very useful at the point of genetic counseling for the couple. If the genetic counseling can be followed-up with a shared discussion of the risks and considerations with all the family members involved, the questions of guilt ("This problem came from your side of the family"; "I should not have waited so long to have a baby," etc.) can be discussed and detoxified. In addition, the grief and fantasy over the loss of the perfect child can begin to be shared by each family member. Sometimes one person (frequently the mother) in expressing her grief may not allow the other family members to experience their sense of loss. Feedback communication between family members is essential at this point for future family well-being.

Dealing with the extended family, which can be of great economic, psychological, and practical support, is an important issue for the family as they formulate coping strategies. Beyond the extended family, there is the question of how to deal with the outside world—the lady next door, the children down the block, the swimming class at the Y—all part of the disabled child's environment. Some families withdraw, erecting impenetrable boundaries around themselves and the outside world and cutting themselves off from any possible means of support as they protect themselves from potential hurt. In such cases, the family structure becomes rigid and attempts to sustain more of the family's needs than it can support.

In California the importance of maintaining a continuous contact with the family has been recognized in the establishment of regional centers that continue to follow a child throughout his lifetime. The general thrust today, which limits institutional placement of children to the more severely handicapped or medically impaired, places an enormous responsibility on the family of origin. The separation that occurs with normal children, and the release of responsibility as a child grows older, is interfered with in the case of the mentally retarded. This does not mean that there is no way for a handicapped child to become less dependent on, or separated from, his family, but that society is not extremely helpful in this respect. Therefore, the normal patterns can become distorted. It frequently is the family therapist's responsibility to help the family normalize these patterns. A very handicapped child of 3.5 years of age may not go off to nursery school, but parents can be helped to take him or her to a peer group of other handicapped children for an hour. The child may never go off to college, but may indeed be directed toward training in a sheltered workshop. Family therapy can be particularly useful, then, as the family reaches transition points that emerge with the child's development. When the family is able to deal with these critical points of change in a positive manner, the severity of emotional disruption, either within the family or within the children, is likely to be lessened.

FAMILY THERAPY AS A TREATMENT MODALITY

In some cases, the family is not able to manage the challenges and problems of the mentally retarded member and serious disruption occurs. Family members may withdraw, or flee from the family into work, too-early marriage, or drugs and alcohol. On the other hand, other families cope with the problem by dedicating themselves to their mentally retarded children. In these families, the handicapped child is perceived as a family "pet," but the care of the child is such an enormous responsibility that no one can leave unless someone else is willing to stay home and be responsible. In this way, the careers of both mother and father can be aborted with eventual anger and regret. Alternatively, or in addition, siblings may become parentified so that they are unable to grow up, leave home, and lead independent lives.

Family therapy is clearly the treatment of choice when the primary symptomatology is family disruption, as in the examples given above. Individual therapy will not approach the real issue and only an intervention involving all family members can resolve the issues.

What is less obvious is that family therapy can also be extremely useful in treating cases in which the mentally retarded child or adolescent, rather than the family, presents most of the symptoms of emotional disorder. In these situations, family therapy alone or in coordination with individual therapy for the child can be very effective. This is true whether or not the emotional disorders can be traced to family patterns of behavior. However, even in those situations in which such links cannot be made, we have found that family therapy can be helpful.

One major advantage of family therapy is that the family can be used as the agent of change, thereby ensuring that the interventions are of greater duration. A drawback of individual or group therapy is that it is likely to be short-term. Because mentally retarded individuals require more experience in order to learn than individuals of normal intelligence, such short-term interventions may be of limited value. By intervening through family members, the duration of ameliorative experience for the mentally retarded individual can be lengthened.

A second advantage is that the mentally retarded child or adolescent may have limited capacities to communicate. His or her difficulties may be expressed more clearly by a family member who knows the child or adolescent well. Similarly, the mentally retarded child or adolescent may not understand some of the issues that arise in treatment. Because the parent may be more capable of explaining certain concepts to the child, the parent can occasionally serve as interpreter. In addition, family members can use concrete situations that occur in daily life to help the mentally retarded child or adolescent understand some of the issues that have been discussed in the family therapy session.

Of course, these advantages of family therapy depend to a great extent on the emotional and intellectual strengths of the other family members. Family members can only serve as agents of change in those cases in which they themselves have developed adaptive responses to the problems of their mentally retarded children. In addition, family members can only act usefully as interpreters when they are able to see themselves and their children independently. In those cases in which identities are fused in the minds of the family member, the use of the family member as an interpreter should be discouraged. In those situations, a family member may speak for the mentally retarded individual, keeping the child from having the opportunity to develop his or her own communicative capacities and sense of independence.

A major advantage of family therapy is that it can allow the family to see the child's behavior both in the context of the family and in other contexts. It is interesting to note that some handicapped children behave individually in a manner that is quite different from their social manner within the context of the family. Some children show more adaptive behavior outside the family context. An observation of this and an analysis of what fosters this maladaptive pattern within the family can be helpful to improve family functioning. On the other hand, some mentally retarded children and adolescents show more pathology outside the family. It is equally important that the family be able to observe these disturbed behavior patterns so that they can deal with the difficulties that the child has in school and/or social situations.

A number of other significant effects accrue from the use of family therapy. The therapist tends to focus on current problems, not spending much time hearing and reevaluating old guilts and previous maladaptive behavior patterns. The family remains responsible for the identified child and is less likely to transfer the responsibility to a medical, psychiatric, or educational system. The significance of nonverbal behavior by other members of the family is a tremendous clue in helping solve the family problems. The case history in its written form and usually narrated by one individual recedes in importance as other members contribute and fill out the picture. The therapist has a chance to model appropriate behavior for the family, set limits, and respond to appropriate behavior patterns in other members of the family. The entrapment of particular siblings in a parentified role is more easily identified by family members in a session. Finally, a session that allows certain flexible boundaries provides an opportunity to bring in support personnel such as extended family, grandparents, physical therapists, social workers, and teachers.

The methods used with a family with a mentally retarded member are similar to those used with other families (Goldenberg & Goldenberg, 1985). Of course, the therapist needs to keep in mind the special problems facing the family that have been outlined earlier in this chapter. In addition, interventions by the therapist may be phrased somewhat more simply than usual in order to ensure that the mentally retarded child understands the communications.

However, in general, the methods are like those utilized with any other family therapy case.

In order to exemplify the use of a therapy with a family with a mentally retarded child, a case example follows. This case is similar to a number of family therapy cases followed in a university hospital setting over the last few years.

Case Example

Sandi was a 16-year-old girl who was admitted to an adolescent psychiatric inpatient unit for depression and psychosomatic illness (projectile vomiting). In addition, she had a controlled seizure disorder and was mildly mentally retarded. Individual and family treatment were provided.

The family consisted of Sandi's parents both in their early 40s and a younger sister, age ten years. Assessment of the family from a systems perspective revealed an extremely close alliance between father and Sandi. Father was also extremely protective of Sandi, which he stated was due to her seizure disorder and retardation. The mother acted overprotectively toward Sandi, who seemed overly dependent on her mother; this relationship was marked by ambivalence from both partners. However, anger and expression of conflict were not tolerated within the family. Thus, mother expressed anxiety and depression about Sandi, which was reinforced by Sandi's intractible vomiting.

Sandi was essentially isolated at home. She had been out of school due to her somatic complaints and had virtually no contact with peers. On the other hand the younger child appeared well adjusted and accomplishing age-appropriate developmental tasks.

In exploration of the marital relationship, it was assessed to be highly stressed and chronically conflicted. However, there was no overt expression of the conflict until later in treatment. Instead, Sandi became the focus of problems in the family. The mother–daughter relationship served as a displacement of the marital conflict. Father directed his attention away from the marriage, to his daughter in the form of overconcern and emotional closeness. The psychosomatic illness served as a focal point for both parents and directed their attention away from the spousal conflict. Sandi was caught, unable to remain neutral with her parents, unable to separate herself from her parents, and unable to resolve the conflict with her mother.

Family treatment focused on disengaging Sandi from the parental conflict, partly by framing and resolving the conflict between mother and Sandi. In addition, specific suggestions were made for Sandi to become more active with peers through organized social activities. Thus, Sandi began to disengage from the family in a developmentally appropriate manner. Consequently, the marital relationship became extremely volatile and separation was threatened. However, the marriage conflict became quiescent again when the younger sister became ill and required much nursing at home.

Marital therapy was offered to the couple, which was refused. Family therapy progressed however to extricate the children from the marital relationship and to contain spousal conflict. Some resolution of the conflict occurred in the family sessions. Family therapy was continued after Sandi's discharge from the ward, to assure that the adaptations achieved during the hospitalization would be sustained.

Assessment. The developmental disability of this adolescent made her vulnerable to a family adaptation that detoured marital conflict into parental overprotectiveness. The social isolation often found in the adolescent retarded was exacerbated by the family dynamics. A therapeutic family systems approach led to resolution of the somatic concerns by containment of the conflict in the spousal relationship and by shifting child-rearing concerns to more developmentally appropriate ones. Because the family systems approach depended on restructuring rather than on insight and verbal ability, this approach was highly effective with this family with a retarded member who was as responsive (if not more so) to systematic changes in the family system. (Courtesy of ML Gottlieb, University of California at Los Angeles. With permission).

In summary, family therapy can be an important means of preventing and/or ameliorating emotional disorders in mentally retarded children. The family is the most important influence on the child and continues to have a strong impact on the mentally retarded individual. It is our hope that interventions with families will be encouraged in order to help adaptation and prevent the development of emotional disorders. On the other hand, there are certain emotional and behavioral problems that cannot be prevented either because of the child's characteristics, the family's traits, or the severe challenges presented by the larger environment. In these situations, family therapy can be a tool for remediation of emotional disorders of mentally retarded children and adolescents.

REFERENCES

Barsch, RH. (1968). *The parent of the handicapped child.* Springfield, IL: Charles Thomas

Cleveland, D, & Miller, N. (1977). Attitudes and life commitments of older siblings of mentally retarded adults: An exploratory study. *Mental Retardation, 15,* 38–41

Cummings, TS. (1976). The impact of the child's deficiency on the father: A study of fathers of mentally retarded and of chronically ill children. *American Journal of Orthopsychiatry, 46,* 246–255

Goldenberg, I, & Goldenberg, H. (1985). *Family therapy: An overview* (2nd ed.). Monterey, CA: Brooks/Cole

Hagamen, MB. (1980). Family adaptation to the diagnosis of mental retardation in a child and strategies of intervention. In LS Szymanski & PE Tanguay (Eds.), *Emotional disorders of mentally retarded persons.* Baltimore MD: University Park Press

O'Hara, DM, Chaiklin, H, & Mosher, B. (1980). A family life cycle plan for delivering services to the developmentally handicapped. *Child Welfare, 59,* 80–90

Olshansky, S. (1970). Chronic sorrow: A response to having a mentally defective child. In RL Noland (Ed.), *Counseling parents of the mentally retarded.* Springfield, IL: Charles Thomas

Payne, JS, & Patton, JR. (1981). *Mental retardation.* Columbus, OH: Charles C Merrill

Roos, P. (1975). Parents and families of the mentally retarded. In JM Kauffman & JS Payne (Eds.), *Mental retardation: Introduction and personal perspective.* Columbus, OH: Charles C Merrill

Wolfensberger, W. (1972). *The principle of normalization in human services.* Toronto: National Institute on Mental Retardation

Author Index

Subject Index

UNIVERSITY OF RHODE ISLAND LIBRARY
3 1222 00308 5407